Veterinary Extension and Rural Development

About the Author

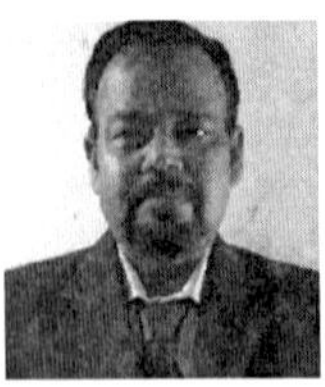

Bhabesh Chandra Das is Assistant Professor, Department of Veterinary and Animal Husbandry Extension, College of Veterinary Science and Animal Husbandry, Odisha University of Agriculture and Technology (OUAT), Bhubaneswar, Odisha. He did his M V Sc from IVRI, and Ph D from NDRI in Extension Education. He has served more than 25 years in many organizations, namely, DANIDA Project, Indo-Swiss Project, DFID, Watershed Mission of Government of Odisha, National Institute of Rural Development and Panchayat Raj (NIRD&PR), Government of India, Odisha Milk Producers' Federation Ltd. (OMFED), Odisha in different positions as an extension education and rural development expert before joining as Assistant Professor in OUAT.

He teaches extension education, rural development and general management in UG and PG classes. He has supervised 14 PG and 02 Ph. D theses and published more than 110 research papers in national and international journals. Dr. Das has authored 10 books and contributed chapters in 7 books.

Veterinary Extension and Rural Development

B.C. Das, Ph.D
Assistant Professor
Department of Veterinary and Animal Husbandry Extension
College of Veterinary Science and Animal Husbandry
Odisha University of Agriculture and Technology
Bhubaneswar-751 003, Odisha, India

NEW INDIA PUBLISHING AGENCY
New Delhi – 110 034

NEW INDIA PUBLISHING AGENCY
101, Vikas Surya Plaza, CU Block, LSC Market
Pitam Pura, New Delhi - 110 034, India
Email: info@nipabooks.com
Web: www.nipabooks.com

For customer assistance, please contact
Phone: + 91-11-27 34 17 17 Fax: + 91-11- 27 34 16 16
E-mail: feedbacks@nipabooks.com

ISBN : 978-93-90175-18-5

Composed and Designed by NIPA.

Preface

Production of desirable changes in the farmers' behavior to adopt new agricultural technologies is one of the greatest concerns for the agricultural scientists, extension workers and administrators of the country. To ensure sustainable income to farmers from farming, besides proven technologies, the role of extension services is very important. The quality of extension services can only be provided if the subject of Extension Education has been understood in the right perspective. The agricultural graduates of different disciplines coming out from agricultural universities should know and realize the importance of Extension Education for agricultural development. Unfortunately, many of us engaged in agricultural development feel that extension education means going to village and discussing with farmers about the improved technologies, conducting meetings or organizing training programmes, etc. This is very narrow vision of a discipline for them who are not rightly exposed to the subject or inadequately trained in it. There is a need to study the subject of extension education, understand it and apply in the right way as it is one of the important pillars of agricultural development. Keeping this in mind, this text book on Veterinary Extension and Rural Development has been written to suit the academic requirements of undergraduate and postgraduate students in the discipline of extension education of Agricultural and other Universities. The information herein have been carefully sorted, analysed, classified, compiled and presented in most easy and understandable manner for benefits of not only undergraduate and post graduate students but also for extension teachers, extension workers, researchers, administrators and planners. This book could be very useful for the students preparing for competitive examinations like UPSC, Sate Public Service Commissions, Bank examinations, etc.

This book contains two sections. First section deals with Extension Education having eleven chapters and second section deals with Rural Development having twelve chapters. Chapters are carefully arranged to keep it interesting while navigating the book for various information. The entire book has been prepared in a simple and clear language so that the contents could be easily followed by the readers. This book is in fact, an outgrowth of my experiences of teaching the subject to undergraduate and post graduate students for several years.

I am highly indebted to my learned colleagues of the discipline for providing me stimulus for writing this book. I am grateful to all those persons and writers whose writings and works have helped me in preparing this book. I am equally grateful to my beloved students who made me understand their needs on the subject and helped me enhance the standard of the book.

I shall feel amply rewarded if this book proves useful in meeting the requirements of the readers. I look forward to suggestions and comments from my esteemed readers for further improvement of the subject contents and presentation of the book.

2020 **B.C. Das**

Contents

SECTION-I: VETERINARY EXTENSION

1

Livestock Extension Education Concept, Principles and Philosophy

1. History of Extension / Extension Education
2. What is Extension?
3. What is Education?
4. Types of Education
5. What is Extension Education?
6. Difference between Formal Education and Extension Education
7. Concept of Extension
8. Need for Extension
9. Objectives of Extension
10. Functions of Extension
11. Basic Elements in Extension
12. Scope of Extension
13. Components of Extension
14. Philosophy of Extension Education
15. Principles of Extension Education
16. Extension Educational Process
17. Suggested Readings and References

History of Extension/Extension Education

> **Extension**
>
> 'ex'-out
> 'tensio'-stretching
>
> First Recorded-Britain in 1840
>
> Father of Extension: **James Stuart**
>
> Extension Education was used formally by Cambridge University first time in 1873

The term extension is more recent in origin, and was first recorded in Britain in the 1840s in the context of 'university extension' or 'extension of the university'. James Stuart, Fellow of Trinity College, Cambridge, who gave several lecturers to women's associations and working man's clubs in the north of England during 1867-68, is considered as father of extension. The term extension was derived from the practice of British universities of having one educational programme within the premises of the university and another away from the university buildings. The programme conducted outside the university was described as "extension education". The expression connoted an extension of knowledge from the university to places and people far beyond. But, the term 'Extension Education' was formally used for the first time in 1873 by Cambridge University of England to describe system dedicated to the dissemination of knowledge to rural people where they lived and worked. Within a short time, the idea had spread to other parts of Britain, Europe and North America. Extension work is an out of school system of education in which adults and young people learn by doing. It is a partnership between the government, the land-grant institutions, and the people, which provides services and education designed to meet the needs of the people (Kelsey and Hearne, 1966). The meaning of the term 'extension' has changed over time, and has different meanings to different countries. The term ''Agricultural Extension'' was adopted in 1914 when the United States Federal Smith-Lever Act of 1914 formalized a nationwide cooperative federal-state-county programme and gave operational responsibility for this to the land grant colleges and Universities. In the beginning, agricultural extension was concerned primarily with the improvement of agriculture, using conventional teaching methods. As time went on, home economics, youth programmes and rural community resource development were included. Agricultural extension spread to tropical Africa, the Caribbean, Asia and Latin America following the involvement of the United States of America (USA) in bilateral AID programmes after the Second World War.

In India, the terms community development and extension became more popular with the launching of Community Development Programme in 1952 and with the establishment of the National Extension Service in 1953. Since then, Community development has been regarded as a programme for an all-round development of the rural people, and extension as the means to achieve this objective.

What is Extension ?

The word 'Extension' is derived from the Latin roots, *'ex'* meaning 'out' and *'tensio'* meaning 'stretching'. Literally it means 'stretching out'. That is stretching out beyond the boundaries of university and research stations to reach the rural people to educate them on various issues.

What is Education ?

Education is the process of developing capabilities of the individuals so that they can respond appropriately to the situations. Or in simple words, it is the process of production of desirable changes in the human behaviour, i.e. bringing out the desired changes in knowledge (things known), attitude (things felt) and skill (things done), either in all, or one or more of them. The education is effective when it results in changes in the following behavioural components as specified by Paul Leagans:

> **Education**
>
> Developing capabilities of individual
>
> Desirable changes in
>
> - Knowledge
> - Attitude
> - Skill
> - Action

i) Knowledge - What an individual knows?

ii) Attitudes -What he thinks?

iii) Skills (both Physical & Mental) -What he can do?

iv) Action - What he actually does?

This aspect is known by the acronym "KASA".

Types of Education

Education may be classified broadly under three categories as:

i) Informal Education

ii) Formal Education

iii) Non-formal Education

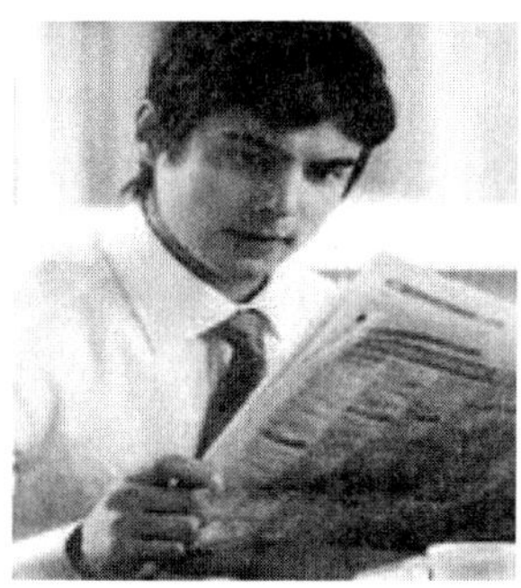

Informal Education is the lifelong process by which every person acquires and accumulates knowledge, skill, attitude and insights from daily experiences and exposure to the environment at home, at work, at play, etc. Example: Reading books, newspaper, etc.

Formal Education is the highly institutionalized, chronologically graded and hierarchically structured education system spanning lower primary school and upper reaches of the university. Example: School Education

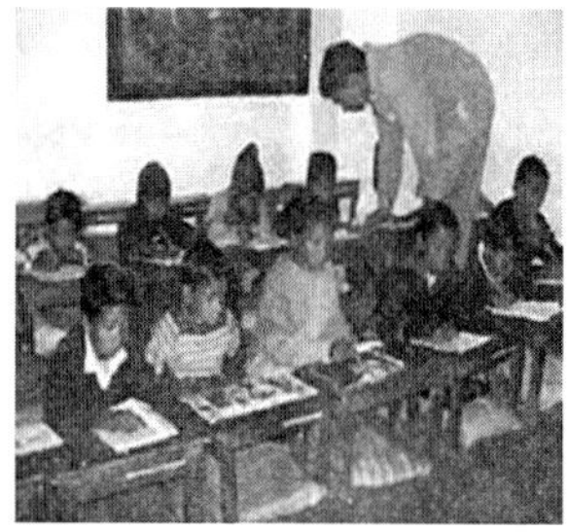

Non-formal Education is an organized, systematic, educational activity carried on outside the frame work of the formal system to provide selected types of learning to particular sub-groups in the population, adults and children according to their needs. Example: Extension Education.

What is Extension Education ?

In continuation to what is being discussed earlier in 'What is Extension', Cumberlage (1956) defined that Extension is education of the rural adults and children outside the school, in matters of their own choice and interest; education for freedom which seeks to help persons to use the liberty of action with which a democratic society is constructed. Whereas, Ensimger (1957) said that extension is education and its purpose is to change attitudes and practices of the people with whom work is done. But, Kelsey and Hearne (1963) explained that extension work is an out-of-school systems of education in which adults and young people learn by doing. Similarly, Rolling (1986) stated that 'Extension' refers to the actual work done by professional extension agents at various levels of management while 'extension education 'refers to the body of knowledge concerning that work or practice. Van den Ban and Hawkins (2002), said that extension involves the conscious use of communication of information to help people form sound opinions and make good decisions.

We may observe from all these definitions that education is the integral part of extension and the type of education imparted to the out of school children and adult is non-formal in nature. However, these definitions do not cover the entire scope of Extension Education which has now attended the stature of a distinct discipline with its own research, methodology, teaching and field (practice) of activities.

Leagans (1961) defines Extension Education is an applied science consisting of content derived from research, accumulated field experiences and relevant principles drawn from the behavioural sciences synthesized with useful technology in to a body of philosophy, principles, contents and methods focused on the problems of out-of-school education for adults and youth.

Extension Education

Educational process to increase knowledge, change attitude, improve skill of the rural people to adopt the improved practices

The National Commission on Agriculture (1976) explains extension education as an out-of-school education and services for the members of the farm family and others directly or indirectly engaged in farm production, to enable them to adopt improved practices on production, management, conservation and marketing.

O P Dahama (1973) defines extension education as an educational process to provide knowledge to the rural people about the improved practices in a convincing manner and help them to take decision within their specific local conditions .

We may say that the extension education is a science which deals with the creation, transmission and application of knowledge designed to bring about planned changes in the behaviour (knowledge, skill and attitude) of people, with a view to help them live better by learning the ways of improving their vocations, enterprise and institutions.From the above definitions, it appears that extension and extension education convey same meanings. They are also found used interchangeable in the extension literatures.

But, in true sense, extension education points out the common fundamental principles, philosophy and procedure which are applied in different technological disciplines or problem areas. Extension education is the core with universal application and extension refers to the actual work done by the extension workers

By definition, extension and extension education are synonymous. They are used interchangeable in the extension literatures.

Difference between Formal Education and Extension Education

Extension education and formal education differs in a number of ways, and some of them are-

S.No	Formal Education	Extension Education
1.	The teacher starts with theory of the subject and works up to practical.	Extension education starts with practical problems of the learners and may take up theory later on.
2.	Teaching is largely confined to the premises of the institutions.	Extension teaching is mostly outside the four walls of the formal institution.
3.	The learners are homogenous with common goals.	The learners (adults) are heterogeneous and have diverse goals.
4.	The learners adapt to the fixed curriculum offered by the institutions.	Extension education has no fixed curriculum. It has to be designed as per the requirements of the farmers.
5	Strict adherence to institutional rules and regulations	Freedom of attendance and choice of subject matters are left to the learners.
6.	Knowledge flows from the teacher to the learners.	Knowledge flows from both teacher to learners and from learners to teacher.
7.	The teacher only instructs the students	The extension agents/workers teach/work a great deal through local leaders/ progressive farmers.

8.	It is more theoretical in nature	It is more practical and problem solving oriented
9.	It is more rigid in nature	It is flexible and accommodative in nature
10	Participation is as per the rules and regulations. Violation attracts penalty	Participation is voluntary

Concept of Extension

> **Basic Elements of Behaviour**
>
> 1. Knowledge and Understanding
> 2. Skill
> 3. Attitude
> 4. Action

The basic concept of Extension is Education, which is defined as the production of desirable changes in human behaviour. The production of desirable changes in human being is possible by changing his/her knowledge, understanding, skill and attitude about any activity. Through extension education either all, or one or more than one of the above is attempted to achieve so that so that a farmer may improve his/her standard of living. Extension is not only attempting to change the behaviour and ensuring adoption of a particular practice but also aims at changing the outlook of the farmer so that they will be receptive to the new ideas and continuously seek means to improve his quality of life. Extension is essentially the means by which new knowledge and ideas are introduced into rural areas in order to bring about change and improve the lives of farmers and their families.

The FAO survey report on Extension in Asia (1975) mentions three important concept of extension, and they are-

i) All-inclusive concept- A number of countries still conceive that extension means the work that is done by the Government departments at village level, including the supplies to the rural farmers.

ii) Service concept-To gain more confidence of the farmers, more work of service nature was also added later.

iii) Educational concept- The ultimate aim is to help people to help themselves through education to bring a change in outlook. But effective education is possible only if there is a separate agency to assume the responsibility for supplies and services enabling the extension workers to devote themselves to the task of training the farmers.

The concept of extension is based on the certain basic premises and they are as follows as mentioned by Hassanullah (1998).

1. People have unlimited potential for personal growth and development.
2. The development may take place at any stage of their lives, if they are provided with adequate and appropriate learning opportunities.

3. Adults are not interested in learning only for the sake of learning. They are motivated when new learning provides opportunities for application, for increased productivity and improved standards of living.
4. Such learning is a continuous need of rural populations and should be provided on a continuing basis, because the problems as well as the technologies of production and living are continuously changing.
5. Given the required knowledge and skills, people are capable of making optimal choices for their individual and social benefits.

Need for Extension

The rural people are to be educated to adopt improved technologies which are being developed in the research stations for their benefits. However, this education process is not simple. The institutions, organizations and extension workers involved in this process should understand the principle and philosophy of adult education. According to Supe (1987), the researchers neither have time nor they equipped for the job of persuading the villagers to adopt scientific methods, and to ascertain from them the rural problems. Similarly, it is difficult for the farmers to always visit the research stations and obtain firsthand information. Thus, there is a need for an agency to interpret the findings of research to the farmers and to carry the problems of the farmers to research stations for solution. This gap is filled by the extension agency.

Objectives of Extension

The literal meaning of the term, objectives, is the expressions of the ends towards which our efforts are directed. In other words, an objective means a direction of movement. The fundamental objective of extension is the development of people by means of education. More specifically stated, the following are general objectives of extension-

> **Objective**
>
> Expressions of the ends towards which our efforts are directed.
>
> **Objective of Extension**
>
> Development of people by means of education.

1. To assist people to discover and analyze their problems, identify the felt needs and taking appropriate decision.
3. Educating people to be able to make similar decisions in future under similar situation.
2. To develop leadership among people and help them in organising groups to solve their problems.
3. To disseminate information based on research work and /or practical experiences in such a manner that the people would accept it and put it in to actual practices.

4. To facilitate the process of farmers' institutions development in the rural areas.
5. To keep research stations informed about the problems of the farmers.
6. Stimulating desirable developments within the framework of the national, economic and social policies involving all the sub sectors of development as a whole.

Basic objective of extension education is to bring desirable changes in the quality of life of the target group which it serves by helping them to change their attitude, knowledge, skill and resources (both natural and man-made) like land, pasture, water, livestock, equipment etc. in a right way. The ultimate objective of livestock extension education is development of livestock farmers by improving their living standards. This could be done by;

- Bringing about desirable changes in the knowledge, attitude and skill.
- Assisting livestock farmers to realize their needs and problems.
- Developing rural leadership, mobilizing people and their resources.
- Providing knowledge about recent technologies and their application

Functions of Extension

The main function of extension is to bring about desirable changes in the human behaviour. Changes may be brought about in their knowledge, skill and attitude towards ideas, innovations, practices, etc. The extension system includes all intuitions like public, private, and non-government development institutions that educate people for their betterment. Extension performs set of functions that induce voluntary change among people for development.

> **Functions of Extension**
>
> Bringing about desirable changes in the human behaviour.

A set of functions of extension includes:

1. Transferring technology for sustainable development
2. Transferring management capacity to mobilize and organize developmental activities by all communities
3. Capacity building of all stakeholders in the developmental process on various aspects like planning, evaluation and implementation of programmes.

Differences between Agriculture Extension and Livestock Extension

Comparison of Crop and Livestock Research

Characteristics	Crops	Animals	Implications for using Animals
Mobility	Stationary	Mobile	Difficult to measure and Control non experimental factors
Life cycle duration	Generally, less than 4 month	Generally over one year	Increased costs, Likelihood of losing Experimental units
Life cycle synchronization	All units synchronized	Units seldom synchronized	Difficult to find comparable units
Multiple Outputs	Only grain/tuber and residue	Multiple outputs: meat, hides, milk, manure, power	Difficult to measure value, treatment effect
Non market inputs and outputs	Few	Many	Difficult to value inputs and outputs
Size of experimental unit	Small, divisible	Large, indivisible	Increased cost, risk to cooperator
Producer attitudes	Impersonal	Personal taboos	Difficult to cull, castrate
Management variability	Low	High	Difficult to isolate treatment effect
Number of observation units	Many	Few	Large statistical variability
Variability of Observations	Low	High	Large statistical variability

Basic Elements in Extension

According to J.P.Leagans (1961), there are three basic elements in extension for rural development which the extension educator must deal with as they are key to his success. These elements are:

1. Main himself-physiological and psychological
2. Men's environment-physical, economic and social
3. Man-created devices for improving her/his welfare

1. A View of Man Himself

An Extension educator should view a man as:

a) Individual human personality possessing many inherited traits, tendencies and capacities that create forces which shape what they think, what they do and how they do it.

b) Possessing extensive mental power to analyze, learn, think, reason, understand, remember, forget, reject, decide, judge, and to do other things.

c) Possessing emotional powers which includes 1) capacity to feel various emotions like love, hate, confidence, fear, sadness, happiness, etc. 2) desire to resists many acts and conditions like innovation, imposition, poverty, strangeness, etc. 3) desire to improve many things like his knowledge and skills level, food, clothing, housing, agriculture production, independence, leadership, etc.

d) Possessing great potential physical skill to improve his condition.

2. Man's Environment

Man is surrounded by other human beings, physical items, social and cultural norms and economic conditions. Environmental forces exert continuous pressure on him and shape his personality accordingly. Some of the major environmental/ external forces facing a typical farmer in an Indian village are:

Low agricultural production
Poor housing and other amenities
Low per capita income
Poor health
Under- employment
Poor educational opportunities
Poor credit system
Poor marketing infrastructure
Low livestock production
Unproductive and uneconomical agricultural implements
Adherence to outmoded customs and traditions, etc.

These are some of the problems, and most of them are men made. Interventions in these areas require proper understanding of the men's environment so that extension programmes could be designed properly to deal these problems.

3. Man-created Devices to Serve Man

In human civilization, man has created various institutions and forces, and developed certain mechanisms to promote his welfare. Man has been always attempting through various institutions-educational, technological, physical, economic, social, administrative, religious, etc.- created by him to minimize the gap between what ought to be and what is in human being. After independence, India has developed various man-created devices to improve the socio-economic condition of the farmers, and few of them are:

Trained personnel
Scientific knowledge

Improved production tools

Improved production materials and methods

Expanded communication media

Policy guidelines

Government aid in money and inputs

Provision of credits

Freedom and encouragement

Promotion of cooperatives, Self Help Groups, Farmers' Organisation, etc.

These three elements lie at the use of extension educator for rural development. The third element, man-created devices are designed to help people to make desirable adjustment between the elements of man and his environment. The methods by which the adjustment is to be made in a free society are education. Only the human element is controlling the progress today. Therefore, the key to rural development lies in the Mind, Heart and Hands of the people and those of their professional leaders (Mathialagan, 2007).

Scope of Extension

> **Scope:**
> Space for action

The dictionary meaning of 'scope' is 'space for action'. The scope is enormous in the present context. The growth and development is required in all sphere of life, and for that, extension plays a very important role. It teaches people how to something efficiently and work out means and ways to meet the different needs of life. Now, extension is an integral part of agriculture and rural development programmes in India. The development, India has made in the fields agriculture, animal husbandry, fishery, forestry, horticulture, sericulture, etc. are largely due to extension services in the particular discipline. Kelsey and Hearne (1967) gave emphasis on nine areas, which indicate the scope of extension, these are:

1. Efficiency in agricultural and allied production
2. Efficiency in marketing, distribution and utilisation
3. Conservation, development and use of natural resources
4. Management on the farm and in home.
5. Family living
6. Youth development
7. Leadership development
8. Community development and rural area development
9. Public affairs

Extension is an integral part of technology transfer or teaching in agriculture, animal husbandry, rural development, social works, etc. The principle, philosophy and methodologies of extension are now being widely used in other fields like health, nutrition, family planning, natural resource management, disaster preparedness, etc. Its application has gained relevance also in the urban areas where teaching, training, motivation and creation of awareness of is required for implementation of various programmes. In view of these, the scope of the extension is very broad and covers many aspects of rural development.

Components of Extension

In the context of rural development, extension has the following three broad components:

- Extension Education
- Extension Services
- Extension Work

Extension Education

Extension education is basically a need based, people's participation based, local resource based and problem-solution based approach, and it is very much interrelated with teaching, extension and research. Here, extension efforts are related to research both in terms of its products, viz. new technologies and process. The extension education role is performed by higher learning institutions, viz. research institutes, universities, and apex level training and extension organisations.

Extension Services

Extension services are the mission and mandate of the various development departments like agriculture, animal husbandry, horticulture, watershed, rural development, health, industry, education, etc. in all the states of the country. It is a programme for development employing the extension process as a means for implementation. Extension service is location specific, input intensive service oriented, and field level professional activities with two objectives (i) transferring new technologies or innovations, and advising the people on improved methods; and (ii) communicating development constraints to research institutes / development organization / policy makers, as feedback for development of solutions to the problems. Thus, extension service serves as a link between researchers, development workers, and people. Extension service also works hand-in-hand with other development departments, credit institutions, NGOs, international agencies, civil society, etc. to multiply their efforts and effects.

Extension Work

Extension work is to assist people to improve their socio-economic condition through educational and service approach. It helps people to take decision in right direction. Through extension work, people are stimulated to make changes that result in more efficient production and marketing, conservation of natural resources, improved livelihood security, health, and more satisfying family and community life. Extension work is location specific and usually susceptible to outside criticism. Extension work is actually to help people to help themselves by taking care of their wellbeing. It is not always doing for them. Extension work ensures the participation of people in developmental works and there after owning the programmes. This is not a work of only providing service rather a work of educating the people to take control of their development. That is way it is an educational process giving more emphasis on developing the capacity of the people rather than only providing services of various kind.

Philosophy of Extension Education

The word "Philosophy" has a wide range of meanings. It is the pursuit of wisdom, a body of general principles or laws of a field of knowledge. Essentially philosophy is a view of life, wisdom or knowledge and its various components. It is a body of general principles of laws of a field of knowledge, activities, etc., such as a philosophy of life or philosophy of extension work. The practical implication is that the philosophy of a particular field would furnish the principles or guidelines with which to shape or mould the programmes or activities relating to that discipline. The philosophy of extension education is based on the hypothesis that the rural people are capable, intelligent and willing to change their situation.

Philosophy

View of life

Wisdom

Knowledge

General Principles

The philosophy of extension education has been interpreted in many ways by various authors and some of them are as follows:

According to Ensminger (1962)

1. Extension is educational for all village people.
2. Extension is changing the knowledge, skill and attitude of the people.
3. Extension is teaching people what to want, as well as how to work out ways of satisfying these wants and inspiring them to achieve their desires.

Extension is

- helping people to help themselves
- learning by doing and seeing is believing
- Self help
- a cooperative effort
- a two-way channel
- educational activities for all

4. Extension is "helping people to help themselves".
5. Extension is "learning by doing and seeing is believing".
6. Extension is development of individual and their society.
7. Extension is living relationship, respect and trust for each other.
8. Extension is working in harmony with culture of the people.
9. Extension is working together to expand the welfare and happiness of people.
10. Extension is a two-way channel
11. Extension is a continuous process educational process in which both learner and teacher contribute and receive.

According to Kelsey and Hearne (1967)

The basic philosophy of extension education is to teach people *how* to think, not *what* to think. Extension's specific job is furnishing the inspiration, supplying specific advice and technical help, and counseling to see that the people as individuals, families, groups and communities work together as a unit to solve their problems. Extension workers work with people to help them develop themselves and achieve personal superior personal wellbeing.

According to Mildred Horton

1. The individual is supreme in a democracy
2. The home is the fundamental unit in a civilization
3. The family is the first training group of the human race
4. The foundation of any permanent civilization must rest on the partnership of man and land (nature).

According to Dahama (1965)

1. Self-help
2. People are the greatest resources
3. It is a cooperative effort
4. It has its foundation in democracy
5. It involves a two-way channel of knowledge and experience
6. It is based on creating interest by seeing and doing
7. Voluntary, co-operative participation in programmes
8. Persuasion and education of the people
9. The programme is based on the attitude and values of the people
10. It is a never ending process

Principles of Extension Education

Principles are generalized guidelines which form the basis for decision and action in a consistent way. These principles are found to be true in delivering results under varying conditions and circumstances. To work with the rural people, we must have knowledge of these principles. Some of these principles related to extension education are mentioned below.

> **Principles**
> Generalized guidelines which form the basis for decision and action in a consistent way

1. **Principle of interests and needs-** People's interest and need should be kept in mind while formulating the extension programme. These needs and interests differ from individual to individual and village to village. So, therefore, extension programme should be need specific. The extension workers should not pass on their interests as those of the people.
2. **Principle of existing environment-** Extension programme should be designed as per the resource availability in the community and capacity of the primary stakeholders. Every social system has its own characteristics, advantages and limitations. Careful examination of issues and problems related to a particular area are required before taking up extension work.
3. **Principle of Participation and co-operation-** Participation of villagers in the programme means involvement of people in identification of problems, planning, implementation and evaluation of the programme. However, this process is hardly followed in any programme execution. Therefore, large numbers of programmes have failed to produce desired outcomes. It has been found that if the villagers take decisions concerning the implementation of the programme, the success rate become very high. Extension workers should involve the community in all aspects while implementing a programme otherwise it would be a viewed by the villagers as a programme implemented by government.
4. **Principle of learning by doing-** The villagers should be actively involved in the programme activities. This will help them to see the result by doing the things which will facilitate the quick behavioural change and develop the confidence to use the practices/ideas in future. The extension worker should keep in mind this important principle of extension that the adults learn maximum by doing things and they should apply this principle liberally in their extension works for better result.
5. **Principle of satisfaction-** The end product of extension work should produce satisfying results for the people. Satisfying results reinforce learning and motivate to seek further improvement.

6. **Principle of leadership-** People believes in local leaders, and work on their advice. Identifying different types of leaders and working through them is essential for extension. The local leaders are to be trained, and used extensively in the extension programme.

7. **Principle of grass roots approach-** Extension programmes should start with local groups, local situations and local problems. Extension work should start with where people are and what they have. Change should start from the existing situation. The objective of starting the extension programme with local people is to demonstrate the value of new practice or programmes so that more and more people would participate.

8. **Principle of democratic approach-** The extension work is democratic both in philosophy and practice. It believes in persuasion and discussion. The people are provided with number of choices and they are free to adopt or not to adopt.

Principles of Extension Education

- Interests and needs
- Participation and co-operation
- satisfaction
- leadership
- grass roots approach
- democratic approach
- culture difference
- indigenous knowledge
- whole family approach
- adaptability
- using existing grass root institutions
- using trained Specialists
- addressing problems of all class of society
- continuous evaluation
- existing environment

9. **Principle of culture difference-** There is cultural difference between the extension agents and the farmers. Differences also exist between group of farmers in different parts of the country in their customs, values, beliefs, attitude and way of life. Extension programme must be carried out in harmony with the prevailing culture for better acceptance and results.

10. **Principle of indigenous knowledge-** People have been solving their problems by application of indigenous knowledge since generations. This knowledge has been part of their social system and people consider it essential for their survival. The extension agent, instead of ignoring the importance of indigenous knowledge, should understand them and their ramification in the life of the people and develop extension programme accordingly.

11. **Principle of whole family approach-** Household is considered as unit of intervention for development. So, extension programme should be developed in such way that it encourages the participation and involvement of entire family members. The goal of development is difficult to achieve without educating the whole family- the male member, the female member and children.

12. **Principle of adaptability-** Extension Programmes should be flexible in nature to accommodate the local conditions. This is required because the people need, resource availability and local situation vary from place to place and time to time.
13. **Principle of using existing grass root institutions/organisation-** At present, there are number of formally established institutions like Gram Panchayat, co-operatives, schools, youth clubs, farmer's associations, Self Help Group (SHG) are working in the village for the development of the villagers. These institutions or organisations know the problems of the village very well than any external agency. The extension agents should utilize the services of good local organisations for promoting the developmental activities.
14. **Principle of using trained Specialists-**Agriculture and allied fields are growing very rapidly due to innovations and adoption of improved practices. Technologies of yester years are becoming obsolete. It is not possible for the extension workers to be abreast of latest developments in various aspects of a particular field. So, the extension worker should use the experts or trained specialists in the programme to recommend the better and latest practice to the farmers to get maximum benefit.
15. **Principle of addressing problems of all class of society-** Extension education programmes is basically democratic in nature. It is expected that the programme benefits the all segments of the society. If the programme favours or ignores any segment or group, the results will be affected.
16. **Principle of continuous evaluation-** Evaluation is a process by which one understands the problems of programme implementation. Accordingly, suitable steps are taken to rectify or speed up the process to reach the target as out lined in the project document. Extension worker should make periodic evaluation of his/her programme to know the extent to which the results obtained are in agreement with the objectives fixed earlier. If there is any deficiency, she/he should take immediate corrective measures to bring the programme in to right track.

Extension Educational Process

Extension educational process involves five essential and integrated steps. The sequence of these steps is discussed on the basis of concept developed by Leagans (1961).

The first step is the **analysis of situation** in which the facts about people, their occupation, interests, need, social customs and habits and economic, social, cultural, physical, technological environment in which they live and work are collected. The facts collected are analyzed to identify the problems.

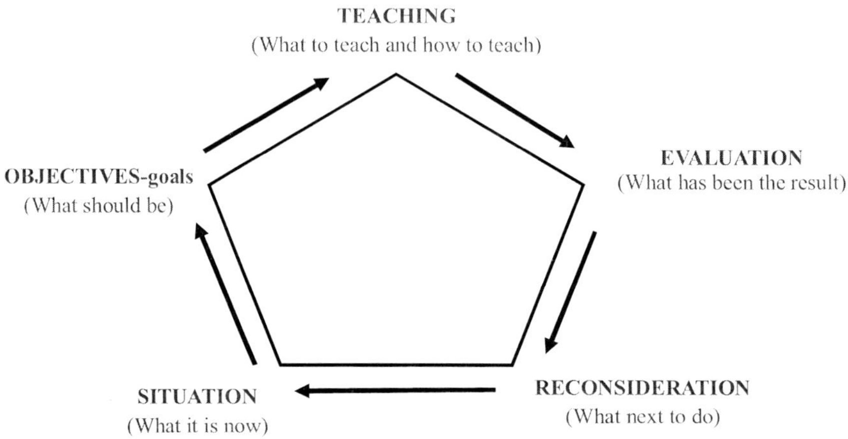

The second step is deciding on **objectives or goals** to be accomplished by the community. A limited number of objectives should be selected by involving the local people. The objectives should be specific, clearly stated and achievable and on completion should produce tangible economic benefit to the people.

The third step is **teaching** which involves what should be taught (content) and how it should be taught (methods). It requires the selection of appropriate methods and aids looking in to the complexity of the contents and objectives of the programme. This phase is very important, and the extension worker's effectiveness is determined on the ability to use extension methods to meet the extension education objectives.

The fourth step is **evaluating the teaching**, i.e. determining the extent to which the objects have been fulfilled. This will also be a test of how accurately and clearly the objectives have been stated and what methodology adopted to reach the goals. The process of evaluation may be simple and informal or it may be formal and very complex. Evaluation not only provides us the reasons of success but also indicate the deficiencies which help to formulate better programmes in future.

> **Extension Educational Process**
>
> Developed by J P Leagans (1961)
>
> **Five steps**
>
> - Situation
> - Objectives
> - Teaching
> - Evaluation
> - Reconsideration

The fifth step is the **reconsideration** of entire extension educational programme on the light of results of evaluation. This step consists of a review of previous efforts and results which reveal a new situation. If this new situation shows the need for further work, then the whole process may begin again, with new or modified objectives.

Hence, the extension education is a continuous teaching- learning process and this process goes on, resulting the progress of the people from a less desirable to more desirable situation. Extension educational process is a continuous process. New problems may emerge which requires the extension teaching process to address it.

Suggested Readings and References

1. Supe S.V. (1987). An Introduction to Extension Education, Oxford and IBH Publishing Co. Pvt. Ltd. New Delhi.
2. Kelsey, L.D. and Hearne, C.C. (1949). Cooperative Extension Work, Vail-Ballou, Inc, Binghamton, New York, U.S.A.
3. Adams, M.E. (1987). Agricultural Extension in Developing Countries, Intermediate Tropical
4. Mani, Gomathi (1994). Adult Learning: Theory and Practice, Sterling Publisher Private Limited, New Delhi-110 016.
5. Dahama, O.P., Bhatanagar, O.P. (1985). Education and Communication for Development, Oxford & IBH Publishing Company, New Delhi.
6. Mathialagan, P. (2007). Textbook of Animal Husbandry and Livestock Extension, International Book Distributing Co. 7, Meerabai Marg, Lucknow, India.
7. Ray, G.L. (2008). Extension Communication and Management, Kalyani Publishers, New Delhi.
8. Reddy, A.A. (1993). Extension Education, Sree lakshmi Press, Bapatla.
9. Sharma, K.R.G. (2008). Veterinary Extension Education, BSPBS Publications, Hyderabad, Hyderabad.
10. Van den Ban, A.W. & H.S. Hawkins, (1998). Agricultural Extension, 2nd Edition. New Delhi, CBS Pub. & Distributors.

2

Teaching-Learning Process in Extension

1. Extension Teaching
2. Requirements of Extension Teaching
3. Principles of Teaching
4. Steps in Extension Teaching
    a) Attention
    b) Interest
    c) Desire
    d) Conviction
    e) Action
    f) Satisfaction
5. Functions of Extension Teacher
6. Nature/Characteristics of Learning
7. Learning Situation
    a) Extension Worker
    b) Learner
    c) Subject Matter
    d) Teaching Materials
    e) Physical Facilities
8. Principles of Learning
9. Learning Experience
10. Types of Learning
11. Laws of Learning
12. Theories of Learning
13. Suggested Readings and References

Extension Teaching

It is now evident that the extension is an educational process which attempts to produce desirable changes in the human behaviour. This educational process is nothing but teaching-learning process and this is explained by Leagans (1961) as follows:

Teaching is the process of arranging situations that stimulate and guide the learning activity towards the goals that specify the desired changes in the behaviour of people. Teaching consists of providing situations in which the things to be learnt are brought to the attention of the learners, their interest is developed, desire aroused, conviction created, action promoted and satisfaction ensured.

Learning is the process by which an individual, through his own activity, changes his behaviour.

Process means a course of procedures, something that occurs in a series of actions or events conducting to the desired end.

Requirement of Extension Teaching

The purpose of extension teaching is not merely informing the people but to bring desired changes in the behaviour. To achieve this, Ray (2008) has explained that extension teaching requires:

a) *Specific and clearly defined teaching objectives*- while formulating the objectives of the extension teaching, the following aspects are to be considered:
    i) people to be taught
    ii) behavioral changes to be developed in the people
    iii) content or subject matter to bring the desired change in behaviour
    iv) the real life situation in which the action is going to take place.

b) *A suitable learning situation*- The learning situation consist of five interrelated elements- (1) Instructor (extension agent), (2) Learners (farmers, farm women, rural youth, etc.), (3) Subject matter (say, clean milk production), (4) Teaching materials (equipments, medicine, audio-visual aids), and (5) Physical facilities (facilities for demonstration, facilities at training site, etc.)

c) *Effective communication process*- Communication involves the transfer of knowledge from a source to one or more receivers. Extension teaching, to be effective must take in to consideration of proper functioning of the elements of communication-communicator, message, channel, treatment and presentation, receiver of message and feedback from receiver.

e) *Well defined content and method-* Extension teaching requires the relevant subject matters to be taught and appropriate teaching methods and aids to deliver the subject matter to intended clients.

d) *Careful planning and designing the programme-*Extension teaching should be properly planned and designed on the basis of relevant data on the situation and available research findings. This is an intentional process and there is no scope for trial and error approach in extension teaching.

e) *Result effective learning-* The extension teaching must produce effective learning, it means that what is taught should be understood and internalized by the learners. An effective teaching experience is one which results in a maximum number of desirable changes in the behavior of the learners.

f) *Educational changes in relation to the subject matter taught-* Desirable changes in the knowledge, skill, attitude, understanding, goal, action, and confidence of the people are to be achieved in relation to the topic being taught.

Principles of Teaching

1. The farmer should understand the purpose of the course.
2. The farmer should want to learn.
3. The extension teacher should keep a friendly and informal atmosphere so that the learners can ask things they do not understand.
4. The physical conditions should be favourable and appropriate
5. The teacher should involve the participants so that they participate and accept some responsibility for the learning process.
6. The teacher should make use of the learners' experience.
7. The teacher should prepare well for the class, should keep hid teaching aids handy and should be enthusiastic about teaching.
8. The method of instruction should be varied and appropriate to the contents and situation.
9. The teacher should be always willing to learn and update his knowledge on the topic or subject.

Steps in Extension Teaching

According to Wilson and Gallup (1955), there are six steps involved in extension teaching process:

1. Attention
2. Interest
3. Desire
4. Conviction
5. Action
6. Satisfaction

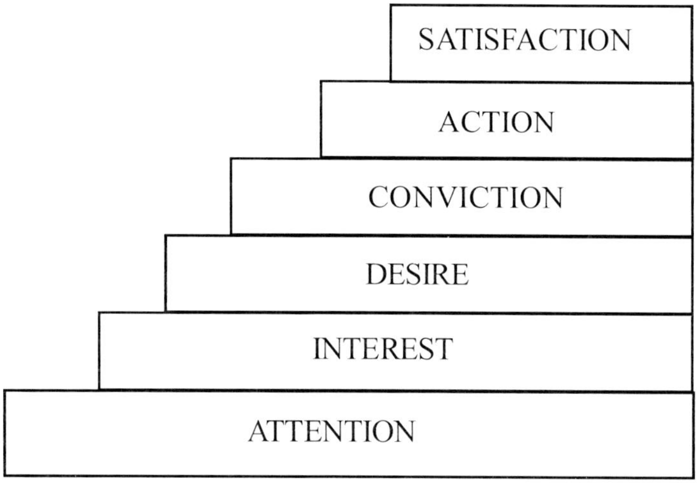

Fig. 1 : Steps in Extension Teaching

Attention

Livestock farmers are not always aware about the improvements or developments in the fields of their interest. The first step in extension education is to make the farmer aware of new ideas or way of doing things. The farmer must know first that there is existence of new ideas and practice. Until the individual's attention has been focused on the change that is considered desirable, there is no recognition of a problem to be solved or a want to be satisfied. Attention is the starting point to the arousing of interest. Mass media methods like television, radio, newspaper, mobile phone etc., and personal contact by extension agent and contact through local leaders are important at this stage. For an example, a livestock farmer's attention is drawn towards a milking machine through these mass media methods. Now, the farmer may be interested to know about the product. He may entre in to the next step of teaching-learning process.

Interest

Once the attention of the livestock farmer has been drawn to the new idea of a milking machine, the extension worker through personal contact, local leader, farm publications, radio, television, etc., to stimulate his interest for enquiring more information about the milking machine. In this stage, the extension worker should provide information to the farmer in such a way that they will be able to understand it and use. It is necessary to present one idea at a time relevant to their needs.

Desire

The continuation of farmer interest on new idea of a milking machine for certain duration becomes desire and motivates him for have a such machine. At this stage, the extension worker should explain to the farmer that the milking machine is suitable to his situation, and having one milking machine will satisfy a significant want or need of the farmer. It will be easier for him to milk the animals. At this stage, extension worker, should emphasize the advantages of the milking machine and its use. To consolidate desire of having one milking machine, the extension worker may conduct demonstrations, organize group discussion, etc.

Conviction

It is a stage of strong persuasion in which extension worker makes the livestock farmer belief that the action is necessary to internalize the practice. He also ensures that the farmer visualizes the action in terms of his own peculiar situation and has acquired confidence in his own ability to do the thing. Visits to result demonstrations to observe the results and weigh the proof of practice under local conditions, participation in method demonstration meeting, slide show, films, television programmes and personal contact by the extension agents are important methods used in this stage.

Action

Unless the conviction is converted in to action, the teaching effort is fruitless. At this stage, the job of the extension worker is to make the livestock farmer to act on the ideas. For this action to happen and thereafter internalize the practice, small scale demonstration may be set up in real life situation by extension worker for the farmers. This provides the opportunity of direct experience on the part of the farmers. At this stage it is required to collect the evidence of change in respect of yields, income, employment, ease in practice, behaviour, etc. Personal contact by the extension agent, demonstration, supply of the critical inputs and ensuring essential services are important at this stage.

Satisfaction

The end product of the extension teaching process is the satisfaction that comes to the farmer as a result of meting a need, solving a problem, acquiring new skill or some other change in behaviour. Satisfaction is a motivating factor to further learning leading to change in behaviour. It is necessary that the extension worker should provide relevant information about milking machine to the livestock farmers on a continuous basis to maintain his level of satisfaction.

Use of mass media, local leaders and personal contact of the extension agent are important at this stage. Availability of critical inputs and essential service are also to be ensured.

These six teaching steps mentioned above are not distinctly separate from each other and often blend with each other and lose their clear-cut identity. There is also overlapping of the extension methods used to advance each of the different steps in extension education process.

Functions of Extension Teacher

The terms "extension educator', 'extension teacher' , 'adult educator', 'instructor', ' animator' and 'change agent' all pertain to ' he/she who assists learning to happen' or 'managing the learning' or 'one who is helping or motivating adults to learn'. The main functions of extension teacher can be broadly classified in to five categories and these are:

1. **The diagnostic function**: Helping the learners to identify their problems in understanding the issues or applying the theory in to practice.
2. **The planning function**: It is organising the teaching and learning activities by extension educators and providing effective learning experiences to learners to attain maximum desirable changes in their behaviour.
3. **The motivational function:** This is creating conditions that will cause learners to want to learn.
4. **The methodological function:** Selecting suitable teaching methods or combination of methods appropriate to the particular learning situation to produce desired results among the learners.
5. **The resource function:** Arranging human and material resources required for the extension teaching programme.

Learning

Learning is a process by which a person becomes changed in his behaviour through self-activity. It is a process that takes within the learner when he feels a need to attain such thing. Learning is a process of progressive adaptation (Skinner, 1961).

> **Learning**
>
> 1 % through taste,
>
> 1.5 % through touch,
>
> 3.5 % through smell,
>
> 11 % through hearing and
>
> 83 % through sight.

Learning results in certain kinds of changes in human being, such as, increase in level of knowledge, improving of a skill or a process, and development of changed attitude. Man gains his ability to substitute the 'good' practice for the 'bad' in the use of his physical and human resources through learning. Research revealed that people learn 1 % through taste, 1.5 % through touch, 3.5 % through smell, 11 % through hearing and 83 % through sight. Dale Edgar s (1964) Cone of experience provides a linkage between learning activity and participants involvement in the process of learning. It illustrates that people tend to remember 10 % of what they read, 20 % of what they hear, 30 percent what they see, 50 percent of what they hear and see, 70 percent of what they say and 90 percent of what they say and do. Learning is most effective when done under the influence of skillfully organised teaching. The result of teaching and learning process is education and these two are actually not distinctly separate process.

Nature/Characteristics of Learning

1. Learning is a fundamental process of life: without learning life cannot exist and no progress can take place.
2. Learning is continuous process
3. Learning is a creative experience
4. Learning is growth
5. Learning is change in behaviour or response
6. Learning is purposive or goal directed
7. Learning is always active
8. Learning takes place within an organism
9. Learning is a process of change
10. Learning is the result of individual activity
11. Learning is determined by conscious as well as unconscious experiences
12. Learning occurs intentionally or unintentionally
13. Learning is transferable
14. Learning is universal. Both animal and human being are subjected to learning.
15. Learning depends upon readiness and motivation
16. Learning is instinctive as well as acquired
17. Learning is positively related to interest
18. Learning is process of improvement with practice
19. Learning may takes place at abstract level or concrete level
20. Learning is not just confined to the formal class room learning

Learning Situation

Extension teaching is basically arranging effective learning situations that stimulate, guide and promote learning activity. An effective learning situation, as per Leagans (1961), consists of five essential elements which are present in dynamic relationship with one another (Fig. 2).

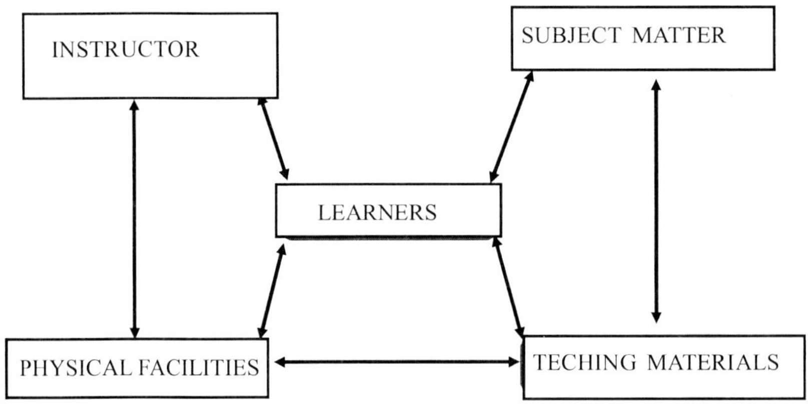

Fig. 2 : The Elements of learning Situation

The Elements of Learning Situation

1. Instructor (Extension Worker)

He is the extension worker who makes effort to motivate the farmers. The quality of learning depends upon how effectively the he creates the learning situation.

The instructor should:

1. have teaching objectives clearly in mind that are significant to learners, that are attainable through the educational process within the mental and physical limitation of the learners.
2. know the subject matter and have it well organised
3. know the techniques of using appropriate teaching methods and aids
4. be able to communicate effectively with learners.
5. be personable, enthusiastic, attractive and interested in the subject matters and learners.
6. react appropriately to the feelings, emotions and attitudes of learners.
7. be able to arrange and manage the learning situations so as to prevent or minimize distractions within and outside the learning situation.
8. be democratic in his leadership
9. be able to encourage participation of the learners.
10. always prepare and use a carefully developed teaching plan.

2. Learners (Livestock Farmers)

Learner is the key element in learning situation. He is the person who is interested to learn and all efforts in the teaching and learning process are directed towards him.

The learners should:

1. have interest on the learning,
2. be capable of learning,
3. have need for the information offered, and
4. be able to use the information once it is gained.

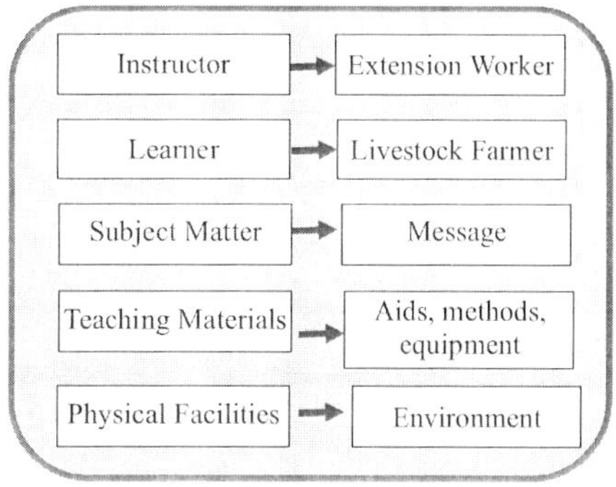

3. Subject Matter (Message)

It is the content or topic of teaching that is intended to pass on to the learners.

The subject matter should be:

1. pertinent to learners' need,
2. proven, correct and based on facts ,
3. applicable to their real life situations,
4. well organised and presented logically and clearly,
5. understandable by the learners,
6. timely and appropriate,
7. consistent with overall objectives of the programme, and
8. challenging, satisfying and significant to the learners.

4. Teaching Materials

These are instructional materials, equipment and aids which are very essential for effective transfer the subject matter. Proper selection and handling of teaching materials facilitate in creating the desirable learning situation.

The teaching materials should be:

1. simple and easy to handle,
2. suitable to subject matter and physical situation,
3. readily available, and
4. each item must be used skill fully.

5. Physical Facilities

It means the physical environment in which teaching and learning takes place.

The physical facilities should be:

1. free from outside distraction,
2. compatible with the objectives,
3. well lighted and ventilated, and
4. adequate and easily accessible.

The nature of each of these elements, their relationship to each other, their role in the education process must be properly understood by the extension worker and should skillfully manipulate these elements in the learning situation to provide satisfactory earning experiences to the learners.

Principles of Learning

The extension education is a teaching-learning process in which an effective learning experience is provided to learners to attain the required changes. To create an effective learning situation for learning to take place, an extension worker should know the principles of learning. However, many principles of learning are well established and have useful application in extension education.

1. Learning should be purposeful

Farmers learn which is required to them and useful in solving the problems. Objectives of the programme must be clear and meaningful to the learner as well as to the instructor. What is to be learned must be important to, and wanted by, a relatively large number of participant in the group, and must be attainable-

a) through the educational process
b) within the time limitation of the extension worker and the participants
c) within the physical and economic resource of the participants, and
d) within the social condition and learning ability of the participants

2. Learning is growth-like and continuous

Extension worker must know the level of understanding, resource position and social condition of the learners and starts teaching at learner's level. New ideas must be related to those already held by the learner and the pace of instruction must be adjusted to the learner's capacity. Ideas must be brought to the attention of the learners repeatedly and over a period of time.

3. Learning must be challenging and satisfying

Learning must provide a sense of satisfaction to the learner. Learning outcome will only be satisfactory if subject matter is need based and useful to them. The ability of the extension worker to create an effective learning situation makes the learning more rewarding to learner.

4. Learning involves appropriate activity by the learners that engages a maximum number of senses

Messages reach the human mind through five senses, namely, seeing, hearing, feeling, testing and smelling. Maximum learning takes place if more than one senses organs are involved in the process. In extension, most of the messages to be learnt reach the mind through seeing, hearing and doing. Learning should be experience centered i.e. farmers should primarily learn by doing, in addition to seeing and hearing.

5. Learning must result functional understanding

Effective leaning does not result from knowledge alone, but from understanding of the knowledge about a phenomenon. Extension education is not only imparting knowledge on a subject but also making the learner to understand how to apply the knowledge in real life situation. Memorizing is one way of gaining knowledge but unless what is learned is applied it will be forgotten and the learning objectives will not be met. For development of functional understanding, it is essential that the farmer understand the whole subject as well as different topics and their interrelationship.

6. Learning is affected by the physical and social environment

The physical and social environment greatly affects the learning situation. The extension worker should take care of physical factors like lighting, ventilation, sitting arrangements, provision of water, temperature, etc., while planning the extension education activity. He should also recognize and utilize the effects of the social environment on learning by involving the learners actively in the learning process. The learning situation should be so designed that the least possible energy is expressed in adjusting it to the physical and social environment.

7. Learning ability varies widely among the learners

Individuals differ in their ability to understand, retain and apply information. Therefore, the level of communication should be in line with the learner's ability, and the subject matter should also be taught at the level of learner's ability to understand apply in its own situation.

8. Learning is a gradual process, and needs multiple exposures for change

Extension teaching is intended to induce learners to adopt new ideas. This usually requires several exposures to new ideas through various ways, and to do this different teaching method must be used from time to time. For example, a new idea may be introduced to a community through television and radio programme and then to village leaders through contact by extension workers. This might be followed by village meeting, followed by demonstration with distribution of reading materials. Research indicates that learners in the extension situation usually must be exposed to ideas from four to eight times, and oveer a period of time, in order to induce a large number of them to take action.

9. Learning capacity remains significantly high throughout normal life

Adult education programmes are based on the assumption that the adults have the capacity to learn. However, the learning ability tends to decline in individual after middle age. The main reasons for this decline among the adults is their less acute vision, less acute hearing, slower reaction, and especially with greater reluctance to learn, increased fear of failure in learning activities.

Some of the implication of these factors for extension workers in teaching adults are :

a) arrange the physical situation properly so that the adults can hear and see clearly
b) use visuals with sharp contrast in the form of charts, poster, diagrams and pictures
c) speak clearly and distinctly
d) repeated presentation of ideas.
e) provide rewards and encouragement to adult learners
f) avoid use of harsh words and nay forms of punishment

10. Learning is an active process

To learn new skill, the learner has to practice them and to lean facts, he has to relate them to each other and to a problem. Similarly, to develop favourable attitude, he has to change his present feelings about things. The extension worker can only create situation that is conducive for learning but the farmer will have to learn by himself.

11. Learning requires effective communication

Communication is the process by which two or more people exchange ideas, facts, feelings, thoughts, or impressions in ways that each gains a common understanding of the meaning and intend of messages. Good communication is the essence of good extension teaching. Better communication can be achieved by integrating suitable visuals in the teaching process.

12. Theory and Practice must be related

Theory and practice are always related. Principles or theory relate to *why* and technique relates to *how*. It is required that the extension worker must know theory behind a good practice. In fact there is no good practice without support of sound theory. Extension workers equipped with an understanding of principles applicable to the work are more likely to be creative than those who pride themselves on just being practical.

Learning Experience

The main objective of livestock extension worker is to create a situation in which a learner gains sufficient learning experience to solve his problems. Leagans (1961) has defined that the learning experience is the mental and/or physical reaction a learner makes to seeing or hearing or doing the things to be learned, through which he gains meanings and understandings useful in solving problems.

From this definition, it can be seen that the learning experience involves far more than being physically present in the learning situation. It is what a learner does in the learning situation that is all important aspect of learning. Learning, therefore, takes place through the experience which has, i.e. through the reactions he makes to the content which is to be learned. It is important for extension worker to know what are the learning experiences required to be attained by the learner to meet the objectives of extension teaching, and accordingly he should design the activities in the extension programme.

Types of Learning

1. **Motor Leaning:** It is characterized by the involvement of muscular activity. There are two types of motor learning (a) Sensory motor learning-which involves in the acquisition of simple habits through sense organs and (b) perceptual motor learning-which involves in the acquisition social habit and complex skills-e.g. cycling, swimming, dancing, etc.
2. **Concept Learning:** It pertains to the acquisition of ideas, concepts and mental associations. In learning a concept, an individual tries to find out some common property in a group of objects. When we acquire knowledge through concrete experience, it leads to generalization or concept formation.
3. **Perceptual Learning:** This types of learning takes place largely or entirely through the senses. Learning through concrete object and spoken or written symbols or drawing the figures or reading, etc. comes under this category.

4. **Verbal Associate Learning:** In most of the cases, learning takes place in human being through involvement of words. Ability to manipulate symbols, as a language, makes it possible for us to learn things.
5. **Attitude Learning:** An attitude is an emotionalized system of ideas, which predisposes an individual to act in a certain way under certain conditions. Much of our learning involves in change in attitudes. Because of our formation of attitude, favourable or unfavourable response is shown to various objects or to persons or to ideas or to situations.
6. **Cognitive Learning:** It pertains to the acquisition of knowledge, concepts and their interrelationships.
7. **Observational Learning:** Interrelationships, insight and imitation are the three important aspects of observed learning. In learning, observation is useful because through it the learner is able to observe the interrelationship among the objects or the things observed.
8. **Problem Solving Learning:** Problem solving learning encourages one to think. In this learning, emphasis is put on the suggestions or possible solutions and reasoning.
9. **Imaginative Learning:** The process of which things of the past, present and future take definite shapes in consciousness is known as imagination and the process by which such things are learned and understood, is called imaginative learning.
10. **Conditioning:** Conditioning is considered to be fundamental form of learning. Ian Pavlov is the pioneer of the study of conditional learning in dogs. His finding is that an organism reacts to a new experience on the basis of identical past experience.

Laws of Learning

Thorndike's four laws of learning are:

1. **Law of readiness:** This law states that when a learner is ready to learn a thing, he or she will learn not only effectively but also quickly. Readiness means preparation for action; it is a kind of 'action tendency' aroused through preparatory adjustments, sets, attitudes and the like. The fulfilling of the tendency is satisfying and its non-fulfillment is annoying. However, the learner will become ready when he feels that the learning the new behaviour will satisfy his motives.
2. **Law of Exercise/ Frequency:** This law is also called as law of use and disuse. It implies the strengthening of stimulus-response (S-R) connections (bonds) with practice and their weakening (forgetting) when the practice is

not continued. It means that the practice is considered necessary for retention of what is learned otherwise it will be forgotten. The teacher must help the learners to practice and review the desirable behaviour as many times as is found necessary. When a response is repeated several times it tends to become habitual i.e. learning is a self-activity.

3. **Law of Effect:** The name stresses the importance of the effect or the consequence of a response on its fixation. This law implies the strengthening or weakening of a behaviour as a result of its consequences. The people learn rapidly and permanently when the learning experience is rewarding, pleasant and enjoyable. The bond between a stimulus and a response is strengthened or weakened because of the satisfaction or annoyance that accompanies the action.
4. **Law of Belongingness:** Belongingness as a law of learning refers to the fact that a connection is more easily learnt if the response belongs to the situation and an after effect strengthen the response. The law of belongingness has a very great implication for organising teaching and learning. It implies the application of only such rewards and punishments to the S-R bonds which are relevant to the situation.
5. **Law of spread:** Thorndike's Law of Spread of Effect principle states that reward strengthens not only the response to which it belongs, but also the responses adjacent (after or before) to the rewarded response.

Theories of Learning

One can organise learning in many different ways. For this, psychologists have grouped learning theories under three broad categories, such as behaviourism, humanism and cognitive process. All most all human behaviour is acquired and learning results in a relatively permanent change in behaviour. Many theorists agree that learning results in relatively permanent change of behaviour, that it takes place within the context of experience, and that ease or rate of learning depends on the ease with which new information is integrated by the learner. Knowledge of theories on learning is essential for the extension worker to understand why certain methods or techniques are applied in a particular situation. There are several theories of learning, and the word 'learning' is used to cover a wide variety of experiences. Some of these theories propounded by psychologists and educationists are discussed below very briefly.

i) Thorndike's theory of Connectionism (Trial and Error)

E.L. Thorndike propounded this theory of Connectionism in his book on 'Animal Intelligence' in 1898. He said that learning implied an association between sense impression, or a stimulus(S) of impulse, to action or a response (R). Such association he called by the name of 'bond' or 'connection'. In the process of learning 'S-R bonds' are constructed, strengthened and organised. Thorndike's theory of learning is based on the three elements:

- the stimulus element which involves an environmental element
- the response elements which indicate a behavioural act
- the formulation of a connection or a bond which implies that every stimulus is inked with some kind of response, and thus makes the building block or structure of behaviour.

When an organism is said to have learned something, according to his views, it is essentially the formation of a connection, or bond or association between a stimulus and a response. He conducted a number of experiments to demonstrate the tenability of such a concept using chicks, cats, fishes, dogs and monkeys as subjects of his experiment. In an experiment, he put a hungry cat in a cage, and a fish was kept outside the cage. The cage was so constructed that if a lever was pressed the cage would open. Initially, the cat was indulged on random movements, exploratory in nature; and in the process cat touched the lever and cage was opened. On subsequent trials it was found that the cat pressed the lever when fish was brought in front of the cage. The cat started learning the right thing by trial and error method. This type of learning is also termed as learning by 'selecting and connecting'. During the process of learning, wrong movements were dropped and movements were strengthened by the cat.

ii) Pavlov's Theory of Classical Conditioning

The Russian physiologist, Ivan Pavlov (1849-1936.) explained for the first time the process of conditioning as a form of learning. Conditioning is the modification of natural response. Pavlov to establish the conditional learning made an experiment with a hungry dog by providing food. When he gave food to a hungry dog, the dog made a simple or unconditioned reflex response of secreting saliva. Here, saliva was produced due to natural physiological process. Pavlov then sounded the bell simultaneously with or before as many times as the dog was given food. Then, after several trails, the dog started secreting saliva at the sound of the bell. (The dog took the sound of the bell as sort of signal that food is coming.) Now this saliva secretion is not natural (or unconditioned) but artificially conditioned by learning experience. Thus, in Pavlov's experiment, dog's learning of the secretion of saliva at bell's sound was termed as learning by Conditioning. Significance of classical conditioning theory is very high in extension education. For example, an extension teacher with his defective methods of teaching or some sort of improper behaviour may condition the farmers not to listen him. On the contrary, caring attitude, sympathetic treatment, encouragement and good behaviour shown to the adults may produce desirable result through the process of conditioning.

iii) Skinner's Operant Conditioning Theory

Operant Conditioning theory was developed by an American Psychologist, B.F.Skinner. This theory is based on certain operations or actions, which an organism has to carry out. An operant is a set of acts which conditions an organism in doing something. Thus, an operant is roughly equivalent to the term 'a behaviour'. Operant conditioning, sometimes referred as instrumental conditioning, is a method of learning that is reinforced by rewards and discouraged by punishment. We can find examples of operant conditioning at work all around us. Consider the case of dairy farmers practicing the steps of clean milk production to earn a reward form extension worker in a district exhibition. In this example the promise or possibility of reward causes an increase in behaviour, but operant conditioning can be used to decrease a behaviour. The removal of an undesirable outcome or the use of punishment can be used to decrease or prevent behaviour. For example, a farmer may be told he will lose the opportunity of free treatment and medicine for his animal if he comes late to the treatment camp. This potential for punishment may lead to a decrease in disruptive behaviour of coming late.

Key Concepts Operant Conditioning

a) **Reinforcement:** It is any event that strengthens or increases the behavior it follows. There are two kinds of reinforcers:

   i) **Positive reinforcers:** These are favorable events or outcomes that are presented after the behavior is manifested. In situations that reflect positive reinforcement, a response or behavior is strengthened by the addition of something, such as praise or a direct reward.

   ii) **Negative reinforcers:** Theses involve the removal of an unfavorable events or outcomes after the display of a behavior. In these situations, a response is strengthened by the removal of something considered unpleasant.

   In both of these cases of reinforcement, the behavior increases.

b) **Punishment:** It is the presentation of an adverse event or outcome that causes a decrease in the behavior it follows. There are two kinds of punishment:

   i) **Positive punishment:** It is sometime referred as punishment by application. It involves the presentation of an unfavorable event or outcome in order to weaken the response it follows.

ii) **Negative punishment**: It is also known as punishment by removal, occurs when an favorable event or outcome is removed after a behavior occurs.

In both of these cases of punishment, the behavior **decreases.**

Skinner's theory is one of the most important contributions to learning. It throws light on habit formation, habit-breaking, role of incentives in learning, etc. Extension worker may apply this theory for modification of behaviour of clients by rewarding them for certain action and not rewarding in case the actions are not performed.

iv) Watson's Behavioural Theory

American Psychologist, John B. Watson is best known for his theory called " Behaviuorism". The subject matter of psychology, according to him is animal and human activity which can be observed and measured in an objective way. Watson was an extreme environmentalist: for him environment was much more important than heredity in determining the behaviour. He identified three emotions-fear, anger and love – and believed that they were caused by environmental effects and not due to any glandular changes in the body. Watson was very much helped by Thorndike's trial and error learning, but he gave it new interpretation. Learning, according to him, is the organisation of new habits formed by right responses and he calls it learning by successful variants.

He lays great importance on environment and its influence on the growth and development of the individual. According to him, all behaviour is learned in the process of interaction with the environment. This principle has tremendous implications for education. It emphasizes the role of school, community, and society in general, and the teachers and the parents, in particular in providing proper environment for development of the learners. The teacher should provide the appropriate situations where the learners can interact with the other objects in the environment and acquire the various skills, habits, attitudes and values.

v) Gestalt Theory of Learning

The basic idea behind the theory is that a thing cannot be understood by studying its constituent parts but only by studying it in totality. The term *Gestalt* has derive from German word meaning 'shape' or 'form', 'whole' or 'configuration'. Gestalts psychologists consider the process of learning as integrated whole. They follow the basic principle that the whole is greater than the sum of its parts. In other words, the whole (a picture) carried a different and altogether greater meaning than its individual components (paint, canvas, brush, etc.). In viewing the "whole," a cognitive process takes place –the mind makes a leap from comprehending the parts to realizing the whole.

The founders of Gestalt theory are Germans Max Wertheimer, Wolfgang Kohler, and Kurt Koffka. These theorists focused on different aspects of Gestalt that have, throughout the 20th century, continued to develop across multiple disciplines. Wertheimer applied Gestalt theory to problem solving. According to Wertheimer, the parts of the problem should not be isolated but instead should be seen a whole. This way, the learner can obtain "a new, deeper structural view of the situation. Wertheimer developed a concept titled *"Pragnanz"*(the German word for "precision"), which states that " when things are grasped as whole, the minimal amount of energy is exerted in thinking".

Koffka applied Gestalt theory to applied psychology and child psychology. His research with infants led to a theory that infants "initially experience organized wholes" as opposed to discrete elements. Kohler's experiments with animal learning led him to conclude that they exhibited insight, where relations among Stimuli and Reponses were learned, rather that simple stimulus response connections critical to behaviorist theory. In these experiments, apes were subjected to different trials of having to obtain food that was just out of their reach. They learned how to construct a way to get the food, whether standing on a box to get it, making a long stick to reach it, through trial and error. Kohler determined that the apes generated an "interconnection based on the properties of the things themselves" and thus developed insight on how to get the food based on the tools they had available at a given time.

According to Gestalt psychologists, learning takes place by insight. The insight is helpful in the development and betterment of the power of imagination, reasoning and thinking; and also plays a significant role in creative activities.

vi) Kurt Lewin's Field Theory of learning or Topological Theory of Learning

Kurt Lewin's (1890-1947) contribution is known as Field Theory or Topological Psychology or Vector-Psychology. Though he was associated with Gestalt psychologists, he was more interested in motivation and personality than in perception and learning. Learning according to Field Theory is the organisation and reorganization of behaviour, which results from any interacting influences on the developing organism acting on its shifting environment. The field theory is based on a thesis that behaviour of an individual is a function of the interacting person in a total environmental situation. Lewin termed the environment of the individual as 'Life Space'. An individual's environment may be three types- natural, social and psychological, and one has to strive in these three kinds of environments all through his life. Learning means resultant changes in understandings of his life space in the context of a dynamic interaction with the environment. Lewin has identified four kinds or aspects of learning:

- Change in cognitive structure (knowledge)
- Change in motivation (learning to like or dislike)
- Change in group belongingness or ideology (example an immigrant coming to term with and integrating in to a new culture.)
- Achieving voluntary control to body musculature (example- speech, skills)

For lewin, the main area of attention was the psychological field, the life space. The life space of a person includes the person and his physical and social environment with which he is psychologically engaged at a juncture of moment or even longer duration. The life space is influenced and altered by the physical and social environment. Lewin said that the teacher must not forget the real world and the life space of the student.

vii) Albert Bandura's Social Learning Theory

Albert Bandura is a Canadian Psychologist; and his theory of learning is based on the fact that observations as well as imitation play a leading role in changing one's behavioural pattern. In his views, all human beings learn by observation and imitation. Individuals whose behaviour is observed and often imitated art called 'Models' and observational learning is referred as 'Modelling' . In society we are surrounded by many influential persons like parents, teacher, film stars, progressive farmers, businessman, sportspersons, etc. We pay attention to some of these people (models) and encode their behaviour. At a later time we may imitate (i.e copy) the behaviour of these people. Imitative learning has been described as special case of instrumental conditioning. People more likely to attend to and imitate those people it perceives as similar to itself. Persons around us response to our imitating behaviour with either reinforcement or punishment. If a person imitates a model's behaviour and the consequences are rewarding, the person is likely to continue performing the behaviour.

According to Bandura, the following process or steps are usually involved in social theory of learning:

1. Acquisition: Here the learner pay attention and perceive the behaviour of the person acting as a model.
2. Retention: Here the internalized representation of the modeled behaviour is registered. It means what the learner observes is fixed in his or her memory in the form of mental image.
3. Performance: Here the memory is converted in to action. It means the performance involving motor responses are produced by imitation. For this, good training, demonstration and practice are essential.

4. Consequence: Here the reinforcement of the limited behaviour takes place. It means, the behaviour of the model that is imitated by the learner is reinforced for proper adoption and also for further continuance.

viii) Jean Piaget's Cognitive Theory of Learning

Jean Piaget (1896-1980) was a Swiss biologist and is considered to be the most famous cognitive theorist. He believed that there is a continuous interaction between the environment and the organism. Piaget, in his work mainly described the process of human thinking from infancy to adulthood. As a biologist, he was interested in how an organism adapts to its environment (Piaget described as intelligence.). He coined the term that adoption to the environment is controlled through mental organizations called 'Schema' that the individual uses to represent the world and designate action. This adaptation is driven by a biological drive to obtain balance between schemes and the environment (equilibration).

Piaget described adaptation is mechanical process of extension and modification of thinking that would result in the formation of a 'Cognitive Structure' for future use and according to him this is done by two processes- assimilation and accommodation. Both of these processes are used though out life as the person increasingly adapts to the environment in a more complex manner.

Assimilation refers to a kind of matching between the already existing cognitive and the environmental needs as they arise. Thus assimilation occurs when new something new is drawn in to the old pattern and becomes part of the inner organisation. But the person's old schema does not change in the process. Accommodation is the process of changing cognitive structures in order to accept something from the environment. Both processes are used simultaneously and alternately throughout life.

Stages of Cognitive Development: Piaget identified four stages in cognitive development:

1. **Sensory-motor stage** (birth to 2 years, Infancy). In this period, intelligence is demonstrated through motor activity without the use of symbols. Knowledge of the world is limited (but developing) because it is based on physical interactions / experiences. Children acquire object permanence at about 7 months of age (memory). Physical development (mobility) allows the child to begin developing new intellectual abilities. Some symbolic (language) abilities are developed at the end of this stage.
2. **Pre-operational stage** (2 to 7 years, Toddler and early childhood). In this period, intelligence is demonstrated through the use of symbols, and memory and imagination are developed, but thinking is done in a non-logical, non-reversable manner. Egocentric thinking predominates in this stage.

3. **Concrete operational stage** (About 7 to 11 years, Elementary and early adolescence). In this stage, intelligence is demonstrated through logical and systematic manipulation of symbols related to concrete objects. Operational thinking develops (mental actions that are reversible). Egocentric thought diminishes at this stage.
4. **Formal operational stage** (11 years and above, Adolescence and adulthood). In this stage, intelligence is demonstrated through the logical use of symbols related to abstract concepts.

Suggested Readings and References

1. Chauhan, S.S. (1979). Innovation in Teaching Learning Process, Vikas Publishing House Pvt. Ltd., 5 Ansari Road, New Delhi-110 002.
2. Mani, Gomathi (1994). Adult Learning: Theory and Practice, Sterling Publisher Private Limited, New Delhi-110 016.
3. Rybash *et al.* (1986). Adult Cognition and Aging: Developmental Changes in Processing, knowing and Thinking, Pergamon Press, Maxwell House, Fairview Park, Elmsford, New York, 1 0523, U.S.A.
4. Skiner, E.C. (1964). Educational Psychology, Fourth Edition, Prentice-Hall of India (Private) Ltd. New Delhi.
5. Aggarwal, J.C. (1989). Adult and Social Education in India: Global Perspective, p.4. Delhi: Doaba House.
6. Government of India (1988). National Literacy Mission, p.14. New Delhi: Ministry of Human Resources Development (Department of Education).
7. Jarvis, P. (1990a). Adult uizd Continuing Educution: Theory and Practice, pp. 29-32. London: Routledge.
8. Shah, S.Y. (1995). Indian Adult Education: A Historical Perspective. New Delhi: Directorate of Adult Education.
9. Mani, Gomathi (1994). Adult Learning: Theory and Practice, Sterling Publisher Private Limited, New Delhi-110 016.
10. Mathialagan, P. (2007). Textbook of Animal Husbandry & Livestock Extension, International Book Distributing Co.7, Meerabai Marg, Lucknow, India.
11. Adams, M.E. (1987). Agricultural Extension in Developing Countries, Intermediate Tropical.
12. Dahama, O.P., Bhatanagar, O.P. (1985). Education and Communication for Development, Oxford & IBH Publishing Company, New Delhi.
13. Ray, G.L. (2008). Extension Communication and Management, Kalyani Publishers, New Delhi.
14. Reddy, A.A. (1993). Extension Education, Sree lakshmi Press, Bapatla.
15. Sharma, K.R.G. (2008). Veterinary Extension Education, BSPBS Publications, Hyderabad, Hyderabad.

3

Extension Teaching Methods

1. Extension Teaching Method
2. Extension Methods
3. Classification of Extension Methods
4. Individual Methods and Group Methods
    a) Individual Methods
        i. Farm and Home Visits
        ii. Office Calls
        iii. Personal Letters
        iv. Telephone Calls
        v. Short Message Services (SMS)
        vi. Electronic Mail:
    b) Group Methods
        i. Method Demonstration
        ii. Result Demonstration
        iii. General Meetings
        iv. Group meetings
5. Mass media methods
    a. Farm Publication
        i. Leaflet
        ii. Folder
        iii. Bulletin
        iv. Newsletter
    b. Circular letter
    c. Extension News article
    d. Campaign
    e. Exhibition
    f. Radio
    g. Community Radio
    h. Television
6. Selection, Use and Combination of Extension Methods
7. Combination of Extension Teaching Methods
    i. Methods useful in different steps of Extension Teaching Process
    ii. Methods useful in different stages of Adoption Process
8. Suggested Readings and References

Extension Teaching Method

The function of extension education is to bring about desirable changes in the behaviour of a human being. The changes in human being are produced by increasing his/her knowledge level, improving skill and changing attitude. For all these to happen, an individual has to be taught, trained and communicated. So, the extension education emphasizes the process of communication, and if you examine, you will find that the extension education is broadly a teaching-learning process in which a learning situation is created by an extension worker/ teacher by which an individual attempt to change his/her behaviour. The learning situation created in extension education process is a condition or environment in which the elements like teacher, learner, subject matter, physical facilities and teaching methods and aids for promoting learning are present in a dynamic relationship with one another. The quality of learning depends upon the conditions created by the **teacher** for learners to learn. However, the **learner** is the key element in the teaching and learning process. His willingness and desire for change are very important. The third element; **subject matter** is the content of the message that the extension worker wants to transfer to the client. Transfer of the subject matter will be easy and effective if it is valid, correct, based on facts, applicable to practical life situation and need based. Effective teaching-learning process is also affected if **physical facilities** like place, light, ventilation, seating arrangements, etc., are not properly provided to both teachers as well as to the learners. Besides all these, the transfer of subject matters to the learners requires the help of suitable **teaching methods, aids and media**. Proper selection and handling of methods and aids facilitate in creating the desirable learning situation. The teaching methods and aids should be simple, easy to handle, suitable to subject matter, readily available, suited to the environment and needs of the learners.

Extension Methods

Effective learning depends upon the effective teaching. Effective teaching and creation of learning environment largely depend upon the teaching methods/ extension methods /extension teaching methods used by teacher. Proper selection and skillful handling of extension methods bring out expected changes in adult. (the words like 'extension method', 'teaching method' and 'extension teaching method' carry the same meaning, and in this book they are used interchangeable.) Then, what is the meaning of extension method? We may understand the meaning of extension method in this way- that the extension methods are the techniques and tools used to create a learning situation in which effective communication can take place between the learners (may be an adult or rural farmer) and the teacher.

The main functions of extension methods are:

i. To create an environment in which communication takes place so that the learner may see, hear and do things to be learnt.
ii. To provide stimulation that causes the desired mental and/ or physical action on the part of the learner.
iii. To take the learner through one or more steps of the teaching-learning process, viz., attention, interest, desire, conviction, action and satisfaction.
iv. To provide an atmosphere to teacher to establish rapport with learner so that communication process becomes easier.

Classification of Extension Methods

The extension methods are broadly classified on the basis of their a) use b) form and c) function.

1. Classification according to use

a) Individual method
- Farm and home visit
- Office calls/ Farmer's call
- Personal letters
- Telephone calls
- SMS
- E-mail

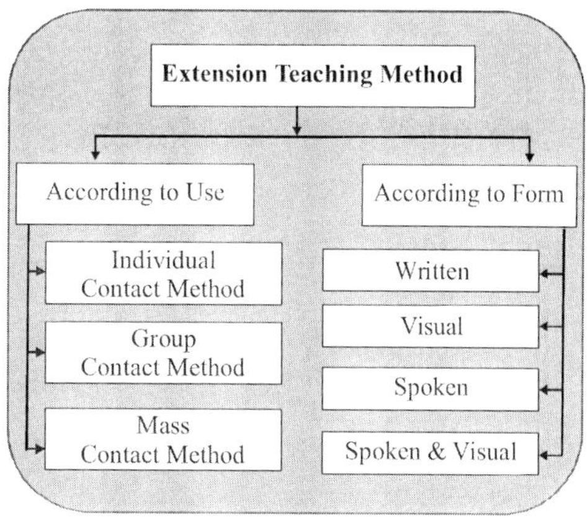

b) Group method
- Method demonstration
- Result demonstration
- All types of Meetings
- Group discussion
- Tours
- Field trips
- WhatsApp

c) Mass media method
- Farm Publications (Leaflets, Folders, Pamphlets, Bulletin, Newsletters, etc.)
- Circular letters
- Campaign
- Exhibition
- Television
- Radio

2. Classification According to Form

a) Written

- Personal letters
- Advisory letter
- News paper
- Circular letters
- Leaflets
- Bulletins

b) Visual

- Result Demonstration
- Posters
- Exhibits
- Slides
- Charts

c) Spoken

- Farm and Home visit
- Veterinary Hospital/Office calls
- Telephone calls
- General meetings
- Radio

d) Spoken and Visual

- Method Demonstration
- Result Demonstration
- Television
- Campaign
- Puppet Show

3. Classification According to Function

a) Telling

- Lecture
- Meetings
- Audio lessons
- Farm & home visit
- Radio talk
- Extension talk

b) Showing

- Exhibition
- Tours
- Motion picture
- Video text
- Internet

c) Doing

- Practical
- Workshop
- Method Demonstration
- Result demonstration
- Do it yourself

(The methods mentioned under each category are not exhaustive)

Individual Methods and Group Methods

Individual Methods

This method is followed when the number of people to be contacted is few and they are located nearer to the extension agent or office of the extension agent. In this method the extension agent communicates with the people individually.

Advantages

i. It provides opportunities to extension agent in building rapport with clients.
ii. Facilitates gaining firsthand knowledge of farm and home.
iii. Helps in selecting demonstrators and local leaders.
iv. Helps in teaching complex practices
v. Helps in changing attitude of the people.
vi. Facilitates transfer of technology.
vii. Facilitates getting feedback information.

Limitations

i. This method is time consuming and relatively expensive.
ii. Coverage of client is very limited.
iii. There is possibility that the extension agent may develop favoritism or bias towards some persons due to his/her frequent interactions.

In individual method, an extension worker contacts directly an individual through various means. The benefits of this method are: (a) closer supervision of clients, with a capability for spotting problems, and doing so quickly; (b) quicker intervention to deal with the problems spotted; and (c) closer interaction with clients, presumably leading to better rapport and to feelings of support. The individual contact may be established through the farm and home visits, office calls, informal contacts, telephone calls, personal letters, etc.

1. Farm and Home Visits

What is it? - It is a face-to-face type of individual contact by the extension worker with the farmer and /or the members of his family on the latter's farm or at his home for one or more specific purpose connected with extension.

Objectives or Purposes

i. Obtain and/ or give firsthand information on matters relating to farm and home conditions.
ii. Give advice or otherwise assist to solve a specific problem; or to teach skills etc.,
iii. Arouse the interest of those not reached by other methods.
iv. Promote good public relations.
v. To sustain interest in adoption of new technology.

Technique

Planning and preparation

- Decide on the client and the objective-whom to meet and what for?
- Get adequate information about the matter you are going to discuss
- Collect relevant publications and materials to be handed over.
- Make a schedule of visits to save time and energy.
- If possible, send advance information.

Implementation

- Visit on the scheduled date and time or according to convenience of the farmer and when the person is likely to listen.
- Create interest of the farmer and allow the individual to talk first.
- Present the message or points of view and explain up to the satisfaction of the farmer.
- Answer to questions raised and clarify doubts. Hand over publications.
- Try to get some assurance for action.

Follow-up

- Keep appropriate record of visit.
- Send committed information or material.
- Make subsequent visits as and when necessary.

Advantages

i. The extension worker gets first-hand information on rural problems.

ii. Helps in rapport building with farmer.

iii. He develops confidence when his ideas are accepted by the farmers.

iv. Helps in locating local leaders and co-operation.

v. Those farmers who could not be contacted by other methods can be contacted by this method.

vi. Percentage of adoption is high.

Limitations

- Only limited number of contacts may be made.
- Requires relatively large amount of time of extension worker
- Comparatively costly method than other methods.
- Attention may be concentrated on a few big and progressive persons; neglecting the large number of small, marginal, tribal farmers, landless labour and backward people; which may prejudice them.

2. Office Calls

What is it? – It is a call made by a farmer or a group to the extension worker at his office for obtaining information and for inputs or other farm-helps needed or for making acquaintance with him.

Objectives or Purposes

i. To get quick solution of problems relating to the problems.

ii. To enable the farmer and homemaker to bring specimens for proper identification of the problem.

iii. To ensure timely supply of inputs and services.

iv. To act as a reminder to the extension agent.

v. To promote close contact between farmers and extension worker.

Technique

Planning and preparation

- Keep the office neat, orderly and attractive.
- Remain present in the office on the days which have been communicated to the farmers in advance.
- Organize an information centre in the office or at least put up a few boards in the office room and display current leaflets, folders, photographs, charts etc. relating to important to important projects and extension activities in the area.

Implementation

- Allow the visitor to talk first and make the point.
- Discuss about his/ her problems and suggest solutions.
- If necessary, take the person to the subject matter specialist.
- Put maximum effort to make visitor satisfied.

Follow-up

- Make a note of the call, if necessary.
- If required, refer the problem to research for solution.
- Supply further information and materials if such commitment has been made.

Advantages

i. Economic use of the extension workers' time and energy.
ii. Farmers likely to be highly receptive to learning.
iii. It develops goodwill and confidence.
iv. It reinforces other methods.
v. It is the sign of confidence that the farmer has in the extension worker and respect for his ability.

Limitations

i. It is not possible to get detailed first-hand knowledge of the farmer's problems and activities.
ii. Limited contact with the farmer.
iii. Waiting for visitors who are not turning up is waste of time.

3. Personal Letters

What is it? – It is a personal and individual letter written by the extension worker to a farmer in connection with extension work.

Objectives or Purposes

i. To answer to queries relating to problems of farm and home.
ii. To send information or seek cooperation on important extension activities.

Technique

- Send the letter in time, or if a letter has already been received, send a prompt reply.
- The content should be clear, complete, to the point and applicable to farmer's own situation.
- Use simple and courteous language.

Advantages

i. To reach more number of farmers at a time
ii. Less costly method.
iii. Easier to seek farmer co-operation for extension work
iv. Useful to educate farmers.
v. The best method to reach farmers who could not be reached by the farm and home visit office call methods.

Limitations

i. It is a time consuming method.
ii. Since majority of the farmers are 'illiterates' this method has limited usage.
iii. It is difficult for the extension worker to answer ' each and every' individual problem.
iv. Only few persons can be contacted.
v. Difficult to teach skill

4. Telephone Calls

What is it? It is the communications between the extension worker and farmers over the telephone on certain matters connected with extension works.

Objectives or Purposes

1. To inform farmers regarding farm problems, supplies, services, etc, in a very short time.

2. To clarify farmers doubt and provide information which are very urgent in nature.

Advantages

1. The communication may be initiated by either farmers or the extension worker.
2. Very useful for giving specific and brief information about various issues of farm practices.
3. Useful means to follow-up extension events and get feed-back of the programme.
4. It is comparatively cheaper than other methods.

Limitations

1. Use of telephone by farmers is very limited in our country.
2. Complex issues and practices cannot be communicated through telephone.

5. Short Message Services (SMS)

What is it? It is an electronic communication service allowing the interchange of short text messages between the users of digital mobile telephone. Both extension worker and farmers should have mobile connections for communication of short text messages.

Objectives or Purposes

1. To communicate with farmers regarding the problems farm, availability or non-availability of supplies, other extension services in a real time.
2. To clarify farmers' doubt and provide information which are very urgent in nature.

Advantages

1. The sending of SMS may be initiated by either farmers or the extension worker.
2. Useful for giving specific and brief information about various issues of farm practices.
3. Useful means to follow-up extension events and get feed-back of the programme.
4. It is very cheap method of extension education.

Limitations

1. Mobile telephone use by the farming community in India is very limited.
2. Complex issues and practices cannot be communicated through SMS

6. Electronic Mail

What is it? It is commonly called email or e-mail. It is the equivalent of a normal physical letter, but it is written on a computer and delivered via the internet. Both the extension worker and farmers should have computer and internet connection to communicate through e-mail.

Objectives or Purposes

1. To communicate with farmers through text, messages, pictures and sound regarding various issues of farm and related practices in a very real time.
2. To clarify farmers' doubt and provide information which are very urgent in nature.

Advantages

1. Both farmers and extension worker can communicate with each other.
2. Useful for giving detail information about various issues of farm practices.
3. Useful means to communicate a large number of farmers in a very short time.
4. Information can be stored in the e-mail and may be reused when it is required.
5. It is less expensive method.

Limitation

1. Use of computer by the farmers is minimal in our country.

Group Methods

In this method, an extension worker communicates with a small number of people in a group. The size of a small group may be from 15 to 25, a medium group from 35 to 50 and a large group from 50 to 100 persons. Examples of group method are result demonstration, method demonstration, group meeting, small group training, field day or farmers' day, study tour, etc.

Advantages

i. Enables the extension agent to have face-to-face contact with a number of people at a time.

ii. Can reach a select part of the target group.

iii. Facilitates sharing of knowledge and experience and thereby strengthen learning of the group members.

iv. Reach fewer people, but offer more opportunities for interaction and feedback.

v. Satisfies the basic urge of people for social contacts.

vi. Motivate people to accept change due to group influence.

vii. More effective than mass method in stimulating action.

viii. Less expensive than individual method due to more coverage.

Limitations

i. Wide diversity in the interest of group members may create a difficult learning situation.

ii. Vested interests, caste groups and village factions may hinder free interaction and decision making by the group members.

iii. Difficult to give attention to all members.

Demonstrations

Farmers like to see how a new idea works, and also what effect it can have on increasing their crop production. Both purposes can be achieved by means of a farm demonstration. A good, practical demonstration is an invaluable method in extension work. The demonstration is a particularly powerful method to use with farmers who do not read easily. A demonstration will give such farmers the opportunity to observe, at first hand, the differences between a recommended new crop practice and traditional practices. The strength of the demonstration should lie in its simplicity and its ability to present the farmers with concrete results. It is based on the principle of "seeing is believing".

There are two principal types of demonstration used by extension agents - method demonstration and result demonstration.

Method Demonstration

What is it? - It is an extension teaching method conducted by an extension worker, or a trained leader or specialist, for a group of persons, to show how to carry out a new skill or to improve an old skill not being properly executed.

In method demonstration, an extension worker shows how to do job step by step such as clean milking procedures. The method demonstration is not concerned with the worth of the practice but with "how-to-do" something. It is not an experiment, but it is a teaching effort. The farmers watch the process and listen to the oral explanation to clear up points. To increase the farmers' confidence in their ability, as many farmers as possible are asked to repeat the demonstration in the presence of the extension worker.

Objectives or Purposes

i. To teach skills and stimulate people to action.
ii. To enable people to improve upon their old skills.
iii. To improve upon the result by doing a job in a better way.
iv. To build up learners' confidence and satisfaction on the practice.
v. To demonstrate a practice to a group of people in short time.

Technique

Planning and preparation

- Select appropriate topic which is important for the client for demonstration
- Select and finalize the target audience and venue of demonstrations.
- Contact subject matter specialists and make necessary arrangements for their participation.
- Collect relevant information and arrange materials and equipments beforehand.
- Identify and list the steps of demonstrations, and practice for its correct presentation.
- Decide on the date and time in consultation with the local leaders and give timely intimation to others.

Implementation

- Reach the demonstration site on the scheduled date and time.
- Explain about the demonstration to the participants
- Conduct operation of the activity step-by step and explaining in each step why it is important. Repeat difficult steps.
- Ask the participants one by one or in small batches to practice the skill. Clarify doubts and answer to their questions.
- When everybody has practiced the skill and has expressed confidence, emphasize on the key points again.

Follow-up

- Keep a record of the participants and maintain contact with them.
- Assist the participants in getting the required materials and equipments.

Advantages

i. It is very effective in teaching new skill.

ii. It stimulates action and builds confidence among the participants

iii. Serves publicity purpose.

iv. It introduces a change of practice at low cost.

Limitations

i. Suited only to the 'skill involving technologies'.

ii. Transporting the materials and equipments to the demonstration plot is difficult.

iii. It requires lot of planning

iv. It causes a setback if whole programme is not properly coordinated.

Result Demonstration

What is it? Result Demonstration method is one which is conducted by a participating farmer on his/her farm, under the guidance of an extension worker, to prove by evidence that the practice being demonstrated is superior to the one in existence. It is a way of showing the farmer the value or worth of a practice whose success has already been proved or established in research stations. In this method the new practice is compared with the old one in farmer's land, and the villagers are asked to see the result on their own eyes and judge the result. Result demonstrations establish proof that the improved practice advocated is applicable locally. It may be conducted for single recommended practice or a series of practices that come in sequence with respect to a problem.

Objectives or Purposes

i. To show the feasibility and applicability of a newly recommended practice in farmer's own situation.

ii. To motivate groups of people in a community to adopt a new practice by seeing its result.

iii. To build up confidence of the farmers and extension agents.

Technique

Planning and preparation

- Analyze farmer's situations and select relevant profitable practices in consultation with research workers and farmers.

- Consult with local leaders and select a demonstrator who is interested in improving his practices and make him ready to do demonstration in his field.
- Select the site of demonstrations where it will be easily visible to a large number of people in the community.
- Prepare a calendar of operations.
- Make wide publicity.

Implementations

- Arrange all necessary materials required for demonstration
- Organize materials and equipments necessary for conducting the demonstrations
- Start demonstration in front of the group of villagers.
- Explain the objectives and steps to the demonstrating farmers.
- Arrange method demonstration where a new skill is involved.
- Put up suitable signboards in prominent places.
- Personally supervise all critical operations.
- Conduct field day or farmers' day to successful demonstration events.
- Help the demonstrating farmers to maintain records.
- Motivate as many farmers as possible to remain present at the time of assessment of the result.
- Let the demonstrating farmers explain to the visitors as far as possible.
- Analyze and interpret the results, and compare them with the farmers' existing practice.
- Emphasize applicability of the new practice in the farmers' own situations.

Follow-up

- Give wide publicity to the results of demonstration
- Use the result of the demonstrations in future extension works
- Utilize demonstrating farmers in farmers' meetings and training programmes.
- Prepare visual aids, particularly photographs, coloured slides, charts etc. on the demonstrations for future extension programmes.

Advantages

- Useful in introducing new practices
- Enhance the confidence of extension workers regarding the suitability of recommended practices in village conditions.

- Successful demonstrator becomes the resource person for the extension worker.

Limitations

- Require lot of time and preparation on the part of the extension worker.
- It is a costly teaching method
- Difficult to find a good demonstrator who will keep record.
- Results may be vitiated by uncontrollable factors like weather.
- It is not suitable for all advocated practices.
- Unsuccessful demonstrations may cause some setback to extension work.

Table : The differences between method demonstration and result demonstration

Particulars	Method Demonstration	Result Demonstration
Purpose	To teach how to do a job involving skill (to teach "doing" skills)	To show locally the worth or value of a recommended practices
Conducted by	Extension worker himself or local leader specially trained for the purpose	Farmer (Demonstrator) under the guidance of extension worker
For the benefit of	Persons present at the demonstration	The demonstrator as well as farmers
Comparison	Not essential	Essential (Not necessary to have replication in the same field
Operation	Easy	Difficult
Maintenance of records	Not necessary	Necessary
Advertisement	Not required	Required
Time Required	Relatively very little	Substantial period
Cost	Relatively cheap	Costly
Interrelationship	Often paves the way for result demonstration	Usually follows observation plots; may involve one or more method demonstrations.

Meetings

Meetings are one of the oldest and the most important group methods of extension teaching. If properly conducted, the benefits are higher compared to other methods in relation to the cost of using methods. The term meeting includes all kinds of meetings held by extension worker. In size, the meeting varies from small committee meeting to large special occasion meetings like *melas* and festival meeting attended by thousands.

Types of meetings

Kelsey and Hearne (1963) identify five general types of meetings involved in extension work:

1. Organization meetings (board of directors' meet, youth clubs),
2. Planning meetings (village planning meeting),
3. Training meetings (rural leaders' training),
4. Special interest meetings (special meeting about dairying), and
5. Community meetings (community meet for general problems).

General meeting

What is it? It is broadly a meeting of heterogeneous participants wherein certain information is passed on for consideration and future action.

The term 'General Meeting' includes all kind of meetings conducted by extension workers. There is a large variety of such meeting in terms of size and form. They may be small committee meetings to those held in special occasions like *melas* or festivals attended by thousands of people. The meetings may be held periodically or sporadically.

Objectives or Purposes

i. To effectively reach and serve large numbers of people.
ii. To prepare the people for the other methods of extension work
iii. To find out the reaction of the people to certain activities.

Technique

Planning and Preparation

- Decide the topic, venue and participants
- Collect relevant information and teaching materials for the meeting
- Inform the resource persons and subject matter specialist
- Arrange social and recreational features
- Advertise meeting in advance

Implementation

- Hold the meeting preferably in a central place having all physical facilities
- Start the meeting on schedule date and time
- State the purpose and objective of the meeting
- Make introduction brief
- Prompt in starting and closing the meeting
- Use appropriate audio-visual materials
- Encourage audience participation when required

- Take advantage of group psychology and employ appeals that arouse interest, create desire and stimulate action.
- Give recognition to all sections and groups participated in the meeting.
- Associate local leaders for welcoming the gathering or thanking the participants if possible.
- Acknowledge the services briefly and then indicate the follow up work, if any.
- Distribute relevant folders and pamphlets at the time of break.

Follow-up

- Remind the members about the decision taken in the meeting and encourage them to take action.
- Facilitate the supply of inputs.
- Sustain interest through personal contact.

Advantages

i. Large number of people can be reached.
ii. Serves as a preparatory stage for other methods.
iii. Group psychology can be used in promoting the programme.
iv. Reactions of the people to a programme can be assessed.
v. Adoption of practices can be accomplished at low cost.

Limitations

i. Meeting place and facilities are not always adequate.
ii. Scope for discussion is limited except possibly for few questions and answers.
iii. Handling the topic become difficult because of mixed composition of audience.
iv. Circumstances beyond control like factions and weather might reduce the attendance.
v. Requires understanding of group dynamics to handle the group by extension worker.

Group meetings

Calling the members of a group or the inhabitants of a local community together for a meeting is the commonest group extension method. Although there may be an air of informality about such meetings, they will nevertheless need to be carefully thought out and planned. The group or community meeting is a useful educational forum where the agent and farmers can come together, and ideas can be openly discussed and analysed. The agent will probably have information about a new government policy, or agricultural idea or practice. He will want to introduce this new information, to seek the opinions of community members and gain their support for extension activities. Indeed, there are a whole range of purposes for such community or group meetings:

Information meetings : The agent calls the group or community together to communicate a specific piece of new information which he feels will benefit them and upon which he seeks their advice. For an example, recently launched dairy scheme of Government.

Planning meetings : The main purpose is to review a particular problem, suggest a number of solutions and decide upon a course of action. For an example, outbreak of Ranikhet disease in poultry birds in villages in spite of timely vaccination against the disease.

Special interest meetings : Topics of specific interest to a particular group of people (e.g., horticulture, bee keeping, or dairy farming) are presented and discussed in detail at a level relevant to those participating.

General community meetings : Men, women and young people of a community are invited to attend to discuss issues of general community interest. It is important to hold such general meetings occasionally so as to avoid any community group feeling that it is excluded from extension activities. For an example, implementation of sanitation programme in a village.

Whatever the case, however, the agent should only call a meeting if he thinks that it can be useful. If farmers feel that their time has been wasted in coming to a meeting, they may refuse to come to subsequent meetings and thus frustrate the agent's work. Once he decides to hold a meeting, the agent should make careful preparations and check a number of important arrangements which will be necessary to ensure a successful meeting.

The basic purpose of the meeting should be agreed and to determine this the agent should consult community or group leaders. Only then can the agent and community leaders consider the content and the best approach to the meeting. It may be useful to write down in a few words what the purpose is, and then to see what are the important aspects to be considered. If it is to be a meeting for providing information, the agent must structure his material in a coherent form and decide in what sequence he is going to present it. If it is to be a general community meeting, then, similarly, he must decide how he will structure the meeting and introduce discussion on the issues he has in mind.

Form of the meeting

Depending upon the nature and purpose of the meeting, the agent must decide the most appropriate form for the meeting and how it can best be conducted. The agent should consider the appropriateness of the different forms the meeting could take and, in consultation with community members, decide accordingly. Ideally, the ingredients should be mixed to suit the occasion.

Smaller meetings are more likely to meet the specific needs of those who attend. When plans are to be made or decisions taken, a small number of representatives will usually achieve more than a large gathering of all community members. On other occasions, it will be important for the meeting to be open to as many people as possible.

A formal meeting, with chairman, agenda and written record of proceedings, is appropriate when specific business has to be dealt with or decisions reached. The chairman keeps the meeting to the central issues, and the decisions of the meeting are recorded accurately so that they cannot be disputed later. In an informal meeting, people feel more able to express their own point of view and less dominated by the structure and formality of the proceedings. However, an open, unstructured discussion, although it allows all to participate, may result in a few people dominating the proceedings.

A lecture or talk allows the agent (or other speaker) to convey a detailed, well-prepared message to his audience on a specific issue; for example, a new piece of technology can be presented in this way, and illustrated by visual aids. It should be remembered, however, thatthe lecture is a particularly tedious approach to meetings and care must be taken to ensure that people will not get bored. Alternatively, in a discussion, many people are able to express points of view and ask questions. Discussions may be completely open and unstructured, or based on a prepared agenda of discussion points.

Planning the meeting

There are two important decisions to make regarding the time and location. A date and time for the meeting must be decided and announced. The time should be convenient to all concerned and should avoid clashes with other events or activities. The meeting-place should be well-known, easy to get to and appropriate for the form of meeting. The meeting-place should also be comfortable and have the facilities necessary for the meeting. An extension agent would never hold a meeting at midday, on a very hot day, in the open sun. Such a meeting could be disastrous, as well as cause considerable discomfort.

After the above two issues have been considered, it may be useful for the agent to draw up a list of other arrangements to be made in preparation for the meeting. Such a check-list could include:

Check-list

- Publicity for the meeting
- Seating arrangements
- Audio-visual equipment and material, or other educational aids
- Agenda, and order of events
- Guest speakers or other specialists who will contribute to the meeting
- Chairman to take charge of the meeting, who should be elected by the community
- Refreshments for speakers and, where necessary, other participants.

Conducting the meeting

Even the most carefully prepared meeting can fail if it is not conducted in the right manner. While the above arrangements are important, the way the actual meeting proceeds will determine whether it will be a success or not. The agent must be conscious that he is dealing with adults who do not want to sit for hours listening to a speaker talk endlessly. The agent should try to vary the agenda of the meeting: for example, a short talk, accompanied by visual aids, followed by comments and questions.

Variety of content, as well as a chance for the farmers to participate, will be important. In addition, the meeting must not go on too long. One-and-a-half hours are probably sufficient for a group or community meeting. It is better to have a highly productive, short meeting than one which rambles on and loses effect.

The agent's role in the meeting should also respond to the circumstances. He should encourage the community to appoint a chairman and should allow the chairman to conduct business. The agent's role should basically be to inform and support, and he should not dominate the meeting. Furthermore, the meeting should not resemble a class-room with the agent as teacher and the farmers as pupils. The agent should make every effort to ensure that during the proceedings the community members feel that it is their meeting and that they have a part to play.

As a guide to the proceedings of the meeting, the agent should keep the following points in mind. He should start the meeting on time. Then he should welcome community members and special guests, explain the purpose of the meeting and the programme to be followed, and begin the programme. Later, the agent should encourage questions and discussion, and be prepared to summarize the main points and note important decisions. The meeting should be closed with thanks to all concerned.

As the most commonly used form of group extension method, the group or community meeting will be most effective if carefully thought out and planned. After each meeting, the agent should make a brief record of the proceedings and the principal decisions taken. He should also take any prompt follow-up action that has been decided.

Mass media methods

The mass media method is followed where a large and widely dispersed audience is to be communicated within a short time. There may be a few communicators such as the extension agent and some subject matter specialists. The size of the audience may be a few hundred in mass meeting, few thousands in campaign and exhibition, and millions in newspaper, radio and television.

Advantages

i. Suitable for creating general awareness amongst the people.
ii. Helps in transferring knowledge and, forming and changing opinions.
iii. Large number of people may be communicated within a short time.
iv. Facilitates quick communication in times of emergency.
v. Reinforces previous learning.
vi. Less expensive due to more coverage.

Limitations

i. Less intensive method.
ii. Little scope for personal contact with the audience.
iii. Little opportunity for interaction with and amongst the audience.
iv. Generalized recommendations hinder application by individuals.
v. Little control over the responses of the audience.
vi. Difficulty in getting feedback information and evaluation of results.

Mass media like farm publications, newspaper articles, circular letters, radio, television, posters, exhibits, etc. disseminate information to a much larger audience at faster rate than the individual or group contact but their impact is less than the other two methods.

1. Farm publications

Extension worker uses various types of farm publications to communicate messages to farmers and some of them are discussed here.

Leaflet: It is a single printed sheet of paper of small size, containing preliminary information relating to a topic. It is made as and when needed and normally distributed free-of-cost.

Folder: It is a single printed sheet of paper of big size, folded once or twice, and gives essential information relating to a particular topic. It is printed as and when required and normally free-of cost.

Bulletin: It is a printed, bound booklet with a number of pages, containing comprehensive information about a topic. It is made as and when necessary. A small price may be fixed on some important bulletins.

Newsletter: It is a miniature newspaper in good quality paper, containing information relating to the activities and achievements of the organization. It has fixed periodicity of publication and normally distributed free-of-cost.

Farm publications are extremely useful to the literate farmers, and even illiterate farmers can make use of them with the help of literate members in their family. Farm publications are used by all types of extension functionaries, input dealers, bank personnel and media-persons.

Objectives or purposes

i. To provide precise and reliable scientific information in simple language
ii. To serve the immediate needs of the farmer in any important issue
iii. To reach a large number of people quickly and simultaneously at a low cost.
iv. To provide accurate, motivating, creditable and distortion-free information.
v. To provide support to other extension methods.
vi. To facilitate use at convenience and to serve as future reference.

Technique

Planning and preparation

- Select a topic of economic and practical importance, for which information is needed by the audience.
- Estimate the time required to prepare the manuscript, print and dispatch, and plan publication in such a way that it reaches the audience in time.
- Check up availability of funds and decide on the number of copies to be printed. It may be useful to have more copies at less cost than a few copies at high cost.

Implementation

- Collect relevant information on the topic from all available sources.
- Contact specialists relating to relevant disciplines.
- Prepare the draft in clear, simple, short and direct sentences, keeping the target audience in view.

- Arrange write-up in short paragraphs, in a logical sequence.
- Give suitable title to the publication and sub-heads to the paragraphs.
- Devote the first paragraph to highlight the economic and other benefits. This may be printed in bold letter.
- Present all weights and measures clearly and directly.
- Put suitable diagrams, photographs and sketch for better understanding
- Go for pre-testing before mass publication.
- Below the press line put the name of the department and the organization under whose authority it is being published.

Follow-up

- Arrange timely dispatch of the publication to the target audience and for the extension programmes.
- Dispatch publications to the media persons and others according to mailing list.
- Attend to requests for publications promptly.
- Try to get feedback information from the users.
- Maintain appropriate records for free distribution and sale of publications.

Advantages

- Can reach a large section of literate people quickly and simultaneously
- Can be read at leisure and preserved for future use.
- Supplement to other teaching methods
- Influence adoption of practices at relatively lower cost.
- Can be used to continue contact with extension agency.

Limitations

- Not suitable for illiterate audience.
- May lose its significance if not carefully prepared and used.
- Periodical version is necessary to keep the publications up-to-date.
- Cannot be used in exclusion to other methods.

2. Circular letter

What is it? It is a letter reproduced and sent to many people by the extension worker to publicize an extension activity or to give timely information on farm activities.

Objectives or purposes

i. To maintain regular contact with farmers.

ii. To communicate some general information which could best be put in the form of a letter?

iii. To stimulate interest in the subject.

Technique

Planning and preparation

i. Determine the place of the circular letter in teaching plan

ii. Determine the specific purpose and the segments of clients to be reached

iii. Plan letter to serve the definite purpose

iv. Have a single purpose and write in simple language.

v. Give complete information.

vi. Be clear in statements which should lead to action.

vii. The letters should be a part of a programme or campaign.

Implementation

i. Write circular letters and get them duplicated

ii. Write appealing immediate personal interest of the clients

iii. Give a cartoon or illustration containing the central idea

iv. State the facts concerning the nature of seriousness of the problem.

Follow-up

- Timely dispatch of the circular letters to the target audience
- Attending the quarries of the clients related to letter promptly.
- Try to get feedback information from the users.
- Maintain appropriate dispatch register.

Advantages

i. Information can reach large number of people in short time.

ii. Preserved and used for future reference.

iii. Comparatively cheap.

iv. Provide accurate information.

v. Easy to make.

Limitations

i. Less useful in low literacy area.

ii. Cannot be use in exclusion of other methods.

3. Extension News Articles (or News Stories)

What is it? This is a piece of write-up on important information about the rural farming and other related issues that interests mostly the farming community.

Objectives or Purposes

1. To develop interest on the subject
2. To inform important developments to farming community
3. To crate favourable attitude towards a product/ practice/use.
4. To reinforce other extension method like meeting and demonstrations.

Technique

1. Write something that has actually happened (e.g. agricultural credit *mela* or inauguration of chilling plant)
2. Write something that is very important for farming community (e.g. declaration of minimum support price by government for cereals).
3. Write something that makes the farmers interested like catastrophe, fight, conflict, competition, new knowledge, etc.
4. News should be recent in nature, timely, accurate, fair and brief
5. Write in simple language and avoid using personal opinion.
6. Use accepted principles of good writing of news items for a newspaper.

Advantages

1. Large coverage in short time.
2. Credibility of news is high due to appearance in print media
3. Reinforces the effect of other methods
4. It is less expensive in comparison to other methods.

Limitations

1. It is of limited use for illiterate farmers
2. Difficult to assess the effects of extension new articles
3. Message may not always reach the intended readers
4. Expertise is required on the part of the extension worker to write good articles.

4. Campaign

What is it? It is an intensive educational activity undertaken at an opportune time for a brief period focusing attention in concerted manner on a particular problem, with a view to stimulate the widest possible interest in a community, block or other geographical area.

The duration of a campaign may be for single day on a theme like 'application of bio-fertilizer', for a few weeks as in family planning, for a few months as in Vanamahostava (tree planting) and for a few years as in 'Grow More Food' campaign. A campaign may be held by involving a small number of people in a few villages, or by involving an entire community or the entire nation over the whole country as in 'Pulse Polio' campaign. Campaign on certain themes (say, environment, disease control etc.) may be organized over the whole world.

Objectives or purposes

i. To draw attention of the large number of people to an important issue

ii. To create mass awareness about an important problem or felt need of the community and encourage them to solve it.

iii. To induce emotional participation of the community at the local level and create a favourable psychological climate for adoption of new practices.

Technique

Planning and preparation

- Identify with the local leaders an important problem or need of the community for campaign.
- List out specialists, local leaders and other persons who could be involved in solving it. Train the required personnel.
- Decide with the local leaders about the time of holding the campaign and its duration.
- Arrange necessary inputs, services and transport.
- Prepare a written programme of the campaign.
- Give wide publicity in advance.

Implementation

- Carry out the campaign as per plan.
- Hold group meeting with the people and discuss about the origin and nature of the problem. Suggest practical and effective solution.

- Arrange method demonstration and training programme for the participants.
- Maintain supply of critical inputs and services.
- Keep close watch on the campaign and take corrective steps, if necessary.
- Arrange mass media coverage.
- Conclude the campaign in time.

Follow-up

- Make individual and groups to find out their reaction.
- Assess the extent of adoption of the practice.
- Publicize the events in newspaper, radio and television.
- Analyze deficiencies and failures.
- Give due recognition to the local leaders.

Advantages

- Especially suited for mass scale adoption of an improved practices
- Successful campaign creates conducive atmosphere for popularizing other methods.

Limitations

- Applicable only for topics of community interest but not suitable to individual problems
- Success depends on cooperation of the community and their leaders.
- Not useful when advocated practice involves complicated technicalities
- Expensive method
- Requires adequate preparation, concerted efforts and propaganda techniques, and uninterrupted of critical inputs.

5. Exhibition

What is it? An exhibition is a systematic display of models, specimens, charts, information, posters, photographs etc. in a sequence so as to be significant in teaching or creating interest in the participating members. An exhibition covers three stages of extension education, viz, arousing interest, creating desire to learn and providing a chance to take a decision (Leagan, 1961).

Farmers' fairs and *krishi melas* held by the agricultural universities, institutes and various other organizations in which field visit, training programmes etc. are combined with exhibition are effective and popular. Exhibitions may also be organized by taking advantage of local fairs and festivals.

Objectives and purposes

i. To prepare visual literacy.

ii. To acquaint people with better standards.

iii. To create interest in a wide range of people.

iv. To motivate people to adopt better practices.

v. To promote understanding and create goodwill towards extension.

Technique

Planning and preparation

- Form an exhibition committee with competent people
- Decide on the theme and distribute the responsibility to the committee members
- Decide on the venue, time and duration.
- Prepare a written programme and communicate to all concerned members of the team in time.
- Get the site ready within the selected date. Make provision for essentials facilities.
- Earmark a stall for display of exhibits to be bought by the farmers.
- Arrange a *pandal* for holding meeting, training and entertainment programmes.
- Display posters at important places. Publicize about the exhibition through mass media.
- Decorate the stalls simply and tastefully and make adequate arrangements for lighting.
- Prepare good quality and colourful exhibits which shall convey the desired message to the visitors. Use local materials as far as possible. Label the exhibits in local language with bold letters.
- Display exhibits about 50 to 60 cm. above the floor of the stall, up to a height of about two meters. Maintain proper sequence. Avoid overcrowding of exhibits.

Implementation

- Organize formal opening of the exhibition by a local leader or a prominent person.
- Arrange smooth flow of visitors.
- Interpreters may briefly explain the exhibits to the visitors so that the intended message is clearly communicated.

- Distribute publications materials to visitors.
- Organize a panel of experts to be present nearby, so that the visitors who would like to know more or discuss some problems could get the desired information.
- Conduct meetings, training programmes etc. as per schedule during the day time.
- Arrange judging of exhibits brought by the farmers and give away prizes and certificates.
- If desired, judge the stalls on the basis of their quality of display, ability to draw visitors and effectiveness in communicating message, and award certificates.
- Keep the exhibits and the premises clean
- Conclude the exhibitions as scheduled by thinking the participants and those who have helped.

Follow-up

- Meet some visitors personally and maintain a visitors' book for comments during the exhibition to get feedback information.
- Talk to the local leaders and assess success of the exhibition.
- Ensure availability of critical inputs and facilities emphasized during the exhibition.
- Look for changes in practice in the community in the coming years.

Advantages

i. Best method to teach illiterates
ii. Create awareness among the visitors about the products
iii. Most fit for festive occasion
iv. Can create market for certain products.

Limitations

- Difficult to represent entire process of a practice
- Requires lot of funds and preparation.
- Cannot be organised frequently.

6. Radio

Radio is an electronic audio-medium for broadcasting programmes to the audience. It is a medium of mass communication and an efficient tool for giving information and entertainment. This medium is cosmopolite in approach and is suitable for communication to millions of people widely dispersed and situated in remote areas. It is suitable for creating general awareness amongst the people. People with no education or very little education and those who are not in a position to attend extension programmes personally, can take advantage of this medium and build up adequate knowledge about a practice. It reaches large number of people with no time and the programmes can be listened by the people while doing work in the field or at home.

Objectives or Purposes

i. To reach large number of people quickly and inexpensively
ii. To build enthusiasm and maintain interest
iii. To motivate farmers by highlighting the achievement of other farmers.
iv. To provide information on extension activities to farmers.

Procedure or Technique

i. Determine radio programme utility in teaching plan
ii. Be clear about the purpose of broadcast and design the programme keeping the interest of the audience.
iii. Decide what treatment to give to your message.
iv. Seek assistance of experts to write message
v. Time the broadcast to synchronize the farmers' leisure hours.
vi. Encourage listener to listen radio programmes and write their views to broadcasting station.
vii. Reply to the queries of farmers.

Advantages

i. Can reach more people quickly than any other means of communication
ii. Especially suited to give emergency and timely information (e.g. weather, disease out-break, etc.)
iii. Suitable to communicate with illiterate people.
iv. Relatively cheap
v. Builds interest on other extension media.

Limitation

i. Limited number of broadcasting stations
ii. Not within reach of all farmers

iii. Generalized recommendations in the programme limit individual application.
iv. No turning back if not understood
v. Difficult to check on results.

Community Radio

The radio broadcasting in India was controlled by the government prior to 2000. However, in 2002 the government took a policy decision to allow the established institutions to set up the Community Radio Stations (CRSs) to broadcast the programmes in their campus. Thereafter in 2006, by further liberalizing the policy, the government allowed the 'non-profit' organisations like civil society and voluntary organisations, etc., to set up the CRS to broadcast the issues relating to development and social change. Now there are 103 operational CRSs broadcasting the programmes in different parts of the country. Out of these 103 CRSs, 71 are run by educational institutions, 23 are run by NGOs and 8 are run by Krishi Vigyan Kendra (KVKs) and State Agriculture Universities (www.mib.nic.in).

Community Radio means radio broadcasting with the objective of serving the cause of the community in the service area by involving members of the community in the broadcast of their programmes. It affords a unique advantage of receiving transmission through low cost, battery operated portable receiving sets and aimed at covering an area of 5-10 Km radius area. The listeners of the programmes are the people living in the coverage zone of the community radio station.

Institutions/Organisation eligible for Community Radio Station

a) Eligibility criteria

i. It should be explicitly constituted as a non-profit organization and should have a proven record of at least three years of service to the community.
ii. The CRS to be created by it should be designed to serve a specific well defined Local community.
iii. It should have an ownership and management structure that is reflective of the Community that the CRS seeks to serve.
iv. Programmes for broadcast should be relevant to the educational, developmental, social and cultural needs of the community.
v. It must be a legal entity i.e. it should be registered under the Societies Act or any other relevant Act for the purpose and having a proven record of at least three years of service to the community at the time of application.

Types of Institutions / Organisations

i. Non-profit organizations like civil Society and voluntary organizations registered under the societies act and having a proven record of at least three years of service to the local community at the time of application.

ii. State Agricultural Universities (SAUs), ICAR institutions and Krishi Vigyan Kendras.

iii. Well established educational institutions.

Community Radio Programmes

The Programmes of Community Radio should be of immediate relevance to the community and focus on issues relating to agriculture, rural development, education, health, environment, etc, At least 50% of content shall be generated with the participation of the local community, for which the station has been set up. Transmission of sponsored programmes shall not be permitted except those sponsored by Central and State governments and other organizations to broadcast public interest information. The CRS shall not broadcast any programmes which relate to news and current affairs and are otherwise political in nature. (Visit the website www.mib.nic.in for more information on Community Radio).

7. Television (TV)

Television is an electronic audio-visual medium which provides pictures with synchronized sound. It is one of the important mass media for dissemination of information in the rural areas. This medium is cosmopolite in approach and can be used to create instant mass awareness. Television combines the immediacy of radio with the mobility of cinema and can carry messages over long distances at a relatively low unit cost. Television is a multi-media equipment as it can include motion picture, recording, slide, photograph, drawing, poster, etc. Television can show recorded as well as live programmes. Television programmes may be broadly classified as commercial and non-commercial. Commercial or general telecasts are revenue earning and include music, dance, drama, serials, cinema and also news, current affairs, etc. Non-commercial or educative programmes are aimed at education and development rather than entertainment. This is a very strong medium to create general awareness amongst the people about agricultural and rural development programmes. In this medium, it is possible to show all the steps of a practice to a large number of viewers either by recording or live. Now-a-days, due to substantial increase of television sets in the rural areas, number of the programmes related to agriculture being telecast by public as well as private channels in the country.

Selection, Use and Combination of Extension Methods

Selection and use of extension methods

The selection and use of teaching method depends upon the objectives of the programme, factors influencing their effectiveness, their nature and characteristics and possibility of their use in combination with others or in media-mix, and the objective to be achieved including the time and the cost involved. The selection of extension methods also depends on the ability of extension worker to use effectively different extension methods. The selection of appropriate method is not an easy task. There is no single thumb-rule for its selection. In order to get more effective results, the extension worker should-

i. Select the appropriate methods;
ii. Have a suitable combination of selected methods; and
iii. Use them in proper sequence so as to have repetition in a variety of ways.

The following considerations should be taken into account in the selection of extension teaching methods:

i. Education level of audience
ii. Size of audience
iii. The teaching objective
iv. The subject matter
v. The state of development of extension organization
vi. Size of the extension staff
vii. Availability of media
viii. Relative cost
ix. Extension worker's familiarity
x. Problems and technological needs of the people
xi. The length of time
xii. The significance of the programme
xiii. General local conditions
xiv. Emergency situation

Ray (2008) has made some suggestions which is presented under table, may serve as guideline for the extension agent for selection of extension methods under different situations.

Table : Use of Extension Methods

Characteristics/ Situations		Extension Methods		
A. Nature of the Audience				
1. Socio-economic status	Low	Individual	Group	
	High			Mass
2.Size	Small	Individual	Group	
	Large			Mass
3. Location	Near	Individual	Group	
	Far			Mass
B. Ecosystem	Friendly	Individual	Group	Mass
	Inhospitable	Individual	Group	
	Hostile	Individual	Group	
C. Teaching objective	Create general awareness			Mass
	Increase Knowledge	Individual	Group	Mass
	Increase skill	Individual	Group	Mass
	Change attitude	Individual	Group	Mass
	Achieve technology transfer	Individual	Group	
D. Extension Programme	National Importance	Individual	Group	Mass
	Local Importance	Individual	Group	
E. Extension Organization				
1. Manpower	Limited			Mass
	Sufficient	Individual	Group	
2. Funds	Limited			Mass
	Sufficient	Individual	Group	
F. Availability time	Limited			Mass
	Sufficient	Individual	Group	
G. Situation	Normal	Individual	Group	Mass
	Emergent			Mass

From the broad categories suggested, the extension agent has to choose a particular method or combination of methods according to specific requirements of the situation. For instance, people with little or no education and low income may respond to personal visits and result demonstrations. The more educated and progressive section of the population may respond well to mass media like farm publications, exhibition, radio and television.

Combination of Extension Teaching Methods

Extension field studies conducted over long period of years show that people are influenced by extension education to make change in behaviour in proportion to the number of different teaching methods with which they come in contact. As the number of methods of exposure to extension increases, the number of farm families changing behaviour increases. For wide spread response, the people may be exposed to teaching methods in several different ways. It is also proved that the combined use of several methods is of utmost important in extension teaching. The percentage of adoption rate is high when more methods are used than single or two methods. The extension worker should know the proper sequence of use of extension methods to get desired result.

Methods useful in different steps of Extension Teaching Process

1. **Attention:** Pictures, Posters, awareness campaign, news stories, displays, exhibits, radio announcement, Television advertisement, banner, leaflet, cartoons, wall painting, hoardings, demonstration, etc.
2. **Interest:** Meetings of various types, film strip and slide show, news articles, radio talks, bulletins and pamphlets, tours, result demonstration, personal contact, etc.
3. **Desire:** Real object, demonstration, circular letters, pictures, models, samples and exhibits, success stories, charts, folders, field trips, etc.
4. **Conviction:** Demonstration, field trips, discussion with scientist, success stories, etc.
5. **Action:** Reminding circular letters, news stories, radio talks, personal contact, campaign, leader contact, etc.
6. **Satisfaction:** Personal contact, news stories, success stories, personal letters, etc.

Methods useful in different stages of Adoption Process

1. **Awareness:** All printed materials, film show, radio, television, local leaders, campaign, banner, leaflets, posters, personal contact, etc.
2. **Interest:** Personal contact, meeting, radio talk, TV/ VCR, meetings, slide, film strips, farm journal, folder, bulletin, etc.
3. **Evaluation:** Demonstration followed by discussion, cassettes, field trips, farmer's experience in any printed form, field day, etc.
4. **Trail:** Personal contact, method demonstration, result demonstration, leaflet, folder, farm journals, field trips, field days, TV/VCR, etc.
5. **Adoption:** Group Discussion, method demonstration, result demonstration, field trips, slide, self-experiences, leaflets, folder, farm journals, training, campaign, etc.

Suggested Readings and References

1. Bains, H.S. (1987). Teaching and Communication in Extension Education. Ludhiana: Sahitya Kala Prakashan.
2. Dale, Edgar (1965). Audio-visual Methods in Teaching. New York: Holt, Rinehart. Kelsey, L.D., and Hearne.

3. G.C. (1963). Cooperative Extension Work. New York: Comstock Publishing Associates.

4. Reddy, A.A. (2006). Extension Education. Bapatla: Sree lakshmi Press.

5. Wilson, M.C., and Gallup, Glady (1955). Extension Teaching Methods. Washington D.C.: SDA.

6. Singh, Ranjit (1987). A Text Book of Extension Education. Ludhiana: Sahitya Kala Prakashan.

7. Mathialagan, P. (2007). Textbook of Animal Husbandiy and Livestock Extension. Lucknow, India: International Book Distributing Co.

8. Ray, G.L. (2008). Extension Communication and Management. New Delhi: Kalyani Publishers.

9. Sandhu, A. S. 1993. Textbook on Agricultural Communication: Process and Method. New Delhi: Oxford and IBH Publishing Co Pvt. Ltd.

10. Van den Ban, A.W., Hawkins, H.S. (1996). Agricultural Extension, (2nd Ed). New Delhi: CBS Publisher and Distributors.

11. Dahama, O.P., Bhatanagar, O.P. (1987). Education and Communication for Development. New Delhi: Oxford & IBH Publishing Company.

12. Supe, S.V. (1994). An Introduction to Extension Education. New Delhi. Oxford and IBH Publishing Co. Lt.

13. Samanta, R.K. (1993). Training Methods for Management and Development, New Delhi, D. Publishing House.

4

Audio-Visuals in Extension Teachings

1. Extension Tools/Aids
2. Classification of Audio-visual Aids
3. Purpose of Audio-visual aids
4. Selection of Audio-visual Aids
5. Advantages of using Audio-visual aids in extension teaching
6. Cone of Experience
7. Cone of Learning
8. The effective Use of Audio-Visual Aids
9. Disadvantages of Audio-visual aids
10. Criteria for Selection and Evaluation of Audio-visual aids
11. Aids currently in use
12. Audio Aids
    - i. Compact Disk Recorder/Player
    - ii. Public Address System (PA System)
    - iii. Telephone/ Mobile Phone
13. Visual aids
    - a) Non-Projected Aids
        - i. Black Board or Chalk Board
        - ii. Bulletin board
        - iii. Flannel Board
        - iv. Magnetic Board
        - v. White Marker Board
        - vi. Pegboard
        - vii. Dust and mud sketching

- b) Graphic Aids
    - i. Flash Cards
    - ii. Charts
    - iii. Graphs
    - iv. Poster
    - v. Photographs and Pictures
    - vi. Map

14. 3-Dimensional Aids
    - a) Models
    - b) Specimen
    - c) Objects
    - d) Diorama
    - e) Puppet Show
    - f) Drama
    - g) Talking Doll
15. Projected Visual Aids
    - a) Direct Projection
    - b) Indirect Projection
    - c) Reflected Projection
    - d) Slides
    - e) Over Head Transparencies
    - f) Filmstrip
16. Audio-Visual Aids
    - a) Motion Pictures
    - b) Video
    - c) Television
17. Suggested Readings and References

EXTENSION TOOLS /AIDS

Audio-visual aids, audio-visual media, audio-visual material, communication technology, educational or instructional media, extension teaching aids, extension tools, extension aids, etc, - all these terms broadly speaking, mean the same thing. The use of the terms like educational technology or instructional technology instead of extension tools/aids in the recent time is primarily due to the dynamic expansion of programmed learning, computer assisted instruction and education television. In this discussion, the term audio-visual aid is used most frequently which is almost same as extension aids.

1 percent of what is learned is from the sense of TASTE.
1.5 percent of what is learned is from the sense of TOUCH.
3.5 percent of what is learned is from the sense of SMELL.
7 percent of what is learned is from the sense of HEARING.
87 percent of what is learned is from the sense of SIGHT.

Livestock Extension workers use different audio-visual aids to communicate the message effectively and efficiently. He makes an effort is to bring the learners very close to direct experience by using appropriate visuals or audio visual aids. These audio-visual aids provide the audience with a situation nearest to the reality and make out the meaning of the spoken words clear. It creates a favourable learning situation through facilitating teaching learning process. The learning will be effective when the dairy farmers were shown the milking machine and it will be more effective when they were taught how to use it and much more effective when they were allowed to practice on using it. Therefore, the audio-visual aids are instructional devices that assist the teacher to teach the learners effectively. The aids can supplement the teachers' teaching effectiveness and help the learners to learn with greater understanding. It helps in stimulating the sensory organs like ears and eyes, and facilitates quick comprehension of the message by the learner. The major ways by which the people learn are seeing, hearing and doing- looking, listening and acting. It has been long recognized the importance of various sense organs in the reception of the message in teaching and learning process. Study conducted by Haas and Packer (1964) showed that learning takes place through the various senses as under:

There is also saying that learners remember:

10 percent of what they HEAR
50 percent of what they SEE
90 percent of what they HEAR, SEE and DO

An old Chinese proverb also says:

> If I hear, I forget,
> If I see, I remember,
> If I do, I know

This proverb suggests that hearing is not sufficient in the learning process. One must hear, see and do things to gain understanding of a practice.

The instructional or communicational devices through which messages can only be heard are known ad AUDIO AIDS. The instructional or communicational devices which help to visualize the messages are known as VISUAL AIDS. The instructional or communicational devices through which the messages can be heard and seen simultaneously are known as AUDIO-VISUAL AIDS.

Classification of Audio-Visual Aids

The audio-visual aids are classified broadly in to three categories as follows.

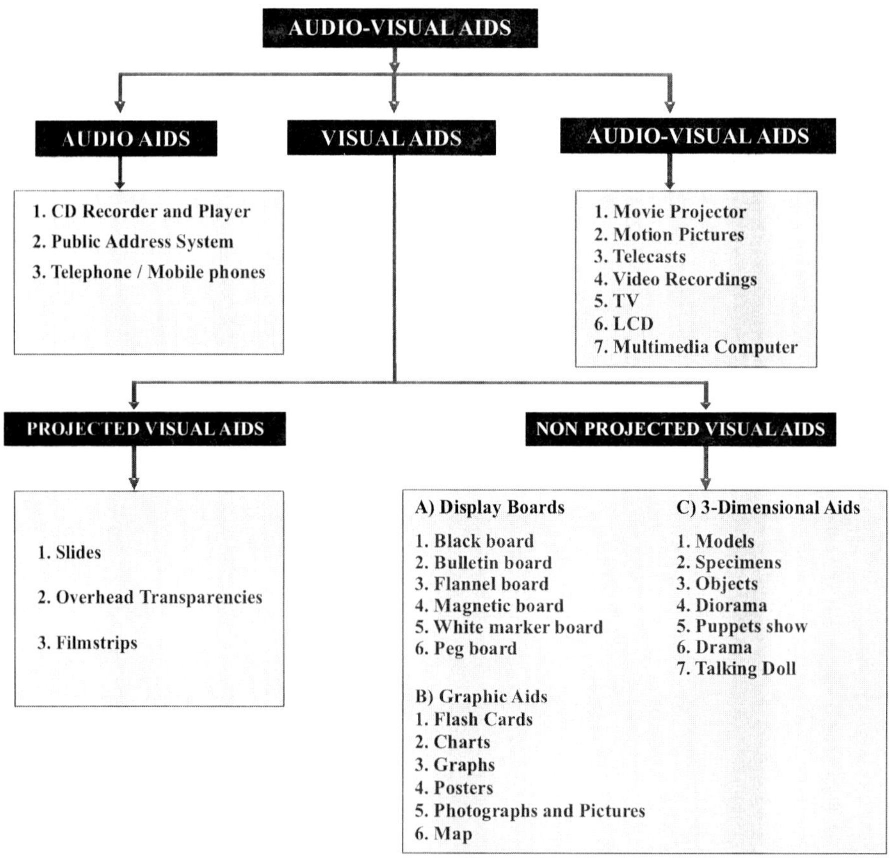

Purpose of Audio-Visual Aids

i. To create an effective learning situation

ii. To increase the concreteness, clarity and effectiveness of the message to be transferred to audience

iii. To involve the most sense organs of the learners to learn

iv. To speed up the process of learning.

Selection of Audio-Visual Aids

Use of audio-visual aids will not automatically increase teaching effectiveness. The structure of the message, its treatment and designing is important while using the aids to support the lesson. Synchronizing the audio and visual channels is very important, otherwise confusion will arise in understanding the facts. In the teaching-learning process, the audio-visual aids are used in single or in combination. However, their proper selection depends upon following factors.

Teaching Objectives: Depending upon the type of behavioural changes expected in the learner, the extension worker may decide the use of teaching aids. He/ she can use films or video show to arouse interest among the farmers towards the adoption of a new practice.

Subject matter: Based on the subject matter to be taught the extension workers can select the aids e.g. to teach the breed characters of a cattle, a colour photograph can be used.

Nature of the learner: According to the age, education, interest, experience, knowledge and intelligence of the learner the extension workers can select the aids, e.g. television for illiterates.

Experience of the teacher: The extension agent, and his familiarity and skill in handling the aid are also important in selection. Depending upon his/her familiarity one may use overhead projector other may use multimedia computer.

Availability: An effective extension agent makes use of indigenous materials. When the teaching aid he would like to use is not available with the extension agent and if there is no power supply in the remote village then he has to choose the non-projected visual aids.

Cost of the aid: Selection of the teaching aids is dependent upon the cost factor. An extension worker should take in to account the resources at his disposal while selecting teaching aids for the programme. However, effective aids need not be necessarily expensive.

Advantages of Using Audio-Visual Aids in Extension Teaching

1. Reduce verbalism
2. Adds variety in the hands of extension teacher
3. The learner can learn faster, learn more, learn thoroughly, and remember longer.
4. Add interest and involvement
5. Stimulate self-activity
6. Develop continuity of thought
7. Clarify idea being presented
8. Impress ideas more indelibly on the mind
9. Overcome the language barrier
10. Attract and hold attention
11. Arouse and sustain interest
12. Stimulate thinking and motivate action
13. Change attitude or point of view
14. Save time because they make learning easier and faster
15. Helps in meeting the different types of needs of the learners
16. Encourages interactions among the learners
17. Act as reinforcers in the teaching learning process.
18. Help the teacher to structure his message in a systematic manner
19. Multiply messages

Cone of Experience

We learn through experiences. Many of our experiences are direct and many are indirect. Similarly, many are concrete and many are abstract. We gain all these experience through our five sensory organs of seeing, hearing, touching, smelling and testing. Using one or more of these organs we gain numerous experiences every day. Edger Dale (1965) has summarized various sources of experiences in pictorial device called "Cone of Experience".

According to Dale, the cone of experience is pictorial representation explaining the inter relationships of the various types of audio-visual materials as well as their individual "position" in the learning process. The source of experience at the pinnacle of the cone is least effective, although most widely used. The more a particular method involves our sensory organs, the more effective it is producing the desired learning. As we go up the cone, we find that the use of sensory organs is diminished. As such the bottom most and the top most sources represent the two extremes in the use of sensory organs. In order to present this proportion in its true perspective, Edger Dale has selected the shape of a cone which has maximum space at the bottom and minimum at the top. The cone device is a visual metaphor of learning experience, in which the various types of audio-visual materials are arranged in order of increasing abstractness as one proceeds from direct experiences. In this cone each division represents a stage between the two extremes of direct experience at the base and pure abstraction at the apex.

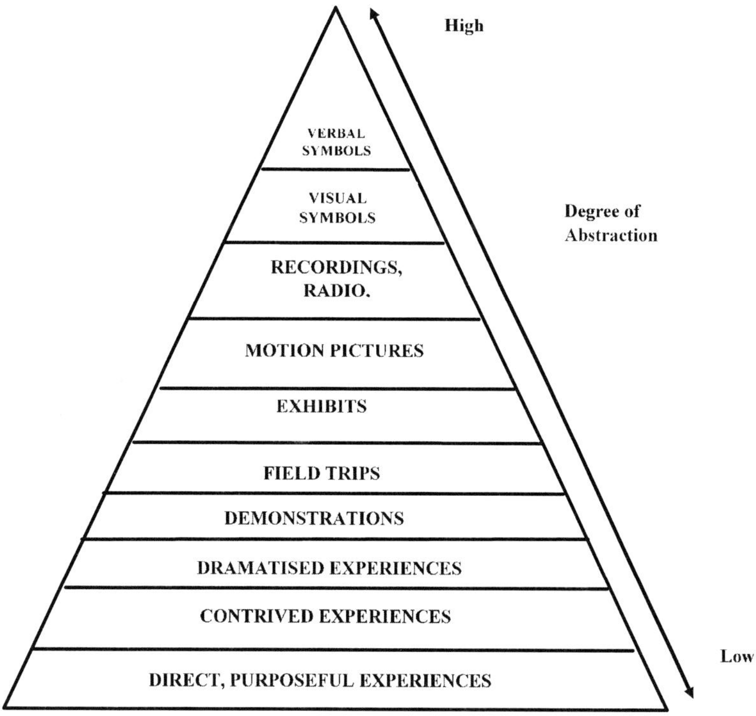

Cone of Experience

A brief description of each of the sources of experience helps in learning process from the bottom of the cone to the top is discussed below.

1. Direct, Purposeful Experience

The base of the cone represents direct reality itself as we experience it at first hand. It is the most effective experiences in terms of achieving the best desired learning results in the learner. It involves maximum number of sensory organs and is the purposeful experience that is seen, handled, tasted, touched, felt, and smelled. These experiences are not only direct; they are purposeful. While a learner is learning to operate a power tiller, all his mental and sensory faculties are actively engaged in the process. Therefore, he is learning by doings which is the best type of learning. This types of learning tends to be permanent and is least likely to be forgotten.

2. Contrived Experience

When it is not possible to see the reality, the reality is presented in a contrived form so that it may be meaningful to viewers. It may not be possible to show a species of high yielding dairy animal, but it may be possible to present it through a model so that one could get a comprehensive idea of about the animal and its external features. A contrived experience differs from the original in size, in complexity, or in both. A contrived experience is, therefore, an "editing" of reality, an editing that becomes necessary when the real thing cannot be clearly perceived directly; when it is too big or too minute, when the things we are interested in are obscured or confused or concealed. In such circumstances the imitation is better for teaching purposes than the reality.

3. Dramatized Experience

There are many things that we may not possibly experience directly in our lives due to restriction of time and place. We also cannot experience directly something that is already in the past. Besides, some of the matters cannot be conveyed by the contrived experience. In these cases, dramatic participation may bring closer to the realty. Dramatization will have much greater impact on the mind since many more faculties will be involved in seeing and hearing rather than merely mental images as in the case of reading.

4. Demonstrations

As discussed earlier, in method and result demonstrations, the learners are not only involved in seeing and hearing but also doing with both hand and mind. This is why the demonstrations are also more effective in terms of producing desired learning than those methods where only seeing and/ or hearing is done.

5. Field Trips

In this case, the participants can only see and occasionally hear someone explain the activities. There is hardly any scope for the use of manipulative skill. This is the reason why field trips are supposedly less effective than demonstration and, as such, are placed above them in the experience cone.

6. Exhibits

These are artificial representation of the reality. They can only be seen and thus employ only one sensory organ. This may account for exhibits being less effective than demonstrations and field trips and their placement above them in the cone of experience.

7. Television and Motion Pictures

Learners are simple spectators before TV and motion pictures. They are in fact different in experience in comparison to direct experience in terms of touching, tasting, handling and feeling of an object. Here, learners are only watching an event, and involved only in imaginative way. That is why; the film and motion pictures present an abstracted version of the real event. But, the film can dramatize the events so efficiently that we feel that we are in the presence of reality. That is why, motion pictures are great educational medium as it arouses and sustain interest on the issues and leave lasting impression on the mind of viewers.

8. Recordings, Radio, Still Pictures

All these employ only one sensory organ. One can only hear or see. This is the reason why are less effective in terms of learning and such placed above other sources in the cone of experience.

9. Visual symbols

Visual symbols are not realistic product of things but an abstract representation. These include the whole gamut of things that we can see with our eyes e.g. posters, charts, flash cards, flannel graph, books, pamphlets, etc. which are very extensively used in teaching and learning process.

10. Verbal Symbols-Pinnacle of the Cone

At the top of the cone are located the verbal symbols which are nothing but words and spoken language. Here all reality has been withdrawn and we are left with nothing but abstractions. They are least effective in terms of producing desired learning. It may sound paradoxical that the verbal symbols are the most commonly used medium of communication not only outside but also inside the class room even though it is least effective.

During the 1960s, Edgar Dale theorized that learners retain more information by what development of the Cone of Experience. The cone of experience is a pictorial device use to explain the interrelationships of the various types of audio-visual media, as well as their individual "positions" in the learning process.

This also proves the gradual progression of the learning ability of the individual with the teaching aids.

(Edger Dale, Audio-Visual Methods in Teaching, 1969)

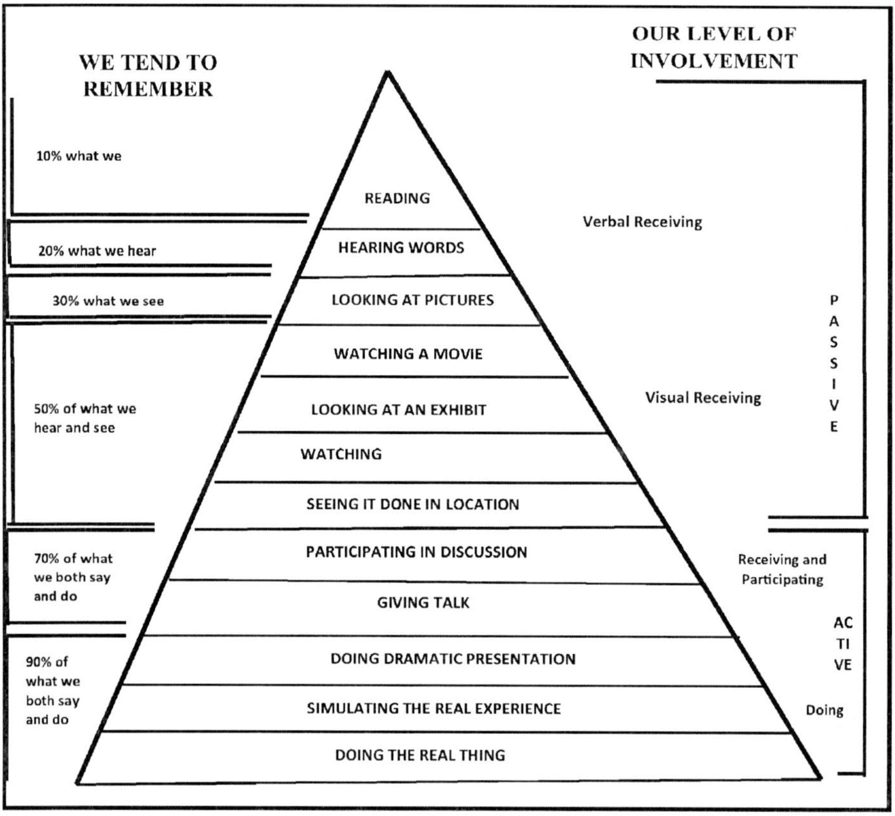

CONE OF LEARNING
(Developed and revised by Bruce Hyland by material from Edger Dale)

The Effective Use of Audio-Visual Aids

The following general procedure may be adopted while using A-V aids in the extension teaching programme.

a) Planning

1. Find out clearly the objectives of the programme
2. Anticipate the size of the audience and make sure the aids are visible and/ or audible to the entire audience.
3. Plan for the use of a variety of colourful visual aids.
4. Determine the appropriate timing for the presentation.

b) Preparation

1. Collect relevant equipments and materials
2. Rehearse and pre-view the audio-visual aids

3. Make sure that all equipments are in good working condition.
4. Check power supply, seating arrangement, darkness of the room, etc.
5. Arrange the audio-visual aids in sequence and have them within easy reach.
6. Keep aids out of sight until actually required for use.

c) Presentation

1. Motivate the audience and stress the key points.
2. Present aids at the right moment and in proper sequence.
3. Display only one aid at a time.
4. Remove all unrelated materials
5. Stand beside the aid, not in front of the aid.
6. Speak to the audience and not to the aids.

d) Follow-up

1. Observe reactions of the audience.
2. Clarify doubts, if any on the spot.
3. Make necessary changes in presentations by improving old materials, if required.

Disadvantages of Audio-Visual Aids

1. Learners are sometime mistaken or distorted impression, unless audio-visuals are supplemented with required explanation.
2. Teaching may be sketchy instead of being complete.
3. Over use of audio-visual aids may make teaching redundant.

Criteria for Selection and Evaluation of Audio-Visual Aids

Evaluation studies on effectiveness of teaching methods, audiovisual aids or combination of methods and aids are very limited in the discipline of extension education. Few studies on the above issues broadly indicate that the combined use of several methods and aids are more useful than the use of one or two methods and aids. However, we may evaluate the usefulness of audio-visual aids by ourselves on the basis of certain criteria suggested below in the table 2. The scoring on the items is also suggested on the basis of your conviction that the audio-visual aid you are employing is going to meet the objective. If you feel that it is 'very much' going to meet the objective than you may award 3 marks, similarly for 'much' -2 marks, 'not so much'-1 mark and 'not at all'-0 mark. The maximum mark one audio-visual aid may score is 21 and lowest is 0 mark. Accordingly, you may decide whether the audio-visual aid is suitable for the session or not. This is an illustration only and the extension teacher may add or delete some items in the table.

Criteria for evaluation of Audio-visual aids

Items	Very much (3)	Much (2)	Not so much (1)	Not at all (0)
The extent to which the audio-visual aid				
i) represents the true picture of the topic				
ii) has the ability to draw attention of the audience				
iii) can arouse interest of the audience				
iv) contributes towards meaningful understanding of the topic				
v) is likely to bring desirable change in the attitude of the audience				
vi) id appropriate to the level of audience				
vi) is worth the time and effort involved				

Source: Ray (2008), pp.140-141

Each type of audio-visual aid has certain advantages as well as limitations. Audio-visuals in combinations are always better than any one type of aid used alone. With the advancements in the means of communication and technology, some of the aids are not in much use. A list of aids that are now mostly used in place of the earlier used aids is given in table .

Aids Currently in Use

Aids getting replaced or becoming obsolete	Aids currently in use
Wall poster	Flexi banners, Collapsible banners, Digital cut outs
Black Board	White marker board/Smart board
Radio	Television
Slide Projector	Multimedia projector/LCD projector
16 mm film projector / film strips	Multimedia projector/LCD projector
Epidiascope	Direct Projector
SLR Camera	Digital Camera
VCP/VCR/Tape Recorder	CD Recorder/ Player
Personal letters	E-mail/ SMS
Land line telephone	Mobile phone

Audio Aids

1. Compact Disk Recorder / Player

Compact Disk (CD) Recorder/Player is an equipment for recording of digital data in an optical disc, which may be played back when needed. Both the functions of recording and playing facilities are available now on a single device. This audio aid is very suitable for use in meeting, training programme, campaign, recording of radio programmes, etc.

Advantages

1. It facilitates on-the-spot recording and playing of the sound
2. Helps in quick duplication of the sound
3. It helps to preserve recorded programmes for future use
4. The recorded CD can be immediately played back without processing.
5. It facilitates editing of sound by adding and deleting unwanted recordings.
6. It can be used for recording the farm broadcasts which may be replayed in convenient time.
7. It is very use to operate.
8. CD can be reused for recording and replaying for several times.

2. Public Address System (PA System)

Public Address System is a set of equipments to amplify and reinforce sound so that it is audible to large audience over a distance. It consists of microphone (mike), amplifier and loud speaker. The microphone is connected to the input terminal of the amplifier and the loudspeaker is connected to the output terminal. This aid is suitable for extension programme involving a large number of people such as mass meeting, training programme, field day or farmers' day, campaign, exhibition, etc.

3. Telephone/ Mobile Phone

Telephone or Mobile phone is electronic equipments through which people can communicate both ways to distant places. The mobile phones or cell phones are very popular due to its superior quality in reception of communication signals, portability in nature and low cost. The increased penetration of mobile phones in the rural areas has helped the extension workers to a great extent to communicate important information instantly to the farmers.

VISUAL AIDS

Non-Projected Aids

A) Display Boards

1. Black Board or Chalk Board

Blackboard

Black board and a piece of chalk prove very useful in illustrating concepts and ideas to the learners. It is probably the most widely used visual aids. It is a simple and unique device which, in spite of new devices and technique in teaching, is irreplaceable at the present moment. The extension worker can sketch diagrams, write important points while making discussion, draw pictures to make presentation interesting, etc. with the use of black board. Normally, two types of black boards are in use in extension teaching. One is rigid type of black board which is more durable and made of woods, plywood, metal, etc. These types of boards are not easily portable due to its size and weight. Other one is roll up type of board which is lighter, compact, portable, and is made of heavy cloth, canvas, oil cloth, etc.

The black-board or chalk board is the most universally used of all the teaching aids. It is one of the cheapest, most effective, most versatile and easiest to use of all the visual aids.

Effective Use of Black Board

1. Black board should be kept clean so that writing on it could be easily read by the learners from all sides.
2. Writing on the black board should be legible. The letters and drawings should be large enough so that they can be easily seen.
3. Writing should be started from the top of the corner of black board.
4. Writing should be in straight line.
5. Materials on the black board should not be covered by standing.
6. Make the materials simple and brief.
7. Get everything needed for black board before the class starts- chalk, ruler, eraser, and other items.
8. Stand one side of the black board.

9. Ensure that the black board is lighted by natural or artificial light.
10. Use colour chalk for emphasis.
11. Erase unrelated materials in frequent interval and keep the chalk board clean.

2. Bulletin board

Bulletin board, also known as "tack board', is surface intended for the posting of message. It may be made of soft insulation board, perforated masonite board or cork to facilitate addition and removal of messages. It can be used in class room as well as in villages to draw attention, develop interest, deliver messages and to promote action. Bulletin boards may be used to display various items like personal news, announcement, leaflets, folders, booklets, brochures, bulletins, charts, diagrams, posters, maps, news paper clippings, drawings, graphs, photographs, pictures, etc.

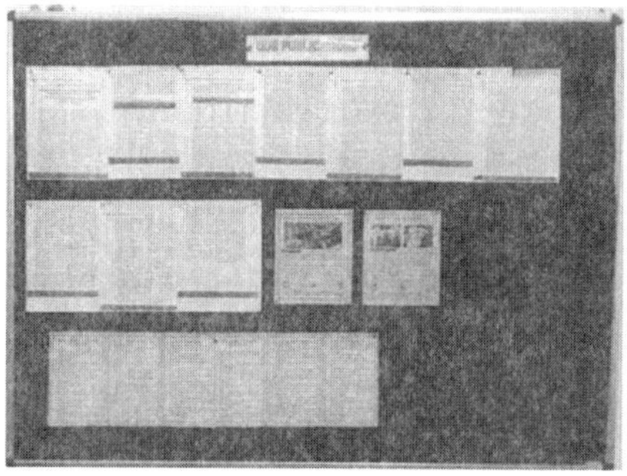

Bulletin Board

How to use Bulletin Board

1. Collect, classify and select suitable materials for display.
2. Remove all old displays and clean the board.
3. Prepare a title and brief description about the subject.
4. Arrange the materials and illustration in an interesting manner.
5. Use colour harmony and balance.
6. Put the board in a place where it would be visible clearly.
7. Observe daily whether materials displayed are in proper order or not.

3. Flannel Board

Flannel board, is also known as 'felt-board', consists of stiff materials and one side is covered with felt materials. Various objects such as pictures, photographs, diagrams, new paper cut-outs, graphs, drawings, text materials, etc. with the similar rough 'flannel like' backing are placed on the board while

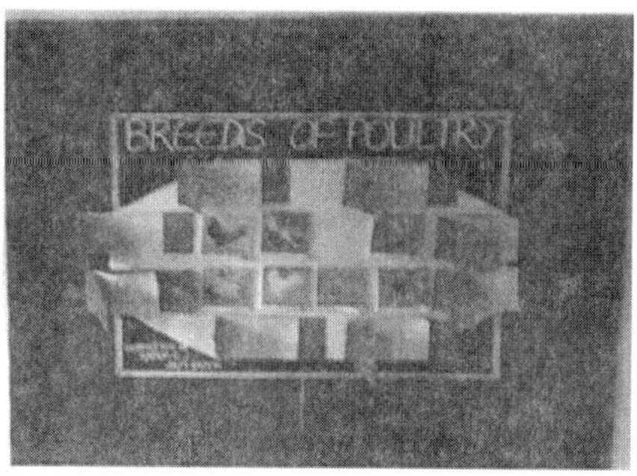

Flannel Board

making on extension presentations. These visuals or set of visuals having flannel like materials on the back and suitable for affixing in the flannel board are called as flannel graphs. These objects placed on the board adhere to it, without the use of tack or tape. This helps the extension worker to construct and develop an idea step-by-step in a very dramatic and impressive manner.

How to use Flannel Boards

1. Plan each steps of presentation.
2. Arrange each part in order.
3. Rehearse the presentation and see that the presentation could be finished in allotted time or not, and accordingly make changes before hand.
4. Make sure that all the flannel board cards are number sequentially.
5. Place the cards nearer to the board before presentation.
6. The flannel board should be placed where it can be seen by all the learners.
7. Stand beside the board, not in front of it.
8. Use cards in a dramatic way to draw attention, but make sure that each point is clearly presented to the group.
9. The title of the topic should be in large letters at the top of the board.
10. Keep the information simple
11. Present information in a step-by-step manner.
12. Leave the materials on the board as long as it is needed by the learners.
13. Avoid excessive changes of cards in the board. It may distract the learners.

4. Magnetic Board

This is like flannel board but it is made of steel on which pictures, charts, letters and other similar materials can be fixed with the help of magnets. This is mostly used in offices in which various information are displayed. The one of the important advantages of this board is that affixed materials can be moved from one place to another place on the board.

5. White Marker Board

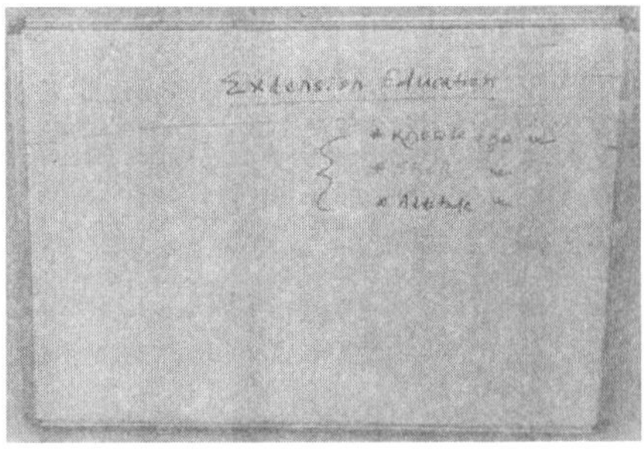

White Board

A whiteboard (also known as marker board, dry-erase board, dry-wipe board and pen-board) is a name for any glossy, usually white surface for nonpermanent markings. Whiteboards are analogous to chalkboards, allowing rapid marking and erasing of markings on their surface. The popularity of whiteboards increased rapidly in recent years and they have become a fixture in offices, meeting rooms, school classrooms, and in other work environments.

6. Pegboard

It is a plywood board, or of other similar material board, which has holes drilled through it at regular intervals of usually 3/4" size. In these holes, different types of metal clips are fixed to hold visual aids such as small posters, books and models. Mostly used in training institutions and offices. It is ideally suited to a lobby display, particularly of publications or other materials.

7. Dust and mud sketching

In sand, dust, soil and mud in which highly elective, inexpensive and readily available visual materials can be drawn using a pointed stick, a sharp stone or one's own finger. It is possible to illustrate many different ideas such as layouts for villages, poultry sheds and equipment sheds.

B. Graphic Aids

Teaching aids are those, which through a combination of drawings, words and pictures, are designed to help an extension worker to communicate ideas and facts clearly and effectively. The commonly used graphic aids are Charts, graphs, posters, flash cards, flannel graphs, flipbooks, cartoons, comics, etc.

Some general principles on the preparation of graphic aids:

- **Simplicity**
- Plain, clear and straight forward messages.
- Limit the materials in the graphics to the minimum.
- **Idea**
- Novel, dramatic or humorous ideas increase effectiveness of graphic aids.
- Keep only one idea in a graphic aid.
- **Colour**
- Proper contrast of colours is necessary to bring out a good graphic aid.
- Try to limit the number of colours to three.
- **Layout**
- Basic composition or arrangement of the elements or constituent parts i.e. the illustration, script, colour and white space within the graphic aid.
- It should be balanced and attractive.

> General principles on the preparation of graphic aids
> - Simplicity
> - Idea
> - Colour
> - Layout
> - Lettering

- **Lettering**
- All good lettering depends on style, colour, size and spacing between letters.
- The letterings should be simple, straight and bold.

Letter sizes for different distances are detailed below

Distance from the farthest viewer (in feet)	Minimum letter height (in inches)
100	3.5
80	2.7
60	2.1
40	1.4
20	0.7
10	0.5

Some of the common graphic aids in use in veterinary extension activities are discussed below

1. Flash Cards

Flash cards are a series of uniform pictorial cards which along with simple verbal explanation when presented before a group in a proper sequence tell a complete story. Flash cards are two dimensional, low cost non projected visual aids used in the presentation of illustrations, diagrams and figures with a title/ caption in a topic. Since it is flashed before the audience it is called as flash cards.

Aim

- To hold the attention to a single point at a time. To tell or inform about one theme through a stepwise story for action.

Principle

- By presenting a systematic set of flash cards the steps in a method demonstration on important animal husbandry practices can be drilled into the minds so that they may not be forgotten. The group easily recognizes the pictorial contents presented in a series.

Materials required for preparation of Flash Cards

- Paper pulp board or any thick material,
- Pencil,
- Eraser and
- Ink.

Preparation

i) Decide the topic which consists of illustration/diagrams

ii) Decide the number of cards required for presentation

iii) Select important captions/topics along with text for each card

iv) Select the size of flash card according to the number of audience. A size of 11"x14"is ideal for 20 people. A size of 22"x 28" is ideal for 30-50 people.

v) The number of flash cards should not exceed 12 per topic. Flash cards should not be used with large gatherings exceeding thirty.

vi) Prepare a rough sketch or layout of each flash card in terms of caption and illustration on a plain paper.

vii) Draw in pencil and then trace with crayon, paint or ink.

viii) Line drawings, cartoons, photos, cutout illustration can be used.

ix) Letter size should be 1" height for clear visibility.

x) Important points of the card should be written on the back side of the card.

xi) Cards should be serially numbered.

How to use Flash Card

i) Check and arrange the cards serially

ii) Keep the cards under the table so that it would not be visible to the audience.

iii) Make verbal presentation of the topic.

iv) Find the mood of the audience and if it is found that they are losing their interest, then flash the card relevant to the topic of discussion going on.

v) Hold the cards with one hand nearer the chest and keep quiet for some time and see that the audience could clearly see the card and then explain the topic.

vi) Flash the card with commentary for required time.

vii) Glance the essential points on the back side of the card while explaining.

viii) Keep the flashed card under the table and go on explaining the left portion of the topic.

ix) Use simple words, local expressions and examples.

x) Display the flash cards on a bulletin board after the discussion.

xi) Other aids can be used with this aid

xii) Ideal size of the audience for the flash card presentation should be less than 30.

Rules for preparation of flash cards

- Know your audience. Try to know the background, interest and problems of the audience to whom you are going to convey some idea through flash cards.
- Choose your subject matter very carefully with clear objectives and these are basic to any presentation.
- Pick up the main points and write down all the important points, which seem good for disseminating to the audience. Now sort out the essential points from these points.
- Draw a picture for each point make simple drawings and have one idea for each card. Do not crowd with more pictures. Too many illustrations should be avoided, further they should be adapted to local conditions.
- Make the illustrations big.
- Use contrast colours for making the presentation attractive.
- Write notes for the presentation. Notes on the back of the cards should be written in the right hand corner on the backside. For the first card the points should be written on the last card and for the second the points should be written on back of the first card and so on.
- Cards should be serially numbered on the top of the backside.
- Before using flashcards in front of the audience rehearse by using them repeatedly.
- Before going to the meeting arrange the cards logically by numbering them at the back.
- See that the cards are clear.
- Hold the card in your left palm on to your chest so that the audience can clearly see the card.
- Do not flash the cards for prolonged period of time.

Communication Characteristics of a Flash Card

i) **Sequence :** Different steps in a topic can be shown in a sequence. This avoids distraction. Attention can be drawn from one step to another.

ii) **Suspense :** When we flash first card during the presentation, suspense is created among the learners to know about what is there in the next card. This helps the audience to remain attentive to the topic.

iii) **Story Telling:** People like to hear stories, and flash cards are developed in such a way that the topic is presented to audience in a story form.

Advantages of Flash Cards

1. They are easy to make
2. They are easy to carry and handle
3. They are cheap
4. They can be used again and again
5. They provide suspense and keep audience attentive to the presentation
6. Suitable to communicate illiterate people due to its story telling quality
7. Logical presentation keeps the audience attentive

Limitations

i) Flash cards are not suitable for all topics

ii) Suitable for only small groups

iii) Extension personnel require skill for its preparation and use.

2. Charts

A chart, is a depiction of pictorial, graphic or numerical information either individually or in combination, explaining relationship between key facts or ideas. Flip charts consist of a series of individual charts, tacked or bound together and hanged on a supporting hand. These individual charts carry a series of related messages in sequences.

Purpose

- To make facts and figures meaningful and clear
- To show hierarchial relationships
- To emphasise proper sequence and relationsips
- To show operational procedure
- To communicate difficult, often dull subject matter in an interesting and effective way.

Principle

- Tells more than a poster
- Gives more detail information of an idea, technique of technology
- Sequencing or steps are crucial importance
- Put chart at a place where people have time to read and study it.
- Teaching with symbols sustains interest among learners.

Materials required

Subject matter, plain charts, pencils, erasers and different colouring materials.

Procedure

- To study the data thoroughly before actually preparing chart.
- Be clear about the concept to be developed and the information to be depicted.
- Develop each chart with only one idea.
- Maintain logical order.

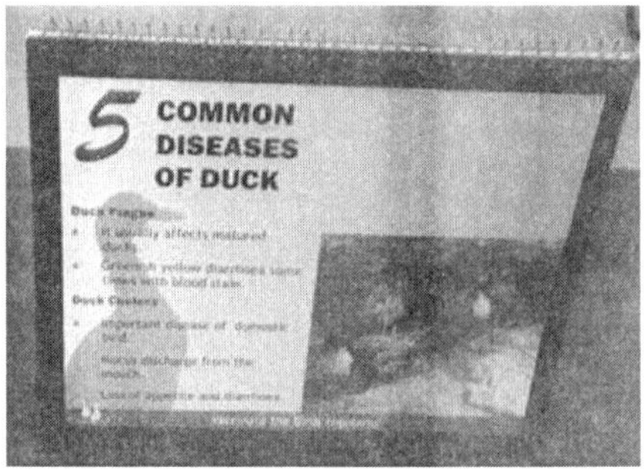

Flip Chart

Points to be considered while preparation

- Charts should be bold and simple lettered.
- Use key words
- Titles and words in charts should be brief.
- Design may be simple.
- Chart should be colourful. Better not more than three colours.
- Don't use more than 8 lines per chart
- Write maximum 8 words per line
- Leave double space between lines
- It must be large enough to be seen.
- Legends and codes should be smaller. All labels should be horizontal.

There are many types of charts are in use in teaching- learning process. Some of the commonly used charts are explained below in brief.

1. **Flip Chart**: Flip chart carries a series of ideas arranged on sequentially on number of chart papers. Individually charts are tagged or bound on one side with a hard card board. During presentation, leaves are turned one after another as the talk progresses.
2. **Pictorial Chart**: Pictorial chart may contain pictures or graphs or combination of both.
3. **Tree Chart**: These are used to show development or growth of things. This chart is developed from a base composed of several roots which lead into a single trunk. The branches in turn represent developments and relationships.

4. **Organizational Chart**: This shows the structure of an Organisation, Department, etc. For an example, Department of Agriculture of a State.
5. **Tabular Chart**: Information presented in a table form in a chart is known as tabular chart.
6. **Outline Chart:** Outline chart depicts main points, sub-points and their relationship in chart.
7. **Flow Chart :** It is made by lines , arrows, boxes, rectangles, etc. to depict the organization or structure of an organization, institutions, association, etc. It can also be used to show the story of a product as to how it has been obtained through a series of processes.
8. **Pull Chart:** the content of the chart is put fully covered with another sheet of paper of same size. While making presentation, we remove the cover and continue with presentation.
9. **Suspense Chart or Strip Tease Chart:** In this type of chart, all the points of chart are covered with a thin strip of paper that can be removed at appropriate time. This technique is very helpful in focusing attention on one point of the topic and also creating suspension about the next point in the chart.
10. **Overlay Chart:** This consists of a number if sheets which are placed one over the other conveniently and form a part of the whole picture. This enables viewer to see not only the different parts but also how they appear when one is placed over the other. After the final overlay is placed, it shows the ultimate product.

Preparation of Chart

1. Decide the topics, collect materials and select important points.
2. Keep title and sub-title to a single line. The title should be the brief statement of the purpose.
3. Make chart simple and present one idea only.
4. Make sure that the lettering, figures, pictures, cartoons, diagrams , etc. are large enough to be seen by the audience. Letter should be simple, of the straight type and bold. Use both upper and lower case letters as per the requirement of the chart.
5. Make proper combinations of colours/ contrast to increase readability.
6. Make presentation logical, direct, clear and accurate.
7. Use short sentences and leave blank lines in between sentences. Sentence should not have more than 8 words.

8. In flip chart, the script describing the pictures or sketches should be written on the back side of the previous page so the presenter can view and make discussion about the chart.

Tips for Presenting Charts

1. Present all the material on chart before discussing
2. Use a pointer to indicate the item being presented
3. Stand at one side of the chart. Never block its view
4. Look to audience as much as possible. Glance chart briefly
5. Avoid too much speech.
6. Try to get learners/ audience to think and discuss.
7. Remove all unrelated materials while using chart.
8. Display charts properly.

Advantages

- Used to present information in an interesting and understandable manner.
- Easy to prepare.
- By using chart, we can communicate even dull subject matter in an interesting way.

Disadvantage

- Improper display of charts creates more confusion than learning.

3. Graphs

Graphs are charts used for visual presentation of numerical or statistical data. It is widely used to show comparisons, trends, developments, relationships, etc. of data. Graphs are more interesting than the tabular information. Facts presented through graph become more comprehensible. There are many types of graphs, and most commonly used graphs in extension presentations are :

1. **Line graph:** This type of graph is used to show trend or relationship between and among various sets of data. It is used only when considerable data are to be plotted or when the data comprise a continuous series, which , over a period of time, clearly shows the progress taking place.
2. **Bar graph**: Bar graphs are used to present and compare data. They are easy to understand, because they consist of rectangular bars that differ in height or length according to their value or frequency. There are two main types of bar graphs: horizontal and vertical. Bar graphs display a change in

magnitude, and not in direction like line graphs. A horizontal bar graph consists of an x-axis, and a vertical bar graph consists of a y-axis. The numbers on the axes are known as the scales. Each bar represents a numeric or categorical variable. Vertical bar graphs are best used for the comparison of time series data and frequency distribution. Horizontal bar graphs are particularly useful when category labels are long; vertical bar graphs do not provide much space for text labels.

3. **Pie graph:** It is a popular form of data comparison, consisting of a circle divided into segments or categories which reflect the proportion of the variables in relation to the whole. Percentages are used to compare the segments, with the whole being equal to 100%. To make a pie chart, draw a circle with a protractor. Then, convert the measures of the variables into percentages, and divide the circle accordingly. It is best to order the segments clockwise from biggest to smallest, so that the pie chart looks neat and the variable are easy to compare. It is also recommended to write percentage and category labels next to each segment, so that users are not required to refer to the legend each time they want to identify a segment. Pie graphs with too many segments look very messy and are difficult to understand; therefore, it is best to use pie charts when there are less than five categories to be compared. Besides, if the values of the categories are very close, the pie chart would be difficult to decipher because the segments would be too close in size.
4. **Pictograph**: Pictographs, also called pictograms, are diagrams that show and compare data by using picture symbols. Each of these symbols corresponds to a specific quantity and is repeated a number of times. While pictographs are easy to understand, they can be misleading because they provide a general representation. Therefore, they are not commonly used by statisticians and scientists who work with very precise measurements.
5. **Area and Solid-figure Graph:** Area graphs consists of squares, circles, or other outline figures of different sizes and pictorially represent two or more related totals. These graphs depend on a comparison of area to represent information, and in consequence are read less easily than other forms.

Solid-figure graphs contain spheres, clubs or other figures developed and used by combining different graphic forms.

Essential Characteristics of Graphs

1. Must be simple
2. Must show comparison or relationship
3. Give approximation rather than precise information

4. Symbols used must be self explanatory
5. Should be brief, with one idea, depicted with a good layout.
6. Number of units should not be more than 4-5.

4. Poster

It is a non-projected visual aids specially designed with pictures/ illustration and few simple words to draw the attention of the passers-by to a single idea. A poster has to be bold in design, simple to understand and attractive in colour. Poster is designed to be both eye-catching and convey information. A good poster should have arresting words, dramatic illustrations and interesting subject matters. It has basically four components and they are: a) picture or illustration, b) the words, c) colour and d) space. Posters generally contain three main features. They are: i) announce a purpose ii) set conditions, and iii) recommend action. It is used in a teaching programme or campaign. It creates awareness among the people. It is useful for making announcement and advertisement of a product.

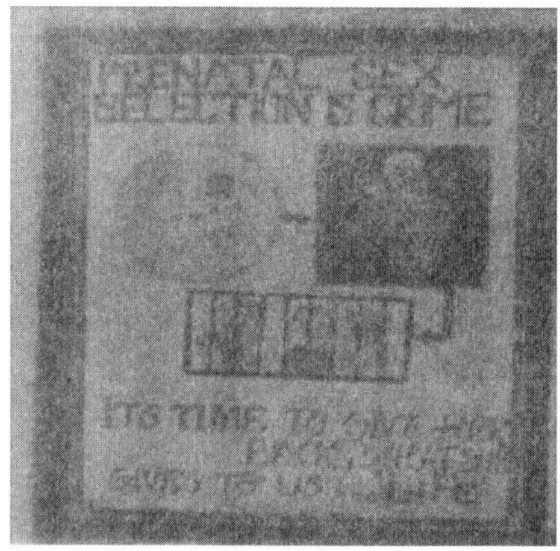

Poster

Example: Poster displaying Clean Milk Production.

Aim

- To create awareness about the extension programme.
- To communicate to a passer-by.
- To implant very quickly in a viewer's mind or to make him recall a single important idea.
- To motivate people to act by repeated reminders.

Principle of a Poster: The poster is generally seen from a distance and the person glancing at it seldom has the time or inclination to stop and read.

- Posters are simple graphic representations with the greatest possible impact. As an advertising medium, they arrest the eye and the mind, remind the public of a message. Posters generally contain *three main features* namely
    - They announce a purpose,
    - They set conditions and
    - They recommend action.

- Posters should be attractive, brief and clear and this is the ABC principle of poster. A hand drawn poster may be used in training programmes, group meetings, farmers' day, etc. printed posters may be used in large numbers in campaigns, exhibitions, etc.

Poster is normally seen at a glance, so the message must be simple and clear. The letters should be bold enough to visible to the passers-by from a distance. Details and wordy sentences should be avoided.

ABC OF A POSTER

A - ATTARCTIVE

B - BRIEF

C - CLEAR

Characteristics of a good poster

i) **Dramatic simplicity**: To attract attention, the prominent features of the poster must stand out clearly. These features may be photographs, drawings, illustration or a striking design. Messages should not be written in vertical order and fancy lettering of text to be avoided.

ii) **Attractiveness:** Poster should have good design, good lettering and attractive colour so that it should be pleasing to eye and interesting to look.

iii) **Brevity :** Minimum number words should be used to communicate the main ideas.

iv) **Self-contained message**: For quick absorption of the message of a poster, the meaning of the text and pictures must be clear and interesting.

v) **Design:** Good composition is one of the principal elements in preparing effective posters. A good poster requires a centre of interest, which must be strong and commanding.

Materials / facilities required

- For handmade posters, paperboards, poster colours, pencil, eraser, scale and good brushes are needed.
- For printed posters computer, litho offset press are required.

Planning

- Decide on the theme of the poster and identify the key points.
- Decide on the size of the poster (10"x 15", 15"x 20", 18"x 22", 20"x 30", 22"x 28"), caption, illustrations and the colours to be used.

- Based on the availability of funds decide on the number of copies to be produced.
- Keep in mind the date by which the posters are to be made ready.

Guidelines for Preparation of a Poster

1. First, decide the target group and then develop the message to communicate.
2. The texts and illustration/picture in a poster express the message simple and clearly.
3. Try to put the message into a few words in the form of a concise, striking and catchy slogan.
4. Use plain, bold lettering and lines.
5. Illustrations or picture is the dominant constituent of a poster. It should be prominent enough to bring out message clearly. Avoid unnecessary detail so that the viewer's attention is not confused.
6. Caption of the poster should be as small as possible. A caption not having more than five words is the best one. Don't write the caption vertically as it creates difficulty in reading. Don't break the caption. The word selected should be arresting words, in slogan form, and printed in plain and bold letters.
7. Effective posters are usually pleasing to eye. Use colour to attract attention and give contrast to poster. But, use of too many colours in extension poster also leads to confusion. It is suggested to use three colours in poster. Don't use odd combinations of colours.
8. Give adequate space between lines, words and illustrations. The poster should not be crowded with words and pictures.
9. Layout of a poster should be well balanced so that the viewer' eyes can travel smoothly and quickly on the message of the poster.
10. Size of the poster must be large enough to be easily seen from a distance. Poster of 28" x 44" size is the most effective size with 2" size of plain letters for caption in slogan form.
11. Prepare a rough sketch of the poster in small scale, i.e 1/3rd or 1/4th of actual size. After the rough lay out is completed, it should be pre-tested with the few people of target group to find out the flaws in poster. Ambiguity or difficulty in understanding the meaning of the poster, if any found, should be removed before going for mass production. The final poster may be made by the help of an artist.

Hints in Preparation of a Poster

a) Promote one idea/point at a time

b) Use dramatic pictures of local demonstrations, exhibits or activities.

c) Must be timely

d) Place the poster where people pass by or where people gather.

Advantage of use of Poster

1. Helps in announcement of important events
2. Creates awareness among the people
3. Covers large number of audience
4. Can be prepared in advance
5. Can be seen from a distance
6. Reinforces messages that viewers receive through other media.

Limitations of Poster

1. Poster used to convey only single idea and con not give detail information.
2. Difficulty in storage of large sized posters for future use without damage
3. Poster designed for one area cannot be useful to other areas because of wide diversities.
4. Production of a good poster is technical in nature and requires intuition, skill, time and money.

Presentation

- Put hand drawn posters in well-lighted places where the visitors are likely to assemble or pass through.
- For printed posters, ensure timely dispatch.
- Display printed posters at prominent places in time. In important places put up a number of posters closely to produce mass effect.

Follow-up

- Watch reaction of the audience.
- Ensure availability of inputs and services and commensurate with the message in the posters.

5. Photographs and Pictures

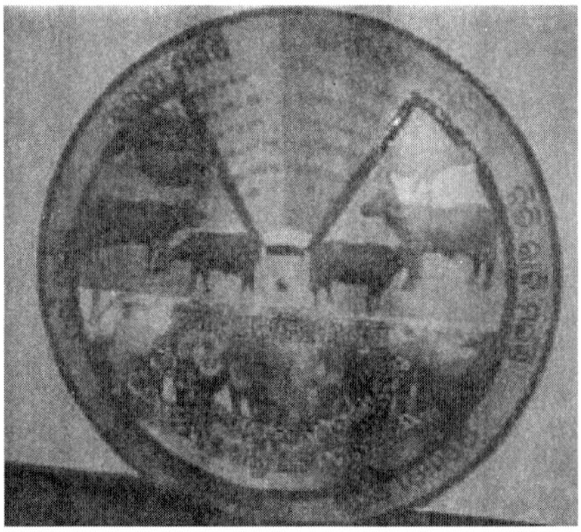

Photograph showing different breeds of buffaloes

The picture or photograph is worth of 1000 words. They speak for themselves. Photograph represent actual recording of things. They have no language barrier. It is very suitable to teaching of illiterates. Photographs could be used in number of ways or indifferent information materials, like farm publications, exhibitions, picture stories, display, etc. Picture and photograph may be black and white or in colour. To be an effective teaching aid, the photograph and picture must tell a story, illustrate one point at a time, show action, have plain and simple background.

Advantages of use of Picture and Photograph

1. Easy to get at moderate cost
2. Can be preserved for long duration
3. Easy to carry
4. Can be used repeatedly
5. Arouses interest and draw attention to the discussion
6. Help in clarifying complex ideas
7. Easy to convey messages to illiterate people.
8. Increases credibility of the message

6. Map

A map is a visual informative diagram of an area. Maps are mostly static two-dimensional, geometrically accurate representation of an area. In map information is presented in abstract form, as such, a higher level of intelligence and education of the audience is required to understand and absorb the information. The rural audience needs assistance from extension worker to understand the message from map.

3-Dimensional Aids

1. Models

Real things may not be available or possible for extension worker to arrange to use in teaching learning process. Sometimes it may be too big, too complex or too small for study. In such circumstances, the model is very useful as it is the miniature replica of an object. When it is not possible to expose the audience to real object, model is used to communicate a reliable idea of the original. Models may be prepared from clay, plaster of paris, wood, light metal, masonite, plastic, etc. Models improve the teaching efficiency because they have the capacity to involve all the sense organs of audience. Scale models, simplified model, cross sectional models, working models (mock-up) , etc. are different types of models used often in training programmes, exhibition, meeting and various demonstrations. Muck-up models are functional device which shows the operations of essential parts of real objects.

Advantages

1. Give three dimensional idea of an object
2. Arouse interest of the audience
3. Save time and money
4. Can be preserved for many years
5. Can be used repeatedly
6. Helps extension workers in effective communication on the topic.

2. Specimen

A specimen is a sample which represents the whole. It may be a part of an object or be a one of group or class to represent the whole group. There are various methods of preserving the specimen: i) dry preservation method e.g. insects, bones , ii) wet preservation method e.g. worms, mummified foetus, etc, iii) live preservation method e.g. tick , fish, birds. The specimens are real and hence appeal to senses and they offer better scope for study. It exposes audience to almost real life situation.

3. Objects

The term objects refer to samples of real things. They are very valuable teaching aids in both formal and informal education. Real objects are the best visual aids as the learners recognize them. The learners can be taken to the field situation to show them the real objects like insect, livestock, paddy field, etc.

4. Diorama

It is a scenic presentation of the original with specimen, model, painting, etc. . The term diorama is derived from a Greek word which means 'to see through'. The diorama may be prepared with a big box having front side open in a semi-circular shape with painting on all side of the box matching as the specimen, model, etc. to be displayed inside it. The objects (specimen, model, etc.) after proper insulation, electric fittings, painting, etc. may be fixed at convenient places in a pattern similar to the natural environment which is needed to be revealed to the audience. The extension personnel must be well trained to communicate messages through demonstration of diorama in front of audience.

5. Puppet Show

In puppet show the dolls are made to perform by control movement of doll by an expert from outside. Extension messages are communicated to the audience through story in puppet show. The impact of the puppetry depends on the process of transformation of puppets which has much in common with magic and with play. It is an interesting aid for communicating with the rural illiterate people. There are different types of puppet such as glove or hand puppet, string puppet, rod puppet, shadow puppet, etc.

6. Drama

It is a theatrical performance by a group of people on a theme. This is a very powerful medium for social mobilization. Enactment of drama requires lot of careful planning and arrangement of materials to make it effective for the purpose of communicating extension message. The extension worker may take the help of experienced artists for the above purpose.

8. Talking Doll

Talking dolls are used to create general awareness about an extension programme. Specialized artist can only perform the play on a topic by having control over the movement of the doll and synchronization of his voice with the movement of doll. Talking dolls are used to communicate the messages on various social themes to the rural mass.

Projected Visual Aids

Visual aids that are used for magnification of image on a screen in dark or semi dark condition are known as projected visual aids. Some of these projected visual aids are slides, transparencies, film-strips, films, etc. The essential principle involved in projection is that when light falls on transparent/translucent/opaque object, it passes through the object or is reflected by it; then, the light is made to pass through convex lens and allowed to fall on a screen at convenient distance, an inverted image of the object appears on the screen. If the object is initially kept inverted before the source of the light, the image will be straight and comprehensible.

Types of Projection

Different kind of equipment materials are used to project visual materials. These equipments use three important method of projection: i) Direct Projection, ii) Indirect Projection, and iii) Reflected Projection.

Direct Projection

In this projection, the rays of light directly comes from the source light, pass through the condenser lens, the object (slide, film or film-strip), the objective lens and finally the enlarged image appears on the screen. In this method, light travels straight and fall on the screen. Loss of light is les, so projection can be done in the semi dark room. The slide projector and film/movie projectors are based on the principle of direct projection.

Indirect Projection

In this method, the rays light coming from a projection lamp, enter one element of a condenser lens unit and are reflected by a plane mirror at an angle of 45^0 with either of the axes of this condenser lens unit. The reflected rays entre the other element of condenser unit, pass through the slide or the transparencies, entre the objective lens and are again reflected by another plane mirror, placed at angle of 45^0 with the axes of the objective lens to form an enlarged image of the material on the screen. The source of light in this is considered to be indirect. The loss of light in this case is more compared to direct projection. The overhead projector is based on the principle of indirect projection.

Reflected Projection

Opaque projector is based on this system of projection. It works on the principle of reflecting light from an opaque surface to the screen. In this method, light indirectly coming from the bulb hits the surface of the object at an angle and consequently the image of the object is reflected on the large mirror fitted at an angle of 45^0 with the axes of the object. The reflected image is made to pass through the objective lens by the rays of light coming all the way from the projection bulb, and finally a magnified faint image appears on the screen. Loss of light is maximum in this type of projection, so complete dark room is required for this projection. Opaque materials such as pictures, book pages, objects and other types of materials can be projected by this method. Opaque projector is also known as epidiascope.

1. Slides

Slides are small pieces of transparent materials on which single pictorial image, scene, graphic or text image has been photographed and are projected by passing light through it for group viewing.

Types of Slide

i) **Lantern Slides:** These were used in the past and presently are not of much use. These slides normally measure 3"x 4"snd mounted on a glass.

ii) **35 mm or 2"x2" Slide:** These types of slides are now commonly used.

Photographs of objects are taken by a 35 mm camera and film is processed. The selected film is cut to individual pictures and mounted on card board or on readymade plastic mounts. The equipment used for projecting the slide is known as Slide Projector. There are two types of slide projector: one is manually operated, in which every time the projected slide is taken out from the slot and pushed by hand in position, and the other one is automatic slide projector in which large number of slides are serially inserted in the magazine slot beforehand and are projected one after another with the help of remote controller. The former one is now almost obsolete.

Operation of Slide Projector

i) Check proper seating, lighting and ventilation arrangements in the room

ii) Arrange the slides in order and insert them in the slide carrier in an inverted position

iii) Set up the projector and connect the cord to electric plug.

iv) Fix the screen and darken the room

v) Turn the switch to on

vi) Focus and centre the image on the screen

vii) Present the slides in the sequence by standing at the back of the projector and support the show with explanation wherever necessary

viii) Slide projection can be combined with recorded commentary using audio tape

ix) After presentation of the slide switch off the projector and make the concluding statement

Advantage of Slide Show

i) Attract the attention of the audience to the topic

ii) Large number of persons can view the slides at a time

iii) Help the extension worker in communication

iv) The story can be told sequentially and in steps

v) Slides can be changed remotely or automatically

vi) Convenient to use

vii) Easy to handle, store and transport

viii) Can be used repeatedly

ix) Less costly and easy to replace

Limitations of slide show

i) It does not show action

ii) It requires 'live' narration

iii) Requires coordination between the projectionist and speaker

iv) It requires semidarkness room for presentation

v) Equipment is costly

2. Over Head Transparencies

Transparencies are popular instructional medium. They are simple to prepare and easy to operate with the overhead projector which is light weight. A 10 x 10 inches' sheet with printed, written or drawn material is placed on the platform of the projector and a large image is projected on a screen behind the presenter. The equipment used to project the information written in transparencies in known as Overhead Projector (OHP). OHP is used generally in a class room situation and it works on the principle of indirect projection. The transparency to be projected is placed on the horizontal glass platform of the projector. The instructor may use a blank transparency and write over it while making presentation. Overhead projection enables the instructor to simultaneously deliver the talk and project instruction materials while facing towards audience. Transparencies may be hand written or hand drawn. Information can be typed or photocopies in transparencies.

Preparation of Overhead Transparencies

a) Materials required

i) Acetate sheets rolls of 10" x10" size (75 microns thickness for writing and 100 microns for photocopying) or cellophane paper or transparent plastic papers

ii) OHP Marker pens

iii) Crayons

iv) Mounts

Common guidelines to use Overhead Transparencies

Guidelines and tips mentioned below about the use of overhead transparencies may seem like commonsense but many presentations fail to produce desired effects because these tips are not consistently applied.

i) Practice your presentation before a group of small audience to find out any problems with the transparencies

ii) Place your overhead projector on a table

iii) Stand on the side of the overhead projector while you face the audience

iv) Place the overhead to your right if you are right handed and to your left if you are left handed

v) Do not face towards the "projected" image on the screen

vi) Cover the transparency when you are not using it

vii) Tape the power cord on the floor to protect the presenter and others from hitting.

viii) Keep always a spare bulb

ix) Store your overhead transparencies in a sturdy box or container.

Using an Overhead Projector

i) Set up the projector at a distance of 2 meters from the screen

ii) Plug the main cord into any 3 pin 5 amps main socket.

iii) Switch on the projector by rotating the control knob to "FAN" position. The fan starts moving. Then rotate the knob further till it just crosses red zone of the arrow, where preheating system comes into play. Allow the knob in this position for about a half minute before moving it on further for the desired light intensity.

iv) Adjust the top mirror tilt knob. A good picture is obtained when the mirror is inclined at an angle of 45^0 to the horizontal plane.

v) Adjust the focus knob till the light on the screen is sharp.

vi) Place the transparency on the projector stage and again adjust the focus knob as required.

vii) Switch of the lamp by bringing the knob to FAN position is not required. This will not only help to increase lamp life but also keep the projector cool.

viii) Before switching off the projector, insure that cool air comes out of the exhaust fan which indicate that the interior of the projector has been cooled.

ix) Use pointer (pencil or pen, etc.) to direct attention to a detail on the transparency. Don't point at the screen as it may cast a shadow on the projected image on the screen.

x) Avoid walking in front of the projector

xi) Other instructional materials can be shown simultaneously with the transparencies.

xii) The presenter should face the audience and maintain eye contact with the audience at all times.

Advantages of using Transparencies

i) Saves time in presenting the talk.

ii) Teacher controls presentation

iii) Easy to prepare the transparencies and can be used repeatedly

iv) Helps the audience to understand the information delivered by the speaker

v) Complex ideas can be presented clearly

vi) Creates interest among the audience

vii) Beneficial for large number of audience

Limitations

i) Effectiveness of the presentation depends on good preparation by the speaker

ii) Opaque materials cannot be projected

iii) Instructor is to stand close to the projector to change the transparency

3. Filmstrip

A film strip is a continuous strip of film consisting of a small number of individual frames of pictures arranged in sequence with explanatory titles. Each strip may contain about 30 to 60 frames of photographs, diagrams, drawings or text materials. The filmstrip has perforation on both the side of the film which facilitates its forward and backward movement of the film. Some of the slide projectors have facility to project filmstrips. Commercial filmstrips are available in the market on various topics. Extension workers may develop his own filmstrip as per his requirement by taking good photographs and assistance of a studio for processing and development. Filmstrips are used in small group discussion and training programmes. Filmstrip projection can be synchronized with the commentary by a voice recorder.

Advantages of Filmstrip use

i) Information can be stored in a condense form

ii) Light, easy to handle and transport

iii) Visuals can be used repeatedly

iv) Less expensive than sound film

Disadvantage of use of Filmstrip

i) The sequence of the picture can be altered

ii) Commercially available filmstrip may not be suitable to our requirements

iii) Development filmstrip is time consuming

Audio-Visual Aids

Motion Pictures

Motion pictures, also called film or movie, is a series of still images taken by a movie camera when projected on a screen, creates an illusion of moving images. Motion pictures are produced by synchronizing movement of picture with sounds. Motion pictures involve two distinct functions: production of the film and projection of the film. Production of film is a highly specialized job and requires different level of expertise. Extension workers are not expected to perform the job of production of film. They are required to project the film for various extension activities. The extension film may be black and white or colour. The films may be 16 mm, 35 mm and 70 mm width but 16 mm film are widely used in extension progrmmes. Movie projector is used to project the motion pictures. Motion pictures are mostly used in campaign, exhibition, demonstration, village meeting, training programmes, etc.

Advantages:

i) Attracts audience and arouse interest

ii) Provides real life experience

iii) Complex matter can be presented effectively

iv) Very useful for illiterate people

v) Can be preserved and repeatedly used

Video

Video is an electronic audio-visual medium for the recording, copying, playback, broadcasting, and display of moving visual media. The video produced can be telecast through TV station to reach the masses. Video lessons produced are used for teaching of small groups of farmers with the help of video projector or through LCD. In motion picture, the image are projected on the screen from outside which requires a darkened place for viewing. In video and television, the images are projected within the receiving set and can be viewed in an ordinary room, preferable with some lights on.

Advantages

i) Video tapes can be prepared in advance

ii) It draws the attention and motivates people to extension programme.

iii) It can be broadcast to large number of people at a time.

iv) Deletion, addition and updating of the video programme is possible.

v) Video programmes can be viewed repeatedly

vi) Besides education, video programme can also be used to entertain the people.

Television

Television is an important audio-visual aid for mass communication. Retention of information is more in TV viewing then radio listening because both the sense organs of eye and ear are involved in former case. It combines both audio and visual impacts, and is very useful in transmitting the agricultural information. The word television comes from Greek word meaning 'far' and a Latin word meaning 'to see. Hence it is 'to see what is far'. It is an effectively medium of dissemination and diffusion of information, entertaining, educating and influencing the thought and the attitude of rural viewers.

Television programme production is a highly specialized job. It involves the stages of planning the subject, preparing a script and issues, specimens and other materials to support the script, recording the programme, editing and telecast.

Advantages

i) It attracts attention of the audience

ii) It helps in creating mass awareness about a programme

iii) It creates interest on the mind of audience about a particular product

iv) TV programmes communicate message to large number of audience in a very short time.

v) Emergency messages can be communicated effectively

vi) Programmes can be repeatedly telecast

Disadvantages

i) It is very expensive audio-visual aid

ii) It requires high degree of professionalism for its production

iii) If editing is not properly, programmes become ambiguous.

iv) Entertainment aspect of the programme may dominate the information content part of the programme.

Suggested Readings and References

1. Karthik, Priyanjan (2005). Audio-Visual Aids and Education, Dominant Publishers and Distributors, New Delhi- 110 002.
2. Adivi Reddy A. (1987). Extension Education, Laxmipress, Bapatla.
3. Chalapathi Rao I.V. (1996). Communication and leadership skills and strategies, Book links corporation, Hyderabad.
4. Kamath H.G. (1969). Writing for farm families, Allied publishers private Ltd., Bombay.
5. Ray G.L. (1996). Extension Communication and management, naya prakash, Calcutta.
6. Ensminger, Douglas (1957). A guide to Community Development, Ministry of Community Development, Government of India, Coronation Printing Works, Fatehpuri, Delhi-6.
7. Kelsey, L.D. and Hearne, C.C.(1949), Cooperative Extension Work, Vail-Ballou, Inc, Binghamton, New York, U.S.A.
8. Dahama, O.P., Bhatanagar, O.P. (1985). Education and Communication for Development, Oxford & IBH Publishing Company, New Delhi.
9. Sandhu, A.S. (1993). Textbook on Agricultural Communication: Process and Method, Oxford and IBH Publishing Co Pvt. Ltd., New Delhi.
10. Van den Ban, A.W. & H.S. Hawkins (1998). Agricultural Extension, 2nd Edition. New Delhi, CBS Pub. & Distributors.

5

Extension Communication

1. Communication and Extension
2. Meaning of communication
3. Concepts / definitions of communication
4. Process of Communication
5. Elements of Communication Process
   a) The Communicator
   b) Message / Content
   c) Channels of Communication
   d) Treatment of the Message
   e) The Audience/ Receiver
   f) Response of the Audience / Feedback
6. Factors affecting communication
7. Models of Communication
   a) Aristotle's model
   b) Lasswell's model
   c) Shannon- Weaver's model
   d) Berlo's Model of Communication
   e) Schramm's model of Communication
   f) Leagan's Model Communication
   g) Rogers and Shoemaker's Model of Communication
8. Model on Extension Communication System
9. Barriers to Communication
10. Types of Communication
    a) Verbal Communication
    b) Written Communication
    c) Oral Communication
    d) Intrapersonal Communication

e) Interpersonal Communication
f) Group Communication
g) Public Communication
h) Mass Communication
i) Non Verbal Communication
j) Visual Communication

11. Functions of communication
12. Suggested Readings and References

Communication and Extension

We spent most of the time in a day by communicating with others. It is impractical to think of a life in which we don't communicate. Communication is a process not only limited to human beings. All creatures of earth communicate with each other for their better existence. In communication, we exchange our ideas, information, feelings, opinions about an issue, emotions, etc. with others throughout our life. It indicates that the communication is inseparable from the existence of life. A hypothetical example on the various kinds of communications that a Veterinary doctor might be using on a normal day is presented below for easy understanding.

A Veterinary doctor goes to office and put his signature in the attendance register (written communication) and greets his staffs (communication through gesture). Then he attends the patients and discuss with the owner (verbal communication). He writes prescription for the ailing animals (written communication). After office works, he may visit and discuss with the villagers about a vaccination programme (group communication) and inform the villagers about the date and time of vaccination. He may sensitize the people about the importance of vaccination through television, radio, newspaper, etc. (mass communication) and develop leaflets/folder/bulletins on different issues for distribution. This brief example suggests that the communication is an inevitable part of our daily life. It may be like that we may not survive without communication.

Meaning of Communication

The word 'communication' comes from the Latin *communis,* meaning common. This implies when we communicate, we are trying to establish '*commonality*' with someone through a message. Communication is the meaningful exchange of information between two or more individuals. The word 'communication' has many different meaning for different persons. According to Webster Dictionary, communication means:

> Communication comes from the Latin word *communis*- meaning common

1. Transmitting
2. A giving, or giving and receiving, of information, signals or messages by talk gestures, writing, etc.
3. The information, messages, etc.
4. A means of communication, especially
   a) A system of sending and receiving messages, s by telephone, telegraph, radio, etc.
   b) A system of moving troops and material
5. The science or art of communicating as a branch of study

However, in this chapter, we will be discussing the various aspects of communication with the faremers to increase their knoweldge and skill to adopt new techonologies.Farmers want knowledge to improve themselves and their ways of living.Extension workers communicate with the farmers to pass the knoweldge and diffuse the tenchnologies among the farmers. Their ommuncation styles motivates the farmers to learn new things and new way of doing things. In real sense, communication involves the transfer of an idea or thought from one's mind to that of another. It is not, therefore, enough if you tell the farm people about a new idea. They must hear it, understand it and remember it. In other words, communication is telling someone something in such a manner that he gets it.

Communication is a process which includes transmission of

information,
ideas,
emotions,
skills,
knowledge
by using
symbols,
words,
gestures,
and visuals
and so on.

Concept/Definitions of Communication

Definitions of communication are many. Few of them are cited for our purpose.

Communication

- anything convey meaning
- message transmitted from source to receiver
- exchange of ideas, facts, feeling, etc.

1. Communication is anything that conveys meaning, that carries a message from one person to another (Brooker 1949)
2. Communication is the process by which the message is transmitted from the source tothe receiver (Rogers, 1983)
3. Communication is a mutual interchange of ideas by any effective means (Thayer 1968)
4. Communication is the process by which two or more people exchange ideas, facts, feelings or impressions in ways that each gains a common understanding of the meaning,intent and use of message (Leagans, 1960)

5. Communication is the transfer of meaning between sender and receiver (Gibson and Hodgets, 6)1980

Therefore, the main purpose of communication is to inform, or to bring around to a certain point of view or to elicit action.

Process of Communication

Communication is a process wherein the act of communication is constantly changing as the communication proceeds. The communication process is dynamic, ongoing and ever-changing and continous in nature. The process has no beginning, end, or fixed sequence of events. It is not static. It is dynamic.The process has at least four elements — acts or action, a continuous change intime, advancement or progress over time, and a goal or result.

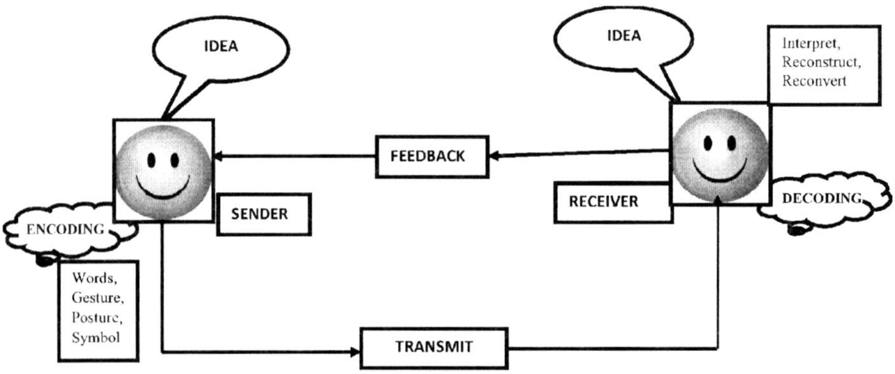

The process of communication involves:

1. The sender who generates an idea in his mind (may be a farmer or extension worker).
2. The idea is then converted into words, pictures, sounds, symbols, actions. This is called 'encoding the idea'.
3. Transmission of encoded idea to the receiver.
4. Receiver receives the encoded message through the senses and perceives it in the mind.
5. Receiver decodes or converts the messages back into meaningful ideas in his / her own mind and understand the meaning of message.
6. Receiver gives feedback to the messages.

The six-stepped equence is illustrated below

Atleast two persons are required to initiate a communication process. One may be you (Extension worker-Sender) and other one may be a livestock farmer

(Receiver). The sender or source conceives an idea, gives it a shape,decides the mode of communication which may be used to convey the idea, and conveys it. Thereceiver receives it, tries to understand it, and finally takes an action which may be either to store theinformation or to send the message to the original source or take any other line of action as requiredby the source. The whole process, thus, may be depicted as follows:

The entire process of communication requires at least the above six steps, i.e., Ideation,Encoding, Transmission, Receiving, Decoding and Feedback. These steps are discussed breifly:

Ideation: The first step in communication is ideation-creative process of genearating, developing and communicating new ideas. Here the sender thinks of an idea whichhe wants to communicate to the other party. This is the content and the basis of the message. He musthave something to say before he really says it. The sender must also keep in mind the sender to whomthe message is intended to be conveyed, and also the channel to be used.

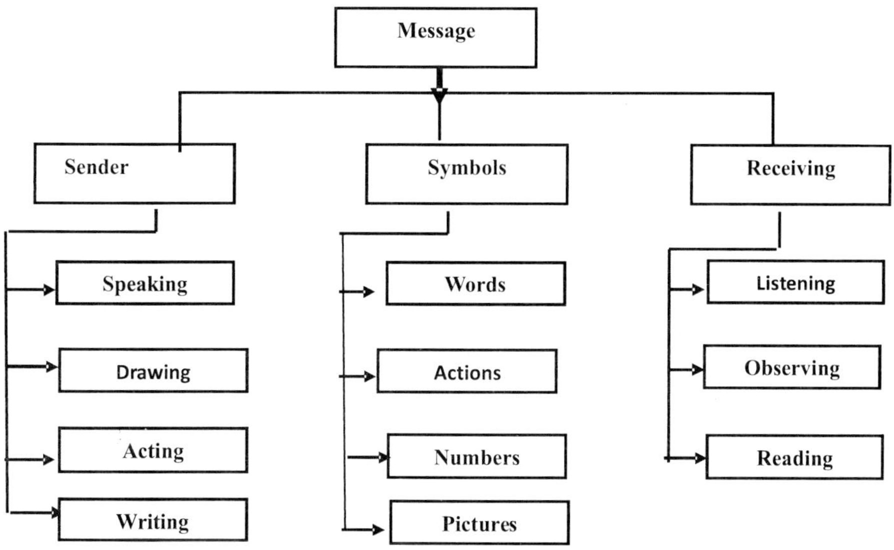

Ideation	Encoding	Transmission	Receiving	Decoding	Feedback
Conceiving of the idea by the sender or source	Encoding the message	Transmission of the message	Receiving of the message by the receiver	Decoding the message	Response or reaction to the message

Encoding: Encoding is the process of turning thoughts into communication. In the process of encoding, the sender (i.e. encoder) uses verbal (e.g. words, signs, images, video) and non-verbal (e.g. body language, hand gestures, face expressions) symbols for which he or she believes the receiver (that is, the decoder) will understand. The symbols can be words and numbers, images, face expressions, signals and/or actions. It is very important how a message will be encoded; it partially depends on the purpose of the Encoding includes selection of the mode of communication. Encoding can be defined as transforming an abstract idea into a communicable message. The wording of the message may be different for different methods of communication to be used. A telegram may be differently worded from a letter. A telephonic conversation may be different from a face to face conversation. A green signal and a whistle from the guard are sufficient signals to the train driver for starting the train, such signals are not sufficient for an aeroplane to take off.

Transmission: The third step is transmission or conveying the message as encoded by thesender. Transmission conforms to the method selected by the sender in the preceding step. Thesender also chooses the channel or path of communication through which the message is to travelfrom the sender to the receiver. The channel may be mass media such as newspapers, radio, television,films etc., or inter-personal involving direct exchange between source and receiver such as telephone,correspondence, or non-verbal symbols like hands or facial gesture, or other body movements. Thesender must consider the effectiveness of the channel in making his selection. A lengthy messagecannot be sent through a telegram. A channel should be such that it minimizes the possibility ofdistortion of the message.

Receiving the message: The next step is the receiving the message by the receiver. The receivermust pay due attention to the message he receives. Any neglect on the part of the receiver may makethe communication ineffective so that the message is lost. Thus, the receiver should be a good listenerin the case of an oral message; however, listening alone is not sufficient, he/she should also be willingto understand.

Decoding: Decoding is the reverse of encoding. It means translation of symbols etc., encodedby the sender into an idea for understanding. The receiver decodes the message by changing thesymbols into a meaning. Understanding the message sent by the sender is the key to the decodingprocess. If the receiver could not decode the message correctly to make it understandable, ormisunderstands it, or pretends to misunderstand it whereas he understands it well, the communicationis rendered ineffective. This happens because perceptions of two persons may be quite different. Decoding is the process of obtaining, absorbing, understanding, interpreting and sometimes using the information that was given throughout a verbal or non-verbal message.

Feedback : It is the response or reaction of the receiver aftre perceiving or understanding the message of the communication. He may ignore the message completely, or may store it, or may act as directed by the sender. He may also senda message to the sender in response to the original message from the sender.

Feedback

Response or reaction of the receiver

The success of any communication effort whether visual, written or spoken depends upon the skill of the communicator to stimulate the audience thinking and to persuade them to action.

Elements of Communication Process

Effective communication requires a skilful communicator sending a useful message through proper channel which is effectively treated to an appropriate audience that responds as desired. There are six major elements of communication and they are briefly explained below:

Elements of Communication Process

- Communicator/ Sender
- Message / Content
- Channel
- Treatment of message
- Audience / Receiver
- Response of the audience (Feedback)

The Communicator

The extension worker is the source of message and he initiates the communication process with a good intention for benefit of the farmers. A veterinary doctor's communication to farmers about the importance of FMD vaccination depends on different factor for acceptance of the message. Livestock farmers may pose several questions regarding your credibility as a communicator. They may try to find out

- Who are you?
- What are your motives?
- How much you know about subject
- Are you a government employees
- What are your attitudes and skills?
- How do you look like?
- How do you act, speak and write?
- Is your purpose to really help the livestock farmers or other things?

Therefore:

Extension worker should know

- The objectives specifically defined
- The people, their needs, interests, abilities, predispositions
- The message- its content, validity, usefulness and importance
- The channels that will reach the people and their usefulness

Extension worker is interested in

- The audience and their welfare
- The results of communication and their evaluation
- The communication channels, their use and limitations
- How to improve further his communication

Extension worker prepares

- A plan for communication
- Communication materials and equipment
- A plan for evaluation of results

Extension worker has skill in

- Selecting messages
- Treating messages
- Expressing messages - verbal and written
- Selection and use of channels
- Understanding audience
- Collecting evidence of results

Message / Content

Extension communication must have a message to convey to the beneficiaries. A message is the information, you wish your livestock farmers to receive, understand, accept and act upon. We communicate for the purpose of promoting a learning and the learning is not possible without a message. Messages for example consist of statements of scientific facts about developmental programme.

Example for messages:

- Benefits of Foul Pox vaccination
- Benefits of Poultry farming

Channels of Communication

A channel may be anything used by senders of message to connect them with intended receivers. It is the binding elements between the sender and the receiver in the communication process. The channel is used by the sender to send the message and similarly by the receiver to send the feedback. Many obstructions can enter in channels. They are often called as noise- i.e. some obstruction that prevents the message from being heard by or carried over clearly to the audience.

Noises emerge from a wide range of sources and causes viz:

- Failure on the part of a communicator to handle channels skilfully.
- Failure to select channels appropriate to the objectives of development.
- Failure to use channels in accordance with audience abilities.
- Failure to avoid physical distraction.
- Failure of audience to listen or read carefully.
- Failure to use enough channels in parallel.
- Use of too many channels in a series.

To become a successful communicator, you should prevent the blockage / noise affecting channels of communication that emerge from one or more of the above conditions.

Treatment of the Message

The treatment aspect of the message deals with how to send the message through channels with maximum probability of reaching their intended destination effectively. Treatment has to do with the way a message is handled to get the information across to an audience. It relates to the technique or details of procedure or manner of performance essential to have expertise in presenting message. Treatment deals with design of methods for presenting messages. The purpose of the treatment is to make the message clear, understandable and realistic to the audience.

The Audience/ Receiver

Audiences (here may be livestock farmers) are the intended beneficiaries of the developmental messages and assumed to be in a position to gain economically, socially or in other ways by responding to the message in particular ways. The more homogeneous an audience, the greater the chances of successful communication. In the attempts to identify audience, it is useful to find out the:

i) Potential audience
ii) Available audience and
iii) Active audience – physical and psychological.

At the primary level there are only two audiences viz:

i) Intended audience
ii) Unintended audience

In the intended audience, there are usually four groups viz.,

i) Listeners or attenders who act on the message

ii) Listeners or attenders who don't act
iii) Listeners and attenders and
iv) Non-listeners and non-attenders

Response of the Audience / Feedback

Goal of feedback is to get confirmation of your massage. This is the terminating element in the communication process. Response by audience to messages received is in the form of action to some degree, mentally or physically. Action, therefore, should be dealt with as an end, not as means.

After receiving a message, it may be generally expected that audience response will be widely varied. The following gives an idea of possible variety in response that may result:

- Understanding vs. Knowledge
- Acceptance vs. Rejection
- Remembering vs. Forgetting
- Mental vs. Physical action
- Right vs. Wrong

Factors Affecting Communication

Effective communication is giving, receiving or exchanging of information, opinions or ideas so that the message is completely understood by everybody involved. There are atleast four important elements in the communication process- Communicator, Message, Channel and Receiver. So, successful communication requires a skillful communicator sending a useful message throughproper channels, effectively treated to an appropriate receiver that responds as desired.

Communicator

In the context of livestock development, extension agent (Livestock Inspector, Veterinary Officer, etc.) is the communicator who starts the process of communication. He is the source, originator or sender of the messages. A communicator may be an individual like you, (Livestock Inspector and Veterinary Officers) or a group (Dairy farmers' association). But, for our discussion, we shall limit our description of the communicator to all those change agents, extension agents, extension workers, etc., those who are communicating to livestock farmers. Your communication performance is likely to be influenced by what you say, or do not say, your status, your position, your credibility, your reputation and livestock farmers' expectations from the communication and past experience of communication of livestock farmers with you.

The characteristics of a good communicator are

The communicator knows:

i. Objectives of communication - have them specifically defined;
ii. Audience – their decoding capabilities, needs, interests, abilities, predisposition;
iii. Message – its concept, validity, usefulness, importance;
iv. Channels that will reach the audience;
v. Organization and treatment of the message;
vi. Professional abilities and limitations of the communicator and organisation.

The communicator is interested in

i. the audience and its welfare;
ii. the message and how it can help people;
iii. the results of communication and their evaluation;
iv. the communication process;
v. the communication channels – their proper use and limitations;
vi. improvement of the communication skill.

The communicator prepares

i. a plan for communication – a teaching plan;
ii. communication materials and equipments;
iii. a plan for evaluation of results.

The communicator has skill in

i. selecting messages;
ii. treating messages;
iii. expressing messages – verbal and written;
iv. the selection and use of channels;
v. understanding the audience;
vi. collecting evidence of results.

Poor communicators, on the other hand

i. Fail to have ideas to present that are really useful to the audience.
ii. Fail to give the complete story and show its relationship to people's problems.

iii. Forget that time and energy are needed to absorb the material presented.
iv. Feel they are always clearly understood.
v. Refuse to adjust to closed minds.
vi. Talk while others are not listening.
vii. Get far too ahead of audience understanding.
viii. Fail to recognize others' view-point.
ix. Fail to recognize that communication is a two-way process.
x. Let their own biases over-influence the presentation.
xi. Fail to see that everyone understands questions brought up for discussions.
xii. Fail to provide a permissive atmosphere.
xiii. Disregard the values, customs, prejudices and habits of the people, and
xiv. Fail to start where people are, with respect to knowledge, skill, interest and need.

Factors which affect Communication Behaviour

1. Communication skill
2. Attitude
3. Knowledge level
4. Position within a socio-cultural system
5. Relationship with the receiver
6. Purpose or Intention
7. Roles and rules
8. Communication Competence

Formula for good communication (J. Pau leagans)

The importance of communication can be stated as

"what is needed is

more people saying the right things

at the right time,

in the right way,

to the right people.

Extension worker should have ability to plan a communication strategy with clear objectives, ability to speak, write, prepare and use teaching aids, properly treat a message for better understanding of the farmers and analyse the feedback receive from the farmers. He should have positive attitudes towards self, subject matter and receivers to communicate effectively. To be a good communicator, the thumb rule is go to the village and listen to the people.

Message

A message is the facts, information, feelings, etc. that a communicator wises to communicate to his/her receivers to receive, understand and act upon. Suppose, you want to discuss about the importance of clean milk production with the dairy farmers, then the information related to clean milk production become message. Information which is relevant to particular set of audiences, constitute the messages, otherwise for them this is 'noise'. A good message clearly state what to do, how to do, when to do and what would be the result. To produce desirable changes in human behaviour, the message must be motivating. Messages which are relevant, interesting, useful, profitable, credible (latest and best, based on research findings) and complete (neither too much, nor too little) are likely to motivate the people.

A good message should be

1. in line with the objective to be attained
2. clear – understandable by the audience
3. significant to the receiver, socially and economically
4. in line with the mental, socio-economic and physical capabilities of the audience;
5. specific- no irrelevant material or vague
6. simply stated – covering only one point at a time;
7. accurate – scientifically sound, factual and current, up to date
8. timely - especially when seasonal factors are important and issues are current;
9. supported by factual material covering both sides of the argument;
10. appropriate to the channel selected;
11. appealing and attractive to the audience – having utility and immediate use;
12. applicable – can apply recommendation to one's own particular situation;
13. adequate – combining principle and practice in effective proportion and
14. manageable – can be handled by the communicator and within the limits of time.

In contrast, poor message often

i. Fall to clearly separate the key message from the supporting content or subject-matter.
ii. Fail to prepare and organize their message properly.
iii. Use inaccurate or fuzzy symbols –words, visuals or real objects – to represent the message.
iv. Fail to select messages that are in line with the felt needs of the audience.
v. Fail to present the message objectively – present the material, often biased, to support onlyone side of the proposition.

vi. Fail to view the message from the standpoint of the audience, and

vii. Fail to time the message properly within a presentation or within a total program.

Treatment of message

Treatment means the way a message is handled, dealt with, so that the information gets across to the audience. It relates to the technique or details of procedure or manner of performance, essential to effective presentation of the message. The purpose of treatment is to make the message clear, understandable, interesting and realistic to the audience. Treatment of the message by the communicator shall depend to a great extent on choice of the channel and the nature of audience. The task cannot be reduced to a formula or recipe. Treatment is creative task that has to be 'tailor-made' for each communication function. For example, treatment of a message will be different when it is conveyed in a meeting or in a face-face to interaction or published in a folder or broadcast. Similarly, there will be difference in treatment of the message according to the level of literacy, socioeconomic status and progressive of the audience. Designing treatment usually requires original thinking, deep insight into the principles of human behaviour and skill in creating and using refined techniques of message presentation. Right treatment of message increases the effectiveness of message.

Channel

The sender and receiver of a message must be connected or tuned with each other so that the message gets through. For this purpose, channels of communication are necessary. They provide the vehicle for getting communication from one person or institution to another. Channel of communication constitutes the medium through which information flows from a sender to one or more receivers. According to Rogers and Shoemaker (1971), communication channel are the means by which message travels from source to receiver. Face-to-face, word-of-mouth is the simplest and yet one of the most widely used and effective means of communication, particularly for the developing countries. As society changes from traditional to modern, the emphasis shifts from oral to media system of communication. Because of the large number of audience or receivers of information and because of physical distance of the communicator and the receivers of information, it is necessary to use different communication channels. Even in interpersonal, face-to-face, word-of-mouth communication, it becomes necessary to use some aids to make communication more effective.

The channels of communication may be classified into a number of ways according to different criteria

a) According to form

Spoken: Farm and home visit, farmer's call, meetings, radio talk etc.,

Written: Personal letter, farm publications, newspaper etc.

b) According to nature of personnel involved

Channels may be localite and cosmopolite depending on the place of origin. Localite channel such as neighbours, opinion leaders/progressive leaders, etc. originate within local system of the receiver. Cosmopolite channels such as extension workers, sale agents, etc., have their origin outside the immediate social system.

Personal localite: They are the local leaders and local people who belong to the receivers own social system. Personal localite channels are important in traditional social system

Personal cosmopolite: These are the channels of communication from outside the social system of the receiver. They are the extension agents of various organizations and are important in changing the farmers from traditional to modern.

According to nature of contact with the people

Individual contact: The extension agent communicates with the people individually, maintaining separate identify of each person. Examples are farm and home visit, farmer's call, personal letter etc.

Group contact: The extension agent communicates with the people in groups and not as individual persons. Examples are group meeting, small group training, field day or farmer's day, study tour etc.

Mass contact: The extension agent communicates with a mass of people, without taking into

consideration their individual or group identity. Examples are mass meeting, campaign, exhibition, radio, television etc.

To help overcome some of the problems of communication, one should take the following factors into account while selecting channels:

i. The specific objective of the message.

ii. The nature of the message – degree of directness versus abstractness, level of difficulty, scope, timing etc.

iii. The audience – size, need, interest, knowledge of the subject etc.

iv. Channels available that will reach the audience, or parts of it.

v. How channels can be combined and used in parallel.

vi. How channels that must be used in a series can be needed to the minimum, and those used made effective.

vii. Relative cost of channels in relation to anticipated effectiveness.

viii. Time available to the communicator and to the audience.

ix. Extent of seeing, hearing or doing that is necessary to get the message through, and

Receivers or Audience

The audience or receiver of message is the intended recipient/consumer of a message. An audience may consist of a single person or a number of persons. It may comprise men, women and youth. An audience may be formed according to occupation groups such as crop farmers, fruit farmers, dairymen, poultry keepers, fish farmers, home makers etc. Audience may also be categorized according to farm size such as marginal, small, medium or big farmers; or according to social criteria whether they belong to scheduled caste, scheduled tribe, etc., Communication to be successful, must be target oriented. The communicator must know the target, their needs, interests, resources, facilities, constraints and even their appropriate number and location.

The attitude of the audience toward the message largely depends upon who gives what message

through which channel; to what extent the content of the message satisfies their needs and intentions; to what measures the suggestions contained in the message are in line with their pre-held experiences and pre-existing preferences; and how far the message is compatible with group norms and value system to which the audience belongs. In case the audience members feel that the communicator is trustworthy, dependable and find the person communicating the message through the medium of their choice, they are likely to receive the message, provided the presentation of the content appear to the audience as interesting and comprehensive.

Audience response/feedback

Response or feedback of the audience/farmers is the ultimate objective of any communication function. Response of an audience to messages received may be in the form of some kind of action, mental or physical. Until the desired action results, extension communication does not achieve its most essential objective. The possible kinds of response to messages received are almost infinite. The following gives an idea of possible variety in response that may result when a useful message is received by a typical village audience

i. **Understanding versus knowledge:** People usually do not act on facts alone, but only when understanding of facts is gained. Understanding is attained only when one is able to attach meaning to facts, see the relationship of facts to each other and to the problem. Communication must promote understanding and knowledge on the subject.

ii. **Acceptance versus rejection:** Audience response may be either way. Communication should lead to understanding and acceptance of the idea or understanding and rejection or not understanding thereby rejection.

iii. **Remembering versus forgetting:** When opportunity for action is not immediately available or action is delayed, the message may be forgotten. Transmitting the right message to the right people at right time is often a crucial factor in successful communication

iv. **Mental versus physical action:** Changes in the minds of the people must always precede changes in the action by hands. People should not only understand and accept the message but shall also act on it; and

v. **Right versus wrong:** The goal of communication is to promote desirable action by the audience as specified in the objective. If the response of the audience is in line with the objective, it is assumed to be 'right' action. However, 'noise' may prevent in getting the desired response from the audience.

The response of the farmers to your message depends upon his/her (i) communication skill (ii) attitudes (iii) knowledge level and (iii) position in a socio-cultural system.

Feedback in Communication

The importance of feedback cannot be overemphasized and needs no specialelucidation. Feedback is the yardstick which measures the effectiveness ofcommunication and is used for evaluation review and to amend the message in thelight of response. Providing feedback therefore needs to be a constructive activity that should be helping to learn. It should not be destructive and critical. Equally important, the recipient should not interpret it as destructive and critical. To be effective, feed back needs to be skilfully given and the receiver must hear, understand, accept and act upon it. However accurate the feedback, if the individual rejects it, the result will be no improvement in performance. Therefore, always consider the human element during feedback.

H - Hear
U - Understand
M - Motivate
A - Acceptable
N – Negotiate

The giving and receiving of feedback are skills which require very careful handling. They require courage, tact, honesty, understanding and respect – both for yourself and for others.

Guidelines for Giving Feedback

You are giving feedback to someone in his/her performance. Your intention must beto improve performance through your feedback.

- Focus Feedback on behaviour rather than on personality
- Feedback should focus on observations rather than inferences.
- Concentrate on change rather than make value judgments
- Feedback is most acceptable when it is describing specific rather than general patterns of behaviour.
- Focus the feedback on the value it may have for the individual
- Focus feedback on the amount of information the individual can use, rather than the amount you feel capable of giving.
- Feedback is most acceptable when it is describing specific rather than general patterns of behaviour.
- Feedback should be well-timed
- Positive feedback followed by negative
- Check the accuracy of the feedback

Guidelines for Receiving Feedback

- Be positive towards the feedback giver
- Listen to the feedback
- Clarify and check understanding
- Check the feedback with others
- Ask for feedback not volunteered
- Describe how to use feedback.
- Explore Options
- Thank the feedback giver

Giving and receiving feedback is a demanding process that requires confidence and respect between the parties involved. The advice offered is necessarily broad and will vary between different individuals and activities. We cannot doubt the value of the feedback in learning. The provision of feedback is especially important for those process skills that occur during learning activities, particularly involving interpersonal skills.

Models of Communication

Models are symbolic representations of structures, objects , operations or event in idealized and abstract form. They are usefultheoretical constructs that are frequently used in social sciences for explanatory purposes. They maybe used to show the size, shape or relationship of various parts or components of an object or process.A model may also be useful in explaining the working of a system.

Aristotle's model

Aristotle (384-322 B.C.) was the first to give the earliest persuasive communication model. In his opinion three elements are essential for a meaningfulcommunication and that we can organize our study of communication processunder the three headings: i) the person who speaks, ii) the speech that he/sheproduces, and iii) the person who listens.

His explanation includes three communication elements

1. Speaker – the person who speaks
2. Speech – the speech that the individual produces.
3. Audience – the person who listens

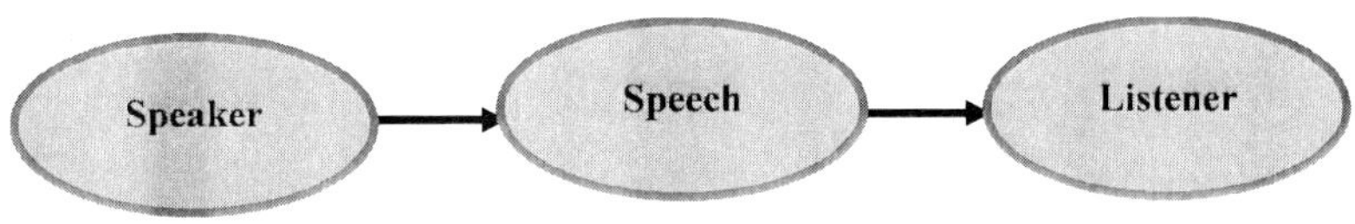

Aristotle's Communication model

Lasswell's Model

Lasswell put forth one of the basic but significant communication models with social scientific background in 1948. This model includes the sequence namely

i) who says
ii) what,
iii) in which channel,
iv) to Whom,
v) under what circumstances, and
vi) with what effects.

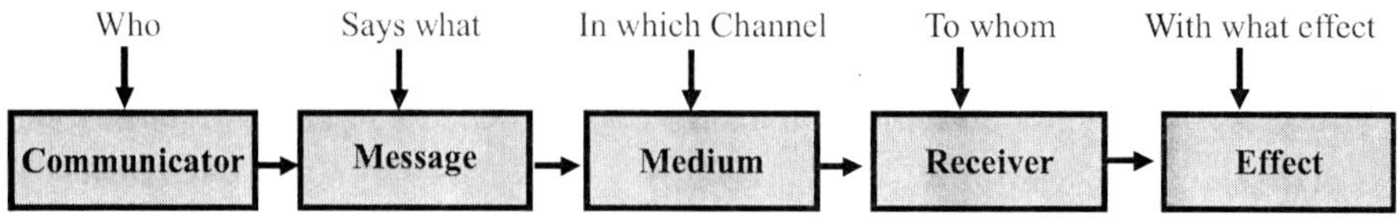

This model provides explanation for linear, one-way communication. This model gives importance to the communicator and his message However, this model had helped improving the understanding about communication among social scientists engaged in communication theories. The model also assumes the communicator wishes to influence the receiver and, therefore, sees communication as a persuasive process.

Shannon- Weaver's model

The Shannon-weaver (1949) provided a communication model in relation to electronic media popularly known as Shannon and Weaver model of communication or 'Mathematical model of communication. According to them, the key components of communication are:

1. Source
2. Transmitter
3. Signal
4. Receiver
5. Destination

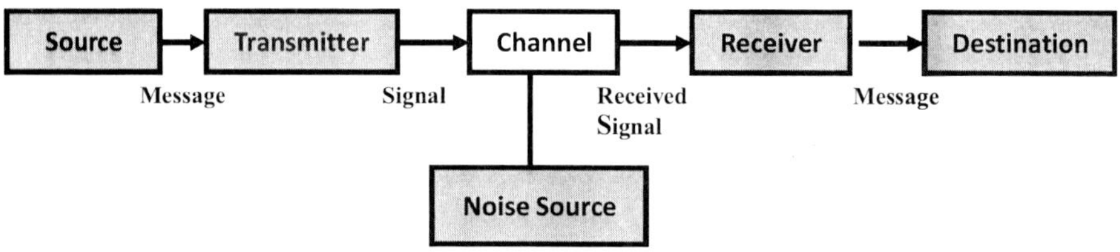

The source produces a desired message out of a set of possible messages, written, or spoken words, pictures, etc. Then the transmitter changes this message into signals suitable for transmission. thereafter, the channel carries signal from the transmitter to the receiver. The receiver, a sort of inverse transmitter transfers the transmitted signals back into a message and the destination is the final consumer of the message. Another important component of their model was 'noise'. They said in the process of transmitting signals, some unwanted disturbances such as sound in the case of radio, television, telephone, etc., may occur or distortion of shape (picture) in television my occur which is called as 'noise'. This model attempted to explain how to overcome noise and how much redundancy is necessary so that the receiver can successfully receive the signal and in turn the right messages.

The three levels of problems in the communication of information indicated in the model are

1. Technical – problems related to the accuracy of transferring information from sender to the receiver, through signals.
2. Semantic - problems related to the interpretation of meaning by the receiver as that of intended meaning of the sender
3. Influential - problems concerned with the success with which the meanings are conveyed to the receiver and the subsequent desired behaviour on his part.

Important Concepts in Shannon and Weaver's Model

Information: The information is viewed as a measure of one's freedom of choice when one selects a message.

Entropy: The information can be measured by entropy i.e one's degree of freedom of choice to select a message. The ratio of the actual to the maximum entropy is called relative entropy.

Redundancy: The amount of information that can be eliminated or added in a noiseless channel, so that the message would still have meaning.

Channel capacity: The amount of information that can be transmitted per unit of time. Beyond optimum level of information would lead to errors.

Noise: Any unwanted sound, distortion that may be added into the channel which are beyond the control of the transmitter or receiver. However, the efficiency of a communication system can be increased by reducing the noise, or by increasing the band width or by increasing the signal power.

Coding process: Whenever we produce or receive a message we use codes. Efficient coding involves best matching the statistical characteristics of the information source and the channel.

Shannon and Weaver's model mainly deals with problems of communication at the technical, semantics and effectiveness levels. From this model, we can learn that for reducing the uncertainty and minimizing the effects of noise by considering the capacity of the sender to encode and that of the receiver to decode messages. Though the model attempts to explain further the process of communication, it is a linear, one-way communication model without any emphasis on feedback.

In this model communication is presented as a linear, one-way process. Shannon and Weaver make a distinction between source and transmitter, and receiver and destination i.e. there are two functions at the transmitting end and two at the receiving end.

Berlo's Model of Communication

Berlo (1960) model is one of the most widely used and is based on behavioural theory and research. His model also focuses on encoding and decoding which happens before sender sends the message and before receiver receives the message respectively. Berlo's Model has mainly, four components to describe the communication process. They are **sender, message, channel and receiver.** Each of the component is affected by many factors. This model of communication is also popularly known as S-M-C-R model.

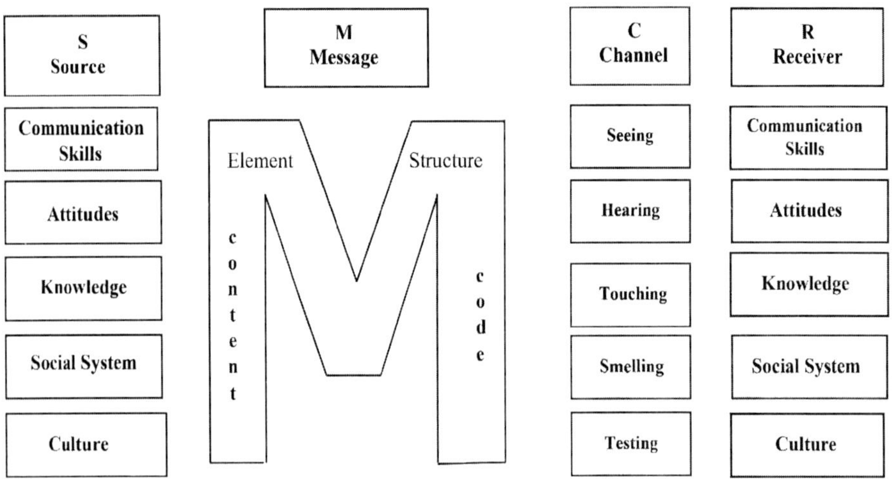

Berlo's Communication Model

Components of Berlo's Model of Communication

S -Source

Sender is the source of the message or the person who originates the message. The source has ideas, needs, intentions, information and a purpose for communication. The following are the factor related to sender and is also the same in the case of receiver.

• Communication Skills

Communication skills of a person is a factor that affects the communication process. If an extension worker is not a skilled communicator than he/she will fail in communicating the message effectively. Communication skills include the skills to speak, present, read, write, listening, etc.

• Attitude

The attitude of the sender and the receiver creates the effect on the message. The person's attitude towards self, the receiver and the environment changes the meaning and effect of the message.

• Knowledge

Familiarity with the subject of the message makes the communicated message have its effect more. Knowledge on the subject matter makes the communicator send the message effectively.

• Social Systems

Values, beliefs, laws, rules, religion and many other social factors affect the sender's way of communicating the message. It creates difference in the generation of message. Place and situation also fall under social systems.

• Culture

Cultural differences make messages different. A person from one culture might find something offensive which is very much accepted in another culture.

M-Message

A message is the substance that is being sent by the sender to the receiver. It might be in the form of voice, audio, text, video or other media. The key factors affecting the message are

• Content

Content is the thing that is in the message. The whole message from beginning to end is the content.

• Elements

Elements are the non-verbal things that tag along with the content like gestures, signs, language, etc.

• Treatment

Treatment is the way in which the message is conveyed to the receiver. Treatment also effects the feedback of the receiver.

• Structure

The structure of the message or the way it has been structured or arranged, affects the effectiveness of the message.

• **Code**

Code is the form in which the message is sent. It might be in the form of language, text, video, etc.

C-Channel

Channel is the medium or carrier used to send the message. The choice of the channel is an important factor in the effectiveness of the communication. In mass communication and other forms of communication, technical gadgets like mobile telephone, internet, etc., may be used as channel.. But in general communication, the five senses of a human being is the channel for the communication flow and it affects the effectiveness of the channel.

- Hearing – We receive the message through hearing.
- Seeing – We perceive through seeing. We also get non-verbal messages by seeing.
- Touching – Many of the non-verbal communication happens from touching like holding hands.
- Smelling – We collect information from smelling.
- Tasting – Taste also provides the information to be sent as a message.

R- Receiver

Receiver, the target of the communication, is the person who gets the message sent in the process. As like source which needs encoder to translate his idea in to message, to express in a code, the receiver needs a decoder to retranslate, to decode the message and to put into a form that the receiver can use. This model believes that the thinking pattern and all other factors mentioned above must be in sync to that of the sender for the communication to be effective. The receiver must also have a very good listening skill. Other factors are similar to that of the sender.

- Communication skills
- Attitudes
- Knowledge
- Social Systems
- Culture

Strengths

i) The idea of 'source' was flexible enough to include oral, written, electronic, or any other kind of "symbolic" generator-of-messages.

ii) 'Message' was made the central element, stressing the transmission of ideas

iii) The model recognized that receivers were important to communication, for they were the targets

iv) The notions of 'encoding' and 'decoding' emphasized the problems we all have (psycho-linguistically) in translating our own thoughts into words or other symbols and in deciphering the words or symbols of others into terms we ourselves can understand.

Criticisms of Berol's SMCR Model

- There is no concept of feedback, so the effect is not considered.
- There is no concept of noise or any kind of barriers in communication process.
- It is a linear model of communication, there is no two-way communication.
- Both of the people must be similar according to all the factors mentioned above.

Schramm's model of Communication

As per Schramm model of communication (1964), there is a source, who encodes a signal, and there is a receiver, who deco des the signal. The sender and receiver must be tuned together and maximum output from communication can be achieved based on the common field experience of both the source-encoder

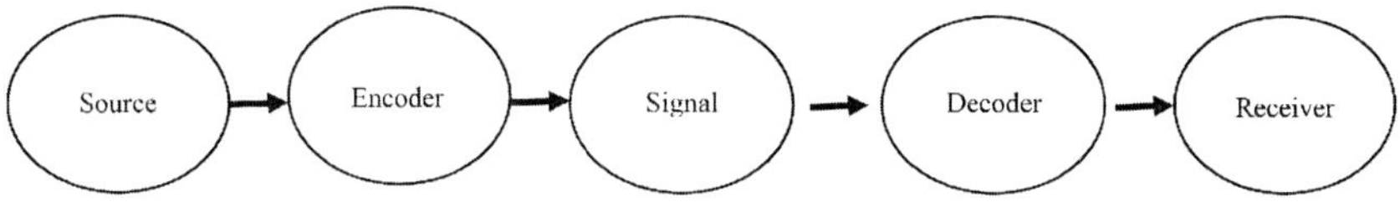

Schramm's Model of Communication

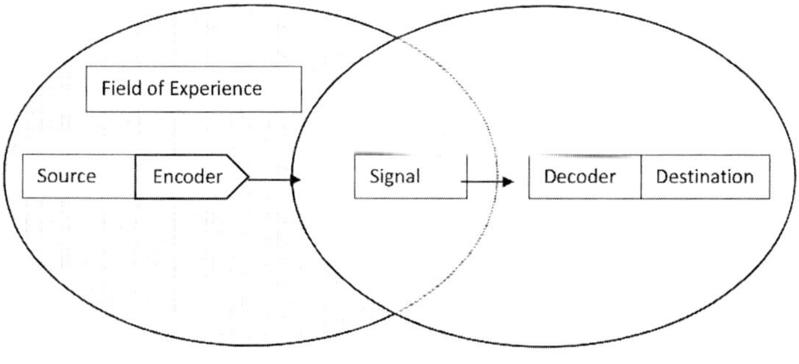

Role of Field Experience in Schramm's Model of Communication

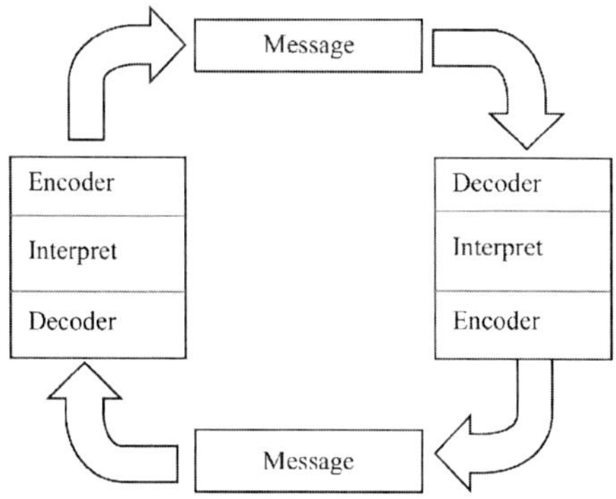

Feedback in Schramm's Communication Model

and the decoder-receiver.

As per this model, both an encoder and a decoder receive and transmit. A person will decode a message, interpret based on past experiences and wisdom, and then encode a response accordingly. Thus, each one is constantly communicating back to the other and the return process is termed as feedback. This model focused on organic nature of communication rather than mere mechanical transfer of message. Schramm (1964) emphasized that communication process is continuous.

Leagan's Model of Communication

According to J P Leagan(1961), communication is a process by which two or more people exchange ideas, facts, feelings, impressions in ways that each gains a clear understanding of the meaning, intent and use of the message. The key elements of the Leagan's model are:

- Communicator
- Message or content
- Channels of communication
- Treatment of message
- Audience and
- Audience response / Feedback.

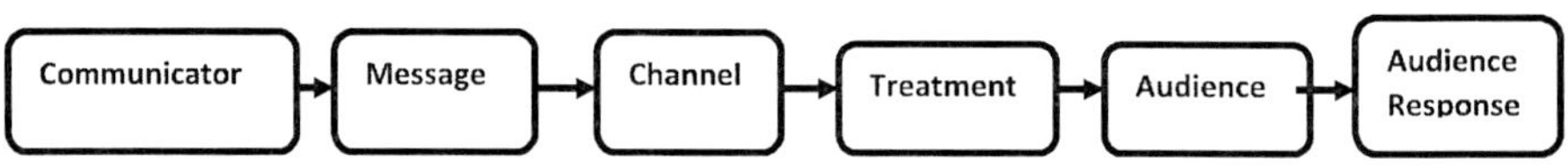

Leagan's Model of Communication

In this model, greater thrust is placed on treatment of message and audience response (Feedback). This model is more popular in agricultural extension, wherein, the focus is on transferring the technology to farmers and bringing desired behaviour and therefore, the communicators fine tune their communication based on feedback.

Rogers and Shoemaker's Model of Communication

Rogers and shoemaker (1971) thought of the communication process in terms of the S-M-C-R-E model, the components of which are –

1. Source
2. Message
3. Channel
4. Receiver
5. Effects

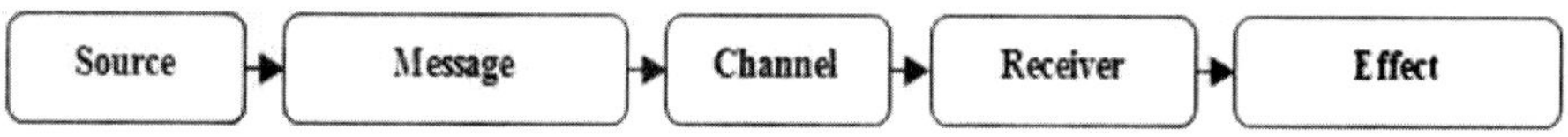

According to them a source (S) and message (M) via certain channels (C) to the receiving individual (R), which causes some effects (E) i.e., changing the existing behaviour pattern of the receiver.

Model on Extension Communication System

Communication in extension may also be thought of as two-way stimulus – response (S-R) situation in which the necessary stimulus is provided by the communicator, the extension agent, in the form of a message which produces certain response on the audience, the farmers and vice-versa. A favourable response by the audience reinforces learning. A diagrammatic representation of the extension communication system on the basis of the model suggested by Leagan's (1963) is presented in the below figure.

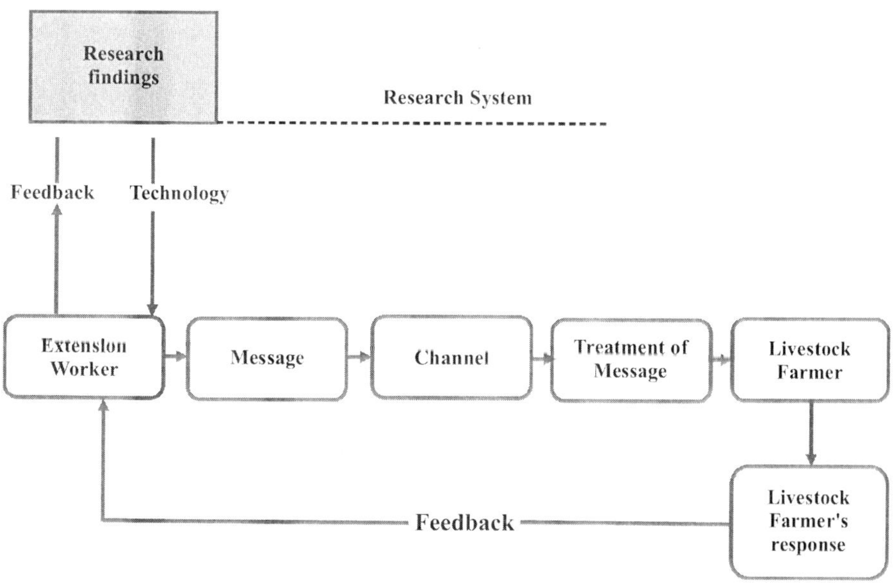

Barriers to Communication

There are many reasons why we do not produce desired results through interpersonal communications. In our communications, the message may not be received exactly in the same way what we intend to communicate. Therefore, it is important that we must seek feedback to know efficacy of our communication. The skills of Active Listening, Clarification and Reflection, may help but the skilled communicator also needs to be aware of the barriers to effective communication. There exist many barriers to communication and these may occur at any stage in the communication process. Barriers may lead to your message becoming distorted and you therefore risk wasting both time and/or money by causing confusion and misunderstanding. Effective communication involves overcoming these barriers and conveying a clear and concise message.

Some common barriers to effective communication include:

- The use of jargon, over-complicated, unfamiliar or ambiguous terms.
- Emotional barriers and taboos.
- Lack of attention, interest, distractions, or irrelevance to the receiver.
- Differences in perception and viewpoint.
- Physical disabilities such as hearing problems or speech difficulties.
- Physical barriers to non-verbal communication.
- Language differences and the difficulty in understanding unfamiliar accents.
- Expectations and prejudices which may lead to false assumptions or stereotyping. People often hear what they expect to hear rather than what is actually said and jump to incorrect conclusions.
- Cultural differences. The norms of social interaction vary greatly in different cultures, as do the way in which emotions are expressed. For example, the concept of personal space varies between cultures and between different social settings. A skilled communicator must be aware of these barriers and try to reduce their impact by continually checking understanding and by offering appropriate feedback.

Types of Barriers to Communication

- **Language Barriers**: Language and linguistic ability may act as a barrier to communication. However, even when communicating in the same local language by you, the terminology used in a message may act as a barrier if it is not fully understood by the receiver(s). For example, a message that includes a lot of English words and abbreviations will not be understood by our farmers who are not familiar with the terminology used. As extension worker, we are especially prone to making this mistake. We must remember to use language that can be understood by the receiver.

- **Psychological Barriers:** The psychological state of the receiver will influence how the message is received. For example, if someone has personal worries and is stressed, they may be preoccupied by personal concerns and not as receptive to the message as if they were not stressed. Stress management is an important personal skill that affects our interpersonal relationships. Anger is another example of a psychological barrier to communication. When we are angry it is easy to say things that we may later regret and also to misinterpret what others are saying. More generally, people with low self-esteem may be less assertive and therefore may not feel comfortable communicating - they may feel shy about saying how they really feel, or read negative sub-texts into messages they hear.
- **Physiological Barriers:** Physiological barriers may result from the receiver's physical state. For example, a receiver with reduced hearing may not grasp the entirety of a spoken conversation, especially if there is significant background noise.
- **Physical Barriers:** An example of a physical barrier to communication is geographic distance between the sender and receiver(s). Communication is generally easier over shorter distances as more communication channels are available and less technology is required. Although modern technology often serves to reduce the impact of physical barriers, the advantages and disadvantages of each communication channel should be understood so that an appropriate channel can be used to overcome the physical barriers.
- **Attitudinal Barriers** Attitudinal barriers are behaviours or perceptions that prevent people from communicating effectively. Attitudinal barriers to communication may result from personality conflicts, poor management, resistance to change, or a lack of motivation. Effective receivers of messages should attempt to overcome their own attitudinal barriers to facilitate effective communication.

Overcoming Barriers

Most of the barriers mentioned above can be overcome by skilful communication.

Active Listening: It is a skill that can be acquired and developed with practice. As an extension worker while communicating with farmers, you must listen very carefully the farmers' views on the issues. Active listening means listening with all senses. If you listen attentively and give freedom to speak, then the speaker will feel more ease and communicate openly and honestly. There are both verbal and non-verbal cues that convey active listening. Non-verbal signs include smiling (if appropriate), making eye contact, nodding at appropriate times, and avoiding distractions. Theses non-verbal cues convey the message that you are interested in what the speaker has to say, and that your attention is not deceptive. Offering verbal signs of active listening can also be useful. Reflecting on something the speaker has said by asking a clarifying question is a terrific way to do this. Paraphrasing involves finding slightly different words to repeat the main idea of the speaker, and is also great way to show active listening.

Using Simple Language: We must use the local language to communicate our ideas. The use of English words, veterinary terminology or jargon, abbreviation should be avoided. Farmers are often intimidated by such language, and can be afraid to admit that they don't understand the message being delivered. While communicating with farmers, communicate slowly, and have pauses. The important information which you want to communicate must be spoken repeatedly in different intervals in your discussion. You must encourage the farmers to ask questions to clarify any points.

Give Constructive Feedback: We must remember that feedback we receive from the farmers help us to improve our communication ability. Therefore, the feedback received should be attended immediately, and we should avoid giving negative/humiliating response to farmers' feedback.

In between the communicator and the receiver, certain barriers considerably affect the quality of information transmission. Some of the major barriers are discussed below.

Filtering

Because of the many other concerns which constantly influence our ability to concentrate on what we hear, the average listener will normally "filter out" certain things that he hears. They will simply ignore a point made by the speaker, as though it had never been presented. This can be deliberate or unintended.

Distortion

For the same reason, the human mind can also distort what it hears. It is an unconscious process. Every person tends to remember best what agrees with his own values.

Communication Overload

Our minds can receive and retain only a limited amount of information without showing strain. This is called channel capacity. This ability can vary with different audiences. Overloading the system will in effect below the mental fuse and defensively shut down the communication process.

Absence of Redundancy

It is the use of repetition. Even under the best condition an audience can have problems grasping or fully appreciating the significance of something new which has been presented to them. By repeating it, or by illustrating it or by restating the same point in different ways a speaker can make it easier for an audience to understand and retain the information passed on by the speaker.

Selective perception

Selective perception means seeing what one wants to see. A person perceives information on the basis of his needs, values, experience, and background. His personal interests and expectations influence the way he decodes information.

Defensiveness

People intentionally attempt to block communication when they feel that the other person is threatening their self-image and prestige. They react in a defensive manner by making sarcastic comments, by passing judgments on others, or by questioning the motives of the other party.

Barriers to communication can be further classified as

- Human/personal
- Semantic and
- Technical barriers.

Types of Communication

Verbal Communication

Human	Semantic	Technical
Personal emotions	World interpretations	Space or geographical distance
Biases	Gesture Decoding	Mechanical failures
Perceptual variations	Language translation	Physical obstructions
Competencies	Signs and symbols	Technological malfunctions
Sensual abilities	Cue meanings	Concrete obstacles
Mental faculties		

On an average, a person spends about 75 per cent of active time on communicating verbally- listening, speaking, reading and writing. In other words, as an extension worker, you spend about 10 or 11 hrs a day on verbal communication.

Non-verbal Communication

It includes the gestures, facial expressions, and movements etc., which make our communication more effective. It is also referred to as body language.

A) Verbal Communication

This mode of communication relies on words to convey a message. Most of the time in our day to day activities, we use this method. The cues we use while communicating verbally include, tone, gestures, and body language. Verbal communication helps in expressing thoughts, emotions and sentiments. A phone conversation, chat with a friend, an announcement made, or a speech delivered are all verbal forms of communication. The two major forms of verbal communication are:

> **Verbal Communication**
>
> On an average, a person spends about 75 per cent of active time on communicating verbally- listening, speaking, reading and writing. In other words, as an extension worker, you spend about 10 or 11 hrs a day on verbal communication.
>
> **Non-verbal Communication**
>
> It includes the gestures, facial expressions, and movements etc., which make our communication more effective. It is also referred to as body language.

i) Written Communication
ii) Oral Communication

i) Written Communication

Written communication is the medium through which the message of the sender is conveyed with the help of written words. Letters, e-mails, reports, SMS, articles, WhatsApp, memos, etc., are some forms of written communication. Unlike some other forms of communication, written messages can be edited and rectified before they are sent to the receiver, thereby making written communication an indispensable part of informal and formal communication. The effectiveness of written communication depends on the writing style, grammar, vocabulary, and clarity.

ii) Oral Communication

The other form of verbal communication is the spoken word, either face-to-face or through phone, voice chat, video conferencing or any other medium. Various forms of informal communications such as the grapevine or informal rumour mill, and formal communications such as lectures, conferences are forms of oral communication. Oral communication finds use in discussions and causal and informal conversations. The effectiveness of oral conversations depends on the clarity of speech, voice modulation, pitch, volume, speed, and even non-verbal communications such as body language and visual cues. Verbal communication makes the process of conveying thoughts easier and faster, and it remains the most successful form of communication.

Verbal communication is further divided into four subcategories:

a) Intrapersonal Communication

This form of communication is extremely private and restricted to ourselves. It refers to communication that transpires inside a person; and this happens all the time. It is like talking to oneself, listening to oneself and relating one to oneself. The individual functions here as the source and receiver. It includes our reflection, contemplation, meditation, our inner monologues, our reflection upon ourselves, and our relationships with others and with our environment. A farmer after exposing to a result demonstration, may think and communicate with himself whether this practice is suitable to his condition, is it going to give profit, etc.

b) Interpersonal Communication

This form of communication takes place between two individuals and is thus a one-on-one conversation or person-to-person contact. Most of the time, we are involved in this type of communication in our office or in daily life. Here, the two individuals involved will exchange their roles of sender and receiver in order to communicate in a clearer manner by means of words, sounds facial expression, gestures and postures. It is considered the most effective type of communication because it is personal, direct, intimate and allows maximum interaction in word, gesture and expression. Immediate feedback can be received in this type of communication and it is possible to influence the other person and persuade him or her to accept your point of view. Since there is proximity between sender and receiver, interpersonal communication has emotional appeal too; it can motivate, encourage and coordinate work more effectively than any other form of communication.

c) Group Communication

This type of communication can take place only when there are more than two people involved in exchange of ideas, information and others. Basically, communication that takes place between many persons in a face to face situation is described as group communication. The degree of directness in this type of communication depends on the size of the group, the place where it meets and also the relationship of the members of the group to one another. Group communication is considered effective as it provides an opportunity for direct interaction among the members of the group and it helps in bringing about changes in attitudes and beliefs.

Office meeting, village meeting, etc,. examples of group communication.

d) Public Communication

This type of communication takes place when one individual addresses a large number of people. Public speeches in a community is example of this type of communication. In such cases, there is usually a single sender of information and several receivers who are being addressed.

e) Mass Communication

Mass communication involves communicating with mass audiences and hence the name mass communication. The channels through which this kind of communication takes place are referred to as mass media. Both mass communication and mass media are generally considered synonymous for the sake of convenience. Mass communication is unique and different from interpersonal communication as is evident from the following definition. Any mechanical device that multiplies messages and takes it to a large number of people simultaneously is called mass communication.

The mechanical devices can be newspapers, magazines, radio, television, websites, social media networks etc. The act of mass communication is much more complex than that of face to face communication. It is addressed to an extremely large audience.

B) Non Verbal Communication

Non-verbal communication is a process of sending and receiving messages without using words. Non-verbal communication uses gestures, body language, facial expressions, eye contact, clothing, tone of voice, and other cues to convey a message. We may raise our eyebrows emphatically when speaking to help make a point, or shake our head to affirm the views of a farmer in a meeting. Nonverbal communication is also known as "silent language." We should avoid use of non-verbal communication with farmers while communicating because it creates ambiguity in mind of receiver if it is not used correctly.

The components of Non Verbal Communication are:

1. **Kinesics** is the interpretation of body language such as facial expressions and gestures - or, more formally, non-verbal behaviour related to movement, either of any part of the body or the body as a whole. Body Language is technically known as kinesics. It is the study of body movements. The aspects of kinesics are face, eye contact, gesture, posture, body movements.

Face: The face and eyes are the most expressive means of body communication. It can facilitate or hamper feedback.

Eye contact: It is the most powerful form of non-verbal communication. It builds emotional relationship between listener and speaker.

Gesture: It is the motion of the body to express the speech.

Posture: The body position of an individual conveys a variety of messages.

Body movement: Used to understand what people are communicating with their gestures and posture. Body movements include gestures, facial expressions and other physical movements. Every body movement conveys a certain meaning. For example, raising an eyebrow conveys disbelief, rubbing the nose indicates puzzlement and shrugging shoulders shows indifference. When a person is eager to hear something, he sits with his feet under the chair, toes pressed to the ground, and leans forward on the desk. When a person is listening carefully, he maintains eye contact and frequently nods his head. Body language coupled with verbal communication gives more meaning to massage.

2. **Proxemics** is the technical term for the personal space aspect of body language. Proxemics is the study of measurable distance between people as they interact. Body spacing and posture are unintentional reactions to sensory fluctuations or shifts, such as subtle changes in the sound and pitch of a person's voice.

3. **Oculesics:** It is the study of the role of eye contact in nonverbal communication. Our eyes are a very significant aspect of the non-verbal signals we send to others. Oculesics is one form of nonverbal communication, which is the transmission and reception of meaning between communicators without the use of words. It can include the environment around the communicators, the physical attributes or characteristics of the communicators, and the behaviour of the communicators

4. **Chronemics** is the study of the use of time in nonverbal Communication. The way we perceive time, structure our time and react to time is a powerful communication tool, and helps set the stage for the communication process. Across cultures, time perception plays a large role in the nonverbal communication process. Time perceptions include punctuality, willingness to wait, and interactions. The use of time can affect lifestyles, daily agendas, speed of speech, movements and how long people are willing to listen.

5. **Haptics** refers to the study of communication by touching. There are six different kinds of touch. These include: positive, playful, control, ritualistic, task-related and unintentional.

6. **Paralinguistics:** It is the study of variations in pitch, speed, volume, and pauses to convey meaning. Interestingly, when the speaker is making a presentation and is looking for a response, he will pause. However, when no response is desired, he will talk faster with minimal pause.

7. **Paralanguage** refers to the non-verbal elements of communication used to modify meaning and convey emotion. Paralanguage may be expressed consciously or unconsciously, and it includes the pitch, volume, and, in some cases, intonation of speech. Sometimes the definition is restricted to vocally produced sounds. Paralanguage refers to voice quality, volume, pitch, speed and non-fluencies (like'ah,''um,'or'uh.') used to convey a message. Sounds are the basis for paralanguage. Paralanguage include t one of voice, power or emphasis, pitch, rhythm, volume, pause or break in sentence, speed of delivery, loudness or softness. Paralanguage can be dividedinto four parts :

   i) **Voice qualities:** Pitch, resonance, volume rate and rhythm

   ii) **Vocal characterisers:** Embracing laughter, coughing, throat clearing and sighing

   iii) **Vocal qualifiers:** Refering to variations in pitch and volume

   iv) **Vocal segregates:** Including the silent sound such as 'ahs'and 'ers' and pauses.

   These languages do much to influence meaning

8. **Physical Appearance:** Physical appearance always contributes towards how people perceive about individuals. Neatly combed hair, ironed clothes and a lively smile will always carry more weight than words. It is believed that physical appearance determines the success a person will attain at every stage of his life.

Nonverbal communication can play five roles

- **Repetition:** It repeats and often strengthens the message you're making verbally.
- **Contradiction:** It can contradict the message you're trying to convey, thus indicating to your listener that you may not be telling the truth.
- **Substitution:** It can substitute for a verbal message. For example, your facial expression often conveys a far more vivid message than words ever can.
- **Complementing:** It may add to or complement your verbal message. As a boss, if you pat an employee on the back in addition to giving praise, it can increase the impact of your message.

- **Accenting:** It may accent or underline a verbal message. Pounding the table, for example, can underline the importance of your message.

C) Visual Communication

This form of communication involves the visual display of information, wherein the message is understood or expressed with the help of visual aids. For example, photographs of exotic milch cows, fodder trees, etc., signs, symbols, maps, posters, banners on animal husbandry practices may help the viewer to understand the message visually. Movies and plays, television shows and video clips are all electronic form of visual communication. Visual communication also involves the transfer of information in the form of text, which is received through an electronic medium such as a computer, phone, etc.

Functions of Communication

- Education
- Information
- Entertainment
- Control
- Counselling
- Social Contact
- Cultural
- Stimulation
- Integration
- Expression of emotion

Functions of Communication

The main function/purpose of communication is to change or guide other people's behaviour. The functions of communication may be categorised as:

a) **Education:** To transfer knowledge for the progress of the society (Example: class room communication)

b) **Information:** To find and explain something new (Example: News media)

c) **Entertainment:** To help pass time and enjoy life (Example: drama, song, films, etc.)

d) **Control function:** To get someone to behave in an appropriate way (Example: management, censorship etc).

e) **Counselling:** To alleviate anxiety and lead to better ways (Example: guidance, consolation etc.)

f) **Social contact:** To help make enjoyable companionship (Example: Friendship, clubs, organizations etc.)

g) **Cultural promotion:** To help foster social values and pass them from generation to generation (Example: Festivals, parties, celebrations)

h) **Stimulation:** To create interest and develop positive thinking /behaviour (Example: Advertisements)

i) **Integration:** To create harmonious relationships among various social groups (Example: Political parties, conferences, meetings etc.)

j) **Expression of emotions:** To communicate feelings or give vent to one's pent up feelings (Example: crying, smiling, Writing poetry, fiction, etc).

Suggested Readings and References

1. Leagans, J.P. (1961). The Communication Process. In: Extension Education in Community Development, Directorate of Extension, Ministry of Food and Agriculture, Government of India, New Delhi.
2. Rogers, E.M. (2003). Diffusion of Innovations, 5th Edition, Free Press, New York.
3. Berlo, D.K. (1960). The process of communication. Holt Rinechart and Winston, New York.
4. Ray, G.L. (1991). Extension Communication and management, Naya Prokash, Calcutta.
5. Singhal, A. and E.M. Rogers (1989). Prosocial Television for Development in India. In R.E. Rice and C.K. Atkin (eds.), Public Communication Campaigns 2nd ed. Newbury Park, Sage, CA.
6. Samanta, R.K. (1990). Development communication for agriculture. B.R. Publishing Corporation, Delhi.
7. MacBride Sean (1982). Many Voices One World, Oxford and IBH Publishing Co., New Delhi.
8. Malhan, P.N. (1992). Communication Media: Yesterday, Today and Tomorrow; Ministry of I&B: Delhi.
9. Hiebert/Ungurait/Bohn (1974). Mass Media: An Introduction to Modern Communication, Longman Inc.,
10. Jay Black, Jennings Bryant (1993). Introduction to Mass Communication, Win. C. Brown Publishers.
11. Parmar S. (1973). Folk music and mass media communication. Publications 95/2, Tatarpur, Tagore Garden, New Delhi.
12. Shankaraih, Chamala (1979). Folk Drama and troupe on wheels. Rural Development Digest 2(1): 46-47.
13. Anand M. (1962). Folk Dances of India Kurukshetra. 10(1): 3-5.
14. Dhama O.P. (1965). Extension and Rural Welfare. Agra, Ram Prasad and Son, pp. 191-215.
15. Dhama O.P. and Bhatnagar O.P. (1980). Education and Communication for Development, New Delhi, Oxford and IBH Publishing Co., pp. 455-456.
16. Kumar K.J. (1981). Mass Communication in India, Jaico Publishing House, Bombay, pp. 169-180.

17. Lent A John (1982). Grass roots Renaissance. Folk media in the third world. Media Asia 9(1): 7.
18. Chalapati Rao I.V. (1999). Communication and leadership, skills and strategies, Book links Corporation, Hyderabad.
19. Kundu, C.L. & Tutoo D.N. (1985). Educational Psychology, Sterling publishers private Ltd., Bangalore.
20. Samuel A. Malone (1997). Mind skills for managers, Gower.
21. ISPA-Indo Swiss Project Andhra Pradesh (Year), Learning Material, Directorate of Animal Husbandry, Hyderabad.

6

Extension Actors

1. Skills and Qualities of an Extension Worker
2. Role of Male and Female Extension Workers
3. Functions/Task of Extension Teacher
4. Rural Women and Livestock Extension
5. Barriers to women's involvement in extension
6. Leadership and Role of Leaders in A H Extension
7. Basic Elements in Leadership
8. Importance of Rural Leadership
9. Role of Village Leader
10. Types of Leader
11. Styles of leadership
12. Identification and Selection of Leaders
    a) Election
    b) Discussion Method
    c) The workshop method
    d) Information ratings
    e) Participative observation
    f) Self-designating method:
    g) Sociometric Technique
    h) Key informants method
    i) Informal Dialogue Method
    j) Discussion with predecessor
    k) Active Participation
13. Advantages of using local leader
14. Problems of working with local leader
15. Suggested Readings and References

Skills and Qualities of A Good Extension Worker

Extension worker should possess the following skills to be effective.

a) Ability to create a learning situation for the farmers
b) Ability to communicate effectively with the livestock owners
c) Know the subject matter clearly which she/he is going to discuss with the farmers
d) Ability to use the teaching aids effectively
e) Ability to demonstrate the practices to the farmers

The skills mentioned are of indicative in nature.

Skills of an Extension Worker

- ability to create learning situations
- ability to communicate effectively
- Know the subject matter
- ability to use teaching aids

Qualities of an Extension Worker

Should be a good listener: You, as an extension worker not only be a good listener but also give respect to the opinions, whatsoever vague it may be, of the villagers.

a) Adjustability to the village conditions: You must carefully observe, study and understand the social systems prevailing in the village. Acquaint yourself to the culture, customs, tradition and way of living in the village.
b) Should be humble, polite and friendly towards the villagers
c) Should be honest, sincere and hard working
d) Should be punctual and adhere to the time given to the villagers for any extension activities
e) Should not lose patience and always seek villagers help in solving the problem
f) Should demonstrate the quality of 'simple living and high thinking'.
g) Should not discriminate individuals on the basis of caste, creed, colour, sex, etc.
h) Should possess sympathetic attitudes towards the villagers.
i) Above all, he should be a good human being to become a good extension worker.

Qualities of an Extension Worker

- Good listener
- Adjustability
- Humble, polite friendly
- Honest, sincere, hard working
- Punctual, adherence to time
- Sympathetic
- Good human being
- Should not lose patience

Role of Male and Female Extension Workers

Extension Workers include all persons working in the field for improving the qulaity of life of people. In our field, Gomitras, Livestock Inspector, VAS, BVO, etc are all extension workers because some way or other they are involved in promotion of livestock activites in the field. The role of extension worker working with rural people is to bring necessary change inindividual and collective behaviour and motivating them. The role of male and female extension worker is not very distinct. However, in some backward communities, the role of the female extension worker to motivate women, is found to be very encouraging. Here, we will discuss the important roles of both male and female Extension workers.

An extension worker should arouse farmers to recognize and take interest in their problems, to overcome these problems, to teach them how to do so, to persuade them to act on his teaching, so that they ultimately achieve a sense of satisfaction and pride in their achievements.

An extension worker should motivate the people so that they may take up the activities which will improve their socio-economic conditions.

Extension worker role is to create self-belief in rural people.

Extension worker should encourage people to have self-dependence.

An extension worker is a person whose primary role is to achieve a transformation of attitudes, behaviour and social organization.

Extension workers are multi-purpose agents serving as links between government and people.

Extension worker is a person who sets in motion a process of change after realizing that certain changes are necessary for the rural society.

Extension worker is an activist whose main role is to help people form their own organizations in order to be able to tackle their problems.

Extension worker is a professional who influences the innovation/decision-making process in a direction deemed desirable by the change agency.

Extesnsion worker role is to develop the close relations between research centre and universities to update his knowleedge and skills on the lateat development.

Functions/Task of Extension Teacher

The terms "extension educator', 'extension worker' 'extension teacher', 'adult educator', 'instructor', 'animator' and 'change agent' all pertain to 's/he who assists learning to happen' or managing the learning' or one who is helping or motivating adults to learn'. The main functions of extension teacher can be broadly classified in to five categories and these are:

1. **The diagnostic function**: Helping the learners to identify their problems in understanding the issues or applying the theory in to practice.
2. **The planning function**: It is organizing the teaching and learning activities by extension educators and providing effective learning experiences to learners to attain maximum desirable changes in their behaviour.
3. **The motivational function:** This is creating conditions that will cause learners to want to learn.

Functions of Extension Worker

- diagnostic function
- planning function
- motivational function
- methodological function
- resource function

4. **The methodological function:** Selecting suitable teaching methods or combination of methods appropriate to the particular learning situation to produce desired results among the learners.
5. **The resource function:** Arranging human and material resources required for the extension teaching programme.

To be a successful Livestock extension worker you should not only know what to teach, but also know how to teach people. In other words, it is not enough that you are equipped with technical knowledge in subject matter fields; but also you should have the ability to successfully communicate your ideas to the people, taking the personal, social and situational factors into consideration. You need to understand not only your own programme and objectives but also the nature of the people with whom you live and work. There is a need to understand the motives of people; why certain people take the new ideas more rapidly than others, why certain people want to take the leadership and why certain others hesitate.

Animal Husbandry Extension involves systematic and organized communication with livestock owners with a view to helping them in such a way that the livestock owners

- obtain a better insight into their present and future position as livestock owners
- acquire sufficient knowledge and skills necessary to increase production or reduce cost of production
- develop positive attitudes of livestock development
- able to choose feasible and optimum objectives
- able to identify problems, look for solutions, solve the problems identified; and

- evaluate the results within the farming system situation in which they are operating.

Rural Women and Livestock Extension

The role of women in livestock and agriculture development is increasingly recognized both at national and local level. There is a growing awareness of the need to reach women farmers and to fully involve them in development programmes. However, extension services still face difficulties in effectively communicating and working with women. Among the reasons for this is the lack of adequate knowledge and understanding of the extension workers on specific issues of women involved in livestock activities. Rural women perform most of the traditional livestock activities.

Some of the common dairy activities are:

- Cleaning of shed
- Gathering dung
- Watering of animals
- Milking of animals
- Feeding of animals
- Grazing of animals
- Collection and feeding of fodder
- Preparing milk products
- Selling of milk and milk products
- Care of new born calf
- Care of sick animals, etc.

Activities in which women involvement is low or limited

- Purchase of animals
- Sale of animals
- Attending meting and training
- Availing of credit
- Purchase of feed and medicine
- Treatment and vaccination of animals

Extension worker must understand the complexity of rural women's work. The variety of works they perform in animal husbandry, agriculture, rural development and household management and implications of their involvement in extension activities.

Women farmers belong, generally, to the small farmer category. They are faced with all the problems common to small farmers. In addition, the cultural, social and economic conditions of women in general, and women farmers in particular, mean that there are a number of specific problems related only to women working in agriculture. It is important to stress that women farmers cannot be considered to be a homogeneous category, sharing exactly the same sort of problems and facing the same constraints. It needs to be recognized that there is considerable diversity between various groups of women like young, old, disabled, married, widow, etc. regarding the extension support. Despite the significance of women's role in agricultural and livestock development, evidence throughout developing countries shows that women's farming productivity and efficiency levels often remain very low. Among the key reasons for this is the lack of technical advice they receive on rearing, production and marketing, cultural practices, skills and technology. Extension services frequently fail to provide adequate information to women farmers through failing to recognize their specific needs. Women farmers face specific constraints not faced by men. In addition to their productive tasks, they are frequently over burdened with household responsibilities which they cannot delegate; they are often less educated than men and have a more limited access to resources such as credit. If an extension programme deals effectively with these constraints, it will be easier for women farmers to get involved in extension activities.

Barriers to Women's Involvement in Extension

1. **Lack of rights to land:** Men and women in our country enjoy equal rights on land. However, due social pressure, women do not exercise their authority on land. Women farmers do not get benefits for land based extension activities due their lack of ownership on land.
2. **Lack of Access to Credit:** Women farmers often face additional obstacles to obtaining credit and consequently are less able to purchase inputs. Statistics show that women have less access to credit than men, despite the generally better loan repayment rates. Women's lower educational levels relative to men's, and their lack of familiarity with loan procedures may also limit their possibilities of obtaining credit from male credit officers or moneylenders.
3. **Lower Levels of Education:** The education level of women is lower than the male counterpart in India. Due to low education, they face difficulty to associate themselves with different livestock extension programme.
4. **Lack of Equipment and Appropriate Technology:** Women farmers generally own fewer tools than men. New technology has also often been developed without consideration of women's needs.
5. **Time Related Problems:** women are more involved than men in routine, time consuming activities and that therefore time availability is more of a

constraint for them. They spent most of the time for household tasks necessary for the well-being of the family (cooking, looking after children, cleaning, repairing household items, etc.). The direct implication of this is that women have less total time available than men to participate in extension activities. Also, their free time may not coincide with that of the men.

6. **Mobility Related Problems:** They are constrained due to –
   - Social or religious restrictions which prevent women from travelling freely;
   - Less cash available to pay for transport;
   - fewer means of transportation available for their use.

Their limited mobility has a noticeable impact on the ability of women to become involved in extension activities.

Other Problems

- Social, cultural and religious restrictions that might prevent male extension workers from contacting and working with women farmers as well as preventing women from joining extension activities planned for a mixed group of men and women.
- Training facilities are very rarely adapted to the needs of rural women (e.g. provision of separate living rooms for overnight courses or separate classrooms);
- The level of education of rural women is frequently lower than that of men, which limits the effectiveness for women of an activity planned for men farmers.
- Women tend to have less secure land tenure and smaller plots which are often of poorer quality and at a greater distance from the household.

These factors could act both as a disincentive to take part in activities and affect the appropriateness of the information provided. If the extension effort does not reach women effectively, the chances of meeting its goals of improving livestock and agriculture production or the living standards of the household are greatly reduced. In some more extreme cases, it can also have some negative unintentional side effects. The extension workers should address the women specific problems while developing any livestock programme.

Leadership and Role of Leaders in Animal Husbandry Extension

Leader and Leadership

Within the power structure of every society, certain vital, integral individuals operate within groups to promote, stimulate, guide, or otherwise influence members to action. Such activity has been called LEADERSHIP, and the individuals have been referred to as LEADERS.

Leader

A person who effectively influences a group to co-operate in setting and achieving goals.

Leader

- Leader is a person who effectively influences a group to co-operate in setting and achieving goals.
- Any one who acts as a model to others is often called a Leader (Sprott)
- Leader is a person who has been spontaneously considered or chosen as being influential (Dahama and Bhatnagar).

Leaders are also known as power holders, man of power, power-centers and power elite. What makes these individuals distinctive is their role in the group, their influence and their possession of social power (Chitamber,1990).

Leadership

Leadership is basically a group phenomenon. A group consists of two or more people who interact together for fulfilment of common goals. In any given group there is pattern of all reactions and interaction among members. Relative strength of interpersonal relationship of the members of a group determines leadership.

Leadership

Process of influencing the behaviour of the individual in a given situation or situations.

Elements in Leadership

- The leader
- The followers
- The situation
- The task

- Leadership is the process of influencing the behaviour of the individual in a given situation or situations.
- It is a process by which an individual directs, guides and influences the thoughts, feelings and impressions of others.
- Leadership is the activity of influencing people to cooperate towards some goal which they come to find desirable
- leadership as an effort to direct the behaviour of others towards a particular and thus it can be said that
    - Leadership is a matter of influencing people in the group.
    - Leader is able to gain cooperation of members in achieving the goal.
    - The decision of people to follow the leader is voluntary.

The Basic Elements in Leadership

1. The Leader - who leads
2. The Followers - who allow themselves to be influenced by the leader
3. The Situation - the cultural context and
4. The Task - the activities performed

Qualities of Leaders

1. He has power to influence the group
2. He is unbiased
3. He makes the decisions only after knowing the problems thoroughly
4. He has the knowledge of basic needs and interests of the group
5. He is committed to work and readily accepts responsibilities and work for the group
6. He respects the right and dignity of the others
7. He understands and adhere the democratic principles
8. He will recognize and praise where it is ought to be.
9. He is optimistic, enthusiastic, and realistic
10. He possesses integrity and also enjoys the trust and confidence of his group.

Importance of Rural Leadership

The utilization of rural leaders is essential because of the following reasons:

- Extension has a long tradition of using leader in extension work. Extension worker as an outsider may not have complete knowledge about different aspects of village community nor they are supposed to have similar perceptions and feelings about village problems as local people may have. Thus, there are good reasons to use such people who belong to the community.
- Leaders by virtue of their influences can convey messages of development more convincingly in the people's language. They can use arguments and styles of presentation most appropriate for the target population. They can also help to get social sanction for development. Besides, they can also serve as mouthpiece of people before extension workers, they can explain elaborately the needs and aspirations of people.
- Number of extension workers is proportionately far less than required. Thus use of leader can help to multiply effects of extension work conveniently and convincingly.

- Leaders can help in enlisting participation of people in programmes of their own development. It is possible to organize people around concrete problems. Leaders can use their influence and skills to bring people together and empower them to take action for their development.
- Villages in India are still haunted by deep rooted beliefs, customs, superstitions and ignorance which influence development negatively. It calls for different types of efforo overcome social barriers. Leaders, if positively inclined, can play prominent roles in master minding development in right earnest.

Role of Village Leader

1. Communication of the new technology to other villages
2. Keeping in touch with the scientists, other institutions, media and sources of information
3. Coordinating the functions of the village organizations and the institutions and channelizing them towards the adoption of technologies for greater production
4. Assisting the villagers in securing the supplies and services required by them
5. Guiding and helping people in getting assistance from government
6. Helping the fellow villagers in the preparation of the action plans
7. Giving constant guidance and acting as the local consultants
8. Focusing on the problems of villager and helping the extension workers and
9. Serving as the demonstrator in the case of agricultural innovations.

Role of a leader in Animal Husbandry Extension

- Adopting improved livestock practices and showing it to others
- Keeping abreast with the latest A H technologies
- Organizing meetings and other discussion groups
- Serving as market advisors
- Supplying the improved A H inputs to the farmers
- Assisting the farmers in getting credits
- Serving the innovative farmers in the village
- Acting as liaison officer between the extension workers and farmers
- Educating the fellow farmers in latest A H technologies

Types of Leader

a) Democratic, autocratic or laissez-faire
b) Formal and Informal
c) Professional and lay (voluntary) leaders
d) Political, Religious, social, academic
e) Elected, selected or nominated
f) Popular and unpopular
g) Traditional and progressive leaders

Traditional and Emergent Leader

There are two broad categories of leaders in villages viz., 'traditional' and emergent leaders. Traditional leaders command influence on the basis of land, wealth or certain inherited status belonging to tradition like caste leaders, land lord, priest. Emergent leaders are those persons who command influence on the basis of their personal qualities, specialization or office of power, political influence or such other acquired traits such as progressive farmers, head of village council (panchayat), cooperatives or member of a voluntary or political organization.

Traditional Leaders

They are respected because they possess wealth or power to conduct social rituals/ceremonies. Thus, they fulfill social and religions needs of the people. They up hold those values. There are many other terms to indicate various types of traditional leaders as given below:

Caste leaders If the influence of some leaders extend to particular caste group, such individuals have interest and active role in social and economic development of their own caste. They are more acceptable by members of their own caste.

Sacred Leaders The term specifically refers to those who officiate in various religions and social ceremonies. They are prominent in sacred or spiritual field such as priests or ojhas (exorcists). Such traditional leaders, however, have influence over a section of society. They are characterized by inherited status due to birth in a family. However, their role in development programme can be limited due to their value orientations and pernicious interests.

Emergent leaders Emergent leaders have come on the rural scene due to new opportunities available in the villages such as village council (panchayat), cooperatives, voluntary organizations, rural branches of political parties etc. Emergent leaders are known by different terms as given below:

Personal leaders Those leaders who are valued due to their specialized skills such as progressive farmers.

Professional leaders They are people who command respect or influence by virtue of their professional status, training etc. such as village extension workers or village school teachers.

Political leaders They are affiliated with an ideology or political party and command respect by virtue of their initiatives in the party.

Social leaders Leaders of various social organizations located in the villages command influence because of their involvement in development of people.

Styles of Leadership

1. Autocratic or authoritarian leadership

Who likes to run the show himself. He takes all decisions himself without consulting the followers. He gives orders and insists on implicit obedience.

2. Participative / Democratic Leadership

- Makes decision in consultation with others
- Decentralizes authority
- Allows the group to discuss and take decision

3. Laissez-faire or Free-rein leadership

- A free-rein leader gives complete freedom to his followers to establish their own goals and policies. He does not lead and avoids power. He lets the group to operate on its own.

4. Paternalistic Leadership

A Paternalistic leader serves as the head of the family and treats his followers like his family members. He assumes a paternal or fatherly role to help, guides and protects the followers.

Identification and Selection of Leaders

There are many ways to locate people with desirable qualities and potential to play leadership role, as given below:

Election

The group members elect the leader. In this method of selection, the livestock extension worker has to explain to the memebrs what type of leader is required to lead the group.

Discussion Method

An opportunity for discussion on real issue gets people in action giving expression to their knowledge, group skill and power of conviction. This is said to be a live laboratory to see display of power and influence in natural condition. The person with sound knoweledge and ability is soon recognised and mere talker easily spotted.

The workshop method

Through this method, where the large group breaks up into smaller unit, leadership emerges, in each group over a period of time, the extension worker can spot certain leaders who come to the fore in taking responsibilities. The extension worker or professional leader in workshop has the position of consultant observer, discussion group leader etc.

Information ratings

In this method, some members of a social system are purposively or randomly selected and asked to designate persons giving advice and information on a general or particular topic. This method is economical and quick as it saves cost and time. However, it is limited to the extent each informant is thoroughly familiar with the social system.

Participative observation

Even though observation is part of both discussion and workshop methods, leaders can be selected through close observation in the community by observer being a part of the scene for a period of time. This provide him enough data regarding conditions of the community opportunities of leadership and skills.

Self-designating method

In this method, each selected person is asked a series of questions designed to determine the degree to which he perceives himself to be a key-communicator. This method has one important advantage in so far as it also measures the individual's perception of his being a key-communicator, which in turn influences his behaviour. However, its accuracy is limited to the extent the respondents can identity and report their self-image correctly.

Sociometric Technique

The term 'sociometry' refers to the pattern of attraction among members of a group. Sociometric technique is meant for determining the extent to which individuals are attarcted or repulsedbetween individuals within asmall group. This helps in revealing the relationship structure within a group. This measure of social distance was adopted by J J Morreno and Halen J Jennings in their study to social attraction of memebrs. This technique can be applied if all the members of the group know each other well. In order to seek preference for leader the specific content is explained to each member and he is asked to give a number of preference (say 1st, 2nd and 3rd,) alongwith rating. Thus people are given a situation narrating whom do you consult from your village if you have problems regarding dairy farming, name three persons from community in order of preference. To take an illustration, suppose it is required to measure the degree of attarction and rejection among 10 dairy farmers in a village, the sociometry method amy be applied. Each dairy farmers would be asked to select three farmers inorde of preference, and number them as 1, 2 and 3. Thus, each of the 10 dairy farmers select only three farmers in order of their preference. When the preferences have been known, they may be arranged either in the form of matrix table or sociogram.Sociometric score is calculated by multiplying number of incoming choices for each person and total of scores obtained in terms of preferences. Thus individuals are ranked on the basis of sociometric score.

CHOSEN

CHOOSING

Name of the Farmer	Bijay	Ramesh	Gyana	Akshya	Prakash	Sontosh	Monaj	Haris	Niraj	Susen	
Bijay		2	1						3		
Ramesh	3		2				1				
Gyana	3			1		2					
Akshya			1		2			3			
Prakash			2	3				1			
Sontosh			1				3	2			
Monaj				1		2			3		
Haris			1			2	3				
Niraj	3	2					1				
Susen			2				3		1		
1st Choice	-	-	4	2	-	-	2	1	1	-	Total 10
2nd Choice	-	2	3	-	1	3	-	1	-	-	Total 10
3rd Choice	3	-	-	1	-	-	3	1	2	-	Total 10
Total	3	2	7	3	1	3	5	3	3	0	

Socio-matrix

From the analysis of the matrix, the following types of relationship can be studied;

1. **Mututal Choice** : In such types of choices, two individual may show preference to each other. The intensity of preference may be same or it may be different. Here, Gyana and Akash have given each other first preference choice. In case of Bijay and Ramesh, the choice is mutual but different in order.
2. **Trangular or Quadrangular Choice:** In the above matrix, we may see that the Gyana has not choosen Ramesh directly, but Gyana has chosen Bijay and Bijay has choen Ramesh, and thus Ramesh and Gyana are mutualy linked through a triangle. When teo persons are connected through four different links the relationship is quadrangular. It may noted here that direct relationship is real and stringer, but as the number of intermediary links increaes , the power of union is reduced.
3. **Clique:**When three or more persons show mutual choice to each other, we say there is establishment of clique relationship. The difference between a trinagular and clique relationship is that where as in the former case the persons are not diirectly connected, in the later case, they show mutual choice for each other and are therefore more closely connected.
4. **Choice star :** Choice star is the person who is chosen by most of the people. Here, Gyana is choice star as he has received maximum choices of 7 among the 10 farmers. They are very popular in the group and usually called as the leader of the group. Next to Gyana, Monaj is the seond best choice in the group as he has received 5 choices from 10 farmers. Most of the farmers in that group go to Gyana to seek his advice for dairy farming. If the extension worker succeds in motivating or influencing " Gyana" to take up certain new practice, it is quite likely that others will be influenced by his behaviour. Hence, it would be much easier for the extension worker to reach other farmers of the community with very less effort.
5. **Secondary choice star :** In this matrix, we may observe that Akshya has received only three choices, and as such can not be said very popular, but if we observe carefully, we could see that he has been given first preference by Choice star of the group-Gyana. The group member who is prefered first by the choice star of the group is known as secondary choice star or aristotle leader. Thus, Akshya may not be very popular in the group directly, but he may be very powerful indirectly as he is pefered by the leade of the group.
6. **Totally isolates:** We may see in the matrix that Susen is not preferred by any member of the group. Such members are very unpopular and friendless in the group. They may create probems in the social gathering. They are mostly lonely and hold no wightage in the group.

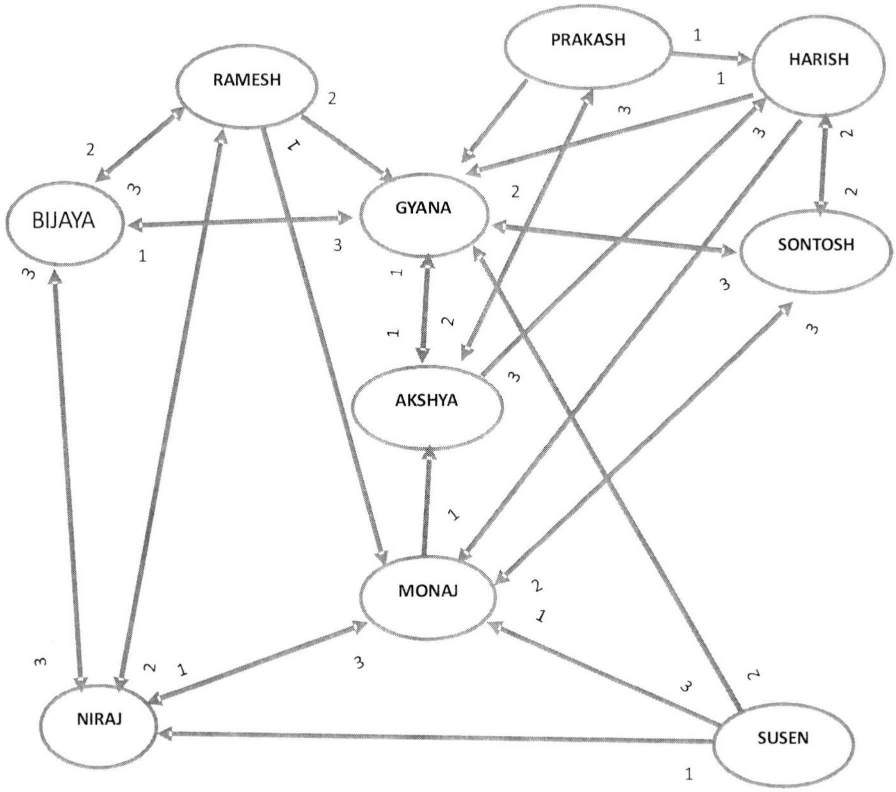

Figure (Sociogram) illustrates this type of test

Key informants method

A community or its members may be asked to indicate opinion leaders in that area. This is cost saving and time saving when compared to sociometric method.

Informal Dialogue Method

The livestock inspector while making informal discussion with clients bringing patient to Livestock Aid Centre (LAC) for treatment, could able to identify the local leader.

Discussion with Predecessor

The Livestock Inspector (LI) may discuss with his collegues who have already worked in that area and esily identfy the leaders for various activities.

Active Participation

The local leaders can be located in the community meetings. Active participation is an indication of their leadership ability.

Advantages of Using Local Leader

- Local leader virtually *plays the role of extension agent* and thereby the area of coverage is increased. By the use of local leaders, extension worker multiplies his work in less time.
- Cost of extension is reduced because local leaders are not paid for their works.
- Local leaders speak in the language of the people and they are better understood by the people.
- Leader of the village can analyse local problem better than a stranger/ extension worker.
- The time of extension worker is used more productively.
- People accept a new idea more readily from a local person who has practically tried it.
- Frequent contact of extension worker with local leader enhances his prestige, which in turn increases the possibility of extensive adoption of new practices.

Problems of Working with Local Leader

- Selected person may not have the qualities and he may not be willing to devote required time for the work.
- Considerable time is required to locate and train local leaders
- Some local leaders use their favoured position with the extension worker for their personal advantage.
- There are chances of misinterpretation and may give wrong advice to their fellow farmers.
- If the extension agent spends too much time on one or more of local leaders, then the issue of favouritism may arise.

Suggested Readings and References

1. Dasgupta (1989). Diffusion of Agricultural Innovations in village India, Wiley Eastern Limited, New Delhi.
2. Rogers E.M., Shoemaker F.F. (1971). Communication of Innovations. The Free Press, New York.
3. Swanson B.E. (1984). Agricultural Extension - A Reference Manual, Second Edition, FAO, Rome, Oxford and IBH Publishing Co. Pvt. Ltd., New Delhi.
4. Domains Czech Conroy And Alistair Sutherland Network Paper No. 133 January (2004). Agricultural Research & Extension Network, Participatory Technology

Development with Resource- Poor Farmers: Maximising Impact Through The Use Of Recommendation.

5. Gonsalves, J., T. Becker, A. Braun, D. Campilan, H. De Chavez, E. Fajber, M. Kapiriri, J. Rivaca-Caminade and R. Vernooy (eds), (2005). Participatory Research and Development for Sustainable Agriculture and Natural Resource Management: A Sourcebook. Volume 1: Understanding Participatory Research and Development. International Potato Center-Users' Perspectives With Agricultural Research and Development, Laguna, Philippines and International Development Research Centre, Ottawa, Canada.
6. Salas Maruja, Jianchu Xu & Tillmann Timmi, July (2002). Field Manual Participatory Technology Development – Linking Indigenous Knowledge and Bio-diversity for Sustainable Livelihood, Yunnan Science and Technology Press, Kunming.
7. Chambers, R; Arnold Pacey and Lori Ann Thrupp (eds.), (1989). Farmer First– Farmer Innovation and Agricultural Research. Intermediate Technology Publications, London, UK.
8. Kumar, B. and Hansra, B.S. (2000). Extension Education for Human Resource Development, Concept Publishing Company, New Delhi. Leagans, J.P. (1961), India's Experience with Training.
9. Baxter M., Slade Roger and Howell John (1989). Aid and Agricultural Extension-Evidence from the World Bank and Other Donors, World Bank Technical Paper Number 87, Washington, D.C. 20433, U.S.A.
10. Kelsey, L.D., and Hearne, G.C. (1963). Cooperative Extension Work, Comstock Publishing Associates, New York.

7

Participatory Extension

1. Participatory Extension
2. Importance of Participation:
3. Steps in Community participation
4. Different Participatory Approaches
5. Rapid Rural Appraisal (RRA)
6. Participatory Rural Appraisal (PRA)
7. Principles of PRA
8. Participatory Tools and Techniques
    i. Social Map
    ii. Resource Map
    iii. Transect walks
    iv. Mobility Map
    v. Time Line
    vi. Trend Analysis
    vii. Livelihood Analysis
    viii. Stakeholders Analysis
    ix. Seasonal Diagram
    x. Causc -Effcct Diagram (Problem Tree)
    xi. Well-being ranking methods
    xii. Venn Diagram
9. Disadvantages of PRA Methods
10. Suggested Readings and References

Participatory Extension

> **Participation**
>
> Involvement of the stake holders in decision making process

Participation means the involvement of the stakeholders in all the activities. In a true sense of participation, the farmers are involved in identifying the problems they face, prioritising the problems, determining ways to overcome them, designing realistic plans by themselves or with others to achieve the goals, and carrying them out. Participation puts emphasis on people's involvement in decision-making processes, implementation of programmes, sharing of benefits of development programmes and involvement to evaluate such programmes. Community participation is an active process by which beneficiary or client groups influence the direction and execution of a development project with a view to enhancing their well-being in terms of income, personal growth, self-reliance, or other values they cherish. Community participation concerns the engagement of individuals and communities in decisions about things that affect their lives. Sometimes you have observed that some people do not want to be involved in decision making process and remain aloof, but it is our responsibility to create a situation so that everyone should have the opportunity to associate with the programme. We should not force people to participate in the project/programme which they perceive that it will affect their livelihood. In that case, we have to create awareness among the people regarding the beneficial effects of the programme. Solutions devised and fulfilled by the people and community in need are far more likely to prove successful than those imposed from outside.

Importance of Participation

- Active participation increases the owning of the programme.
- Active participation of farmers improves democratic and service accountability.
- It enhances social cohesion because communities recognize the value of working in partnership.
- It helps the formulation of policy according to the need of the farmers.
- It gives participants the opportunity to develop the skills and networks that are needed to address other problems.
- It promotes sustainability because community members have ownership of their programme and can develop the confidence and skills to sustain developments once the external agency withdraws from the programme/ project.

Steps in Community Participation

- Needs assessment: Expressing opinions about desirable improvements, prioritizing goals and negotiating with agencies
- Planning: Formulating objectives, setting goals, criticizing plans
- Mobilizing: Raising awareness in a community about needs, establishing or supporting organizational structures within the community
- Training: Participation in formal or informal training activities to enhance communication, construction, maintenance and financial management skills
- Implementing: Engaging in management activities; contributing directly to construction, operation and maintenance with labour and materials; contributing cash towards costs, paying of services or membership fees of community organizations
- Monitoring and Evaluation: Participating in the appraisal of work done, recognizing improvements that can be made and redefining needs.

Steps in Participatory Approaches

a) **Rapport building:** The first most requirement of participatory approach is rapport building and environment creation for free and frank interaction with the villagers. The project team members during the study period may stay, eat and participate in the social function with local people. The workers should have patient to get along with the villagers.

b) **Do-It Yourself:** The team members should make efforts to perform the activities that the villagers are doing such as sowing the seeds, transplanting, harvesting, threshing, feeding the animals, milking, chaffing the fodder, etc. This helps not only in rapport building but provides practical ideas and feelings of complexities of activities in the field conditions. This provides learning opportunities to the field workers.

c) **Consultations with the villagers and outsiders:** The selection of the village should be informed to the officials such as District Collector, Block Development Officers, Sarpanches, before initiating the process. The choice of the village must be agreed upon by the top leadership of the District and civic leaders. The site should accessible for ease of supervision.

d) **Secondary Data Collection:** Secondary data refers to information gathered from reports, newspapers, leaflets, pamphlets, library sources, folklore and other classified documents. This information is derived from researchers, NGO, departmental reports and documentaries. It is advisable to gather information on a community before going to the field to conduct the actual diagnosis. The data collected and synthesized by the multidisciplinary team can be used and background information to the Action Plans to be developed by the village residents. Furthermore, this data can be used to validate information obtained from the semi-structured interviews.

e) **Training of Trainers:** Training of a core team of facilitators is an important phase in PRA activities. It equips the trainers with the knowledge and skills to train other extension workers and farmers, and ensures capacity building for sustainability.

f) **Diagnosis:** Diagnosis is an examination and analysis of any given situation. In the context of PRA diagnosis examines the farmers' practices, opportunities, the problems they encounter, and their causes. This crucial information is obtained using various tools such as secondary data, mapping, transect, Venn diagram and semi structured interviews etc.

Different Participatory Approaches

Organisations and Institutions which believes in participatory process of engagement with community, have developed a number of techniques for effective interaction with communities. They emphasise a re-orientation in the relationship between the outsider and the villagers. Some of them are mentioned below and all these approaches are closely related to each other.

1. Rapid Rural Appraisal (RRA)
2. Participatory Rural Appraisal (PRA)
3. Participatory Learning Methods (PALM)
4. Agro-Ecosystem Analysis (AEA)
5. Participatory Action Research (PAR)
6. Participatory Assessment, Monitoring and Evaluation (PAME)
7. Farming Systems Research (FSR)
8. Participatory Rural Appraisal and Planning (PRAP)

These participatory approaches are widely used by both public and private agencies including NGO. Here we will discuss about RRA and PRA.

Rapid Rural Appraisal (RRA)

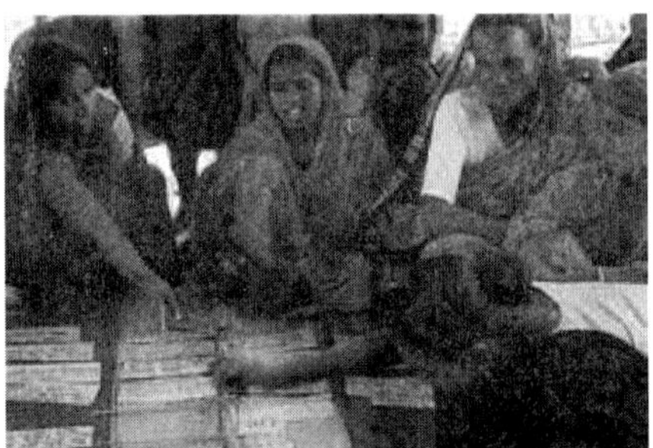

RRA is a social science approach that emerged in the early 1980s for applications in development cooperation. The basic idea of RRA is to rather quickly collect, analyse and evaluate information on rural conditions and local knowledge. This information is generated in close co-operation with the local population in rural areas. In RRA, a multidisciplinary team makes use of simple, nonstandard methods and the knowledge of local people to quickly elicit, analyze and evaluate information and hypotheses about rural life and rural resources that are of relevance for taking action. A main reason for developing RRA was to find shortcuts in the search for relevant information on rural development issues in order to avoid costly and time consuming research procedures. It is a tool which can be used in a lot of different situations to achieve very different objectives.

RRA essentially consists of the following:

- an activity carried out by a group of people from different professional fields or disciplines which usually aims to learn about a particular topic, area, situation, group of people or whatever else is of concern to those organising the RRA
- it usually involves collecting information by talking directly to people "on the ground"
- it uses a set of guidelines on how to approach the collection of information, learning from that information and the involvement of local people in its interpretation and presentation
- it uses a set of tools - these consist of exercises and techniques for collecting information, means of organising that information so that it is easily understood by a wide range of people, techniques for stimulating interaction with community members and methods for quickly analysing and reporting findings and suggesting appropriate action.

Participatory Rural Appraisal (PRA)

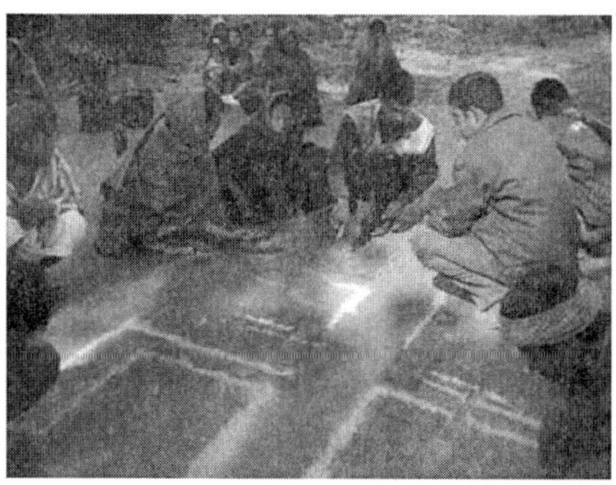

The word "appraisal" in PRA has a much broader connotation than its dictionary meanings as "estimation of the value of asset/goods" or "an act of estimation/assessment of nature, quality and importance of asset". During the 1980s, PRA was firstly developed in India and Kenya, mainly supported by NGOs operating at grass-roots level. PRA is a further evolutionary stage of the RRA approach. In it, emphasis is placed on empowering local people to assume an active role in analysing their own living conditions, problems and drawing up plans, with outsiders mainly acting as "facilitators". Here it is no longer the external experts but rather the local people themselves who "own" the results of the study. PRA is a way of enabling local (rural and urban) people to analyze their living conditions, to share the outcomes and to plan their activities. It's a "handing over the stick to the insider" in methods and action. The outsider's role is that of a catalyzer, a facilitator and convenor of processes within a community, which is prepared to alter their situation.

RRA and PRA methods are used

- In order to ascertain needs ("felt needs")
- To establish priorities for development activities
- Within the scope of feasibility studies
- During the implementation phase of projects
- Within the scope of monitoring and evaluation of projects
- For studies of specific topics
- For focusing formal surveys on essential aspects; and
- To identify conflicting interests between groups.

In **RRA** information is more elicited and extracted by outsiders whereas in **PRA** it is more shared and owned by the local people.

RRA leads to learning by outsiders in a cost effective way.

PRA, on the other hand enables rural people to unravel and analyse their own situation in ways, they do not normally do, and in optimal cases to plan and act on their own premises. (Robert Chambers, 1992).

Potential Differences between RRA and PRA

RRA	PRA
1 Responding to needs of development workers and agencies	Responding to needs of communities and target groups
2 More emphasis on efficient use of time & achievement of objectives	More emphasis on flexibility to adapt to time frame of community
3 Communication and learning tools used to help outsiders analyse conditions and understand local people	Communication and learning tools used to help local people analyse their own conditions and communicate with outsiders
4 Focus of RRA decided by outsiders	Focus of PRA decided by communities
5 End product mainly used by development agencies and outsiders	End product mainly used by community
6 Enables development agencies and institutions to be more "participatory"	Enables (empowers) communities to make demands on development agencies and institutions
7 Can be used purely for "research" purposes without necessarily linking to subsequent action or intervention	Closely linked to action or intervention and requiring immediate availability of support for decisions and conclusion s reached by communities as a result of the PRA

Areas of application

- Natural resource management
- Agriculture
- Poverty alleviation/women in development programmes
- Health and nutrition
- Preliminary and primary education
- Village and district-level planning
- Institutional and policy analysis.

Principles of PRA

Chambers (1997) has listed the following principles.

Listening and Learning

PRA is based on the principle of listening and learning through participatory interactions. The local people have their knowledge, their experience, their history and culture, their views and ideas and their priorities and preferences. Listening to local people helps in understanding their views. We should be mentally prepared to listen, learn from local people and show respect to their views. This would help us to do the work jointly without conflict. PRA relies heavily on participation by the communities, as the method is designed to enable local people to be involved, not only as sources of information, but as partners with the PRA team in gathering and analyzing the information.

Key Principles of PRA

- Listening and Learning
- Offsetting Biases
- Utilization of precious Community Time
- Teamwork
- Triangulation /Cross checking
- Optimal Ignorance
- Flexibility

Offsetting Biases

PRA aims at offsetting biases, which generally accompany a "rushed" appraisal by professionals for quick results. Professionals tend to appraise samples at convenient times when the weather is favourable; consult would-be-beneficiaries (mostly men) who are generally better off; and professionally tend to look at those aspects which they think are important. In order to offset such biases, PRA, encourages relaxed listening and learning, seeking participation from people who are relatively worse off, visiting remote and interior locations and visiting local communities at their convenience. This process should try to have involvement-of those who would otherwise never get a chance to speak, here may be some initial hesitation, but the local people start enjoying it as new facts about the poorest people, women, disadvantaged groups in remote areas etc. still important is that the team must refrain from any value judgment about others.

Utilization of precious Community Time

About learning from local people, PRA is based on the principle of utilizing precious community time in the best possible way. Local community members are busy in pursing local livelihoods and it is important to keep track of their time and learn as much as time permits. This also implies that community members are requested to spare their time for interaction at their convenient time. The learning should also be focused so as to make proper utilization of such time.

Seeking Diversity

PRA involves learning from diverse conditions and different actors. It consults with more of difference rather than looking for representativeness of results or data collected. It is looking for diverse events, different processes and forces, which help in understanding of issues from different perspectives. For any analysis, greater the diversity, better is the understanding of "reality".

Triangulation /Cross checking

Triangulation is adopted as a principle to improve trust worthiness of data. It will be done by changing the team composition, the sources of information and the techniques applied. There is need that each activity or phenomenon is considered from different viewpoints and studied using different techniques. The process of cross checking is an important principle of PRA for minimizing errors and doing mid-way corrections. Since there are different sources from which information can flow it is important to cross-check the reliability and validity of the data by putting it to different tests. There exist different ways to check the validity of the data in PRA such as changing methods, locations, timing, groups, teams, etc.

Optimal ignorance and appropriate imprecision

In order to minimize cost and time, the principle of optimal ignorance is a handy principle for PRA facilitators to keep in mind. It means knowing what is worth knowing and knowing enough to serve the purpose and not knowing the rest or not trying to find out more. Associated with this is seeking appropriate imprecision or avoiding precision of information that is not necessary.

These principles of PRA help in making learning iterative, in facilitating participatory sessions, in making such processes interactive, innovative and informational and in making effective use of time.

Multi-disciplinary Team

The scientific team conducting PRA must have fairly broad base, meaning there by inclusion of scientists of all important disciplines relevant to the area of study. It is also important to have female scientists in the team so that rural women could be effectively involved in the appraisal exercise. The team should identify among themselves one member who should work as Team Leader/Facilitator. Another member should be identified to work as Process Recorder or Content Recorder. While interacting with the villagers he/she should not jump directly to the objective of the study but first develop rapport with them. The responsibility of rapport building may be assigned to one member of the team who could work as Environment Controller.

Participatory Tools and Techniques

Participatory approaches in extension activities emphasise the involvement of local people in the selection, design, planning and implementation of programmes and projects that will affect them. The PRA approach is particularly useful as it enables vulnerable groups in a community to have a voice and impart their views on issues of transportation and access from which they are most often excluded. Hence, participation by different groups such as women, the elderly, disabled and even school children, researchers and other professionals are able to paint a realistic picture of community life which facilitates the effective project formulation and implementation by the villagers.

PRA Tools and Techniques

1. Social Map

A social map is drawn by the residents and which shows the social structures and institutions found in an area. It also helps us to learn about social and economic differences between the households. Social mapping is the most popular method in PRA. The focus here is on the depiction of habitation patterns and the nature of housing and social infrastructure: roads, drainage systems, schools, drinking-water facilities, etc. Social map is different from other

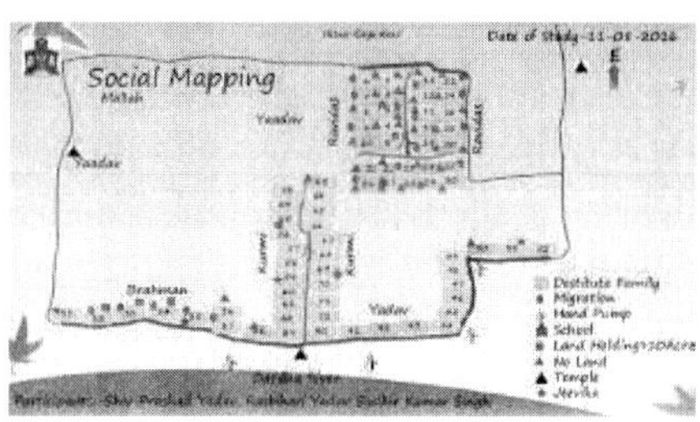

regular maps in significant ways. For one, it is made by local people and not by experts. For another, it is not drawn to scale. It depicts what the local people believe to be relevant and important for them. Thus it reflects their perceptions of the social dimensions of their reality with a high degree of authenticity. Social Mapping helps in developing a broad understanding of the various facets of social reality, viz., social stratification, demographics, settlement patterns, social infrastructure, etc.

The diverse applications of social maps include:

- Developing a comprehensive understanding of the physical and social aspects of village life.
- Collecting demographic and other required information household-wise
- Providing a forum of discussion in which to unravel the various aspects of social life
- Serving as a guiding instrument during the process of planning interventions
- Serving as a monitoring and evaluating tool.

Resource Map

The Village Resource Map is a tool that helps us to learn about a community and its resource base. The primary concern is not to develop an accurate map but to get useful information about local perceptions of resources. The participants should develop the content of the map according to what is important to them. the resource map focuses on the natural resources in the locality and depicts land, hills, rivers, fields, vegetation, etc. A resource map may cover habitation as well. At times, the distinction between the resource map and social map may get blurred. A resource map in PRA is not drawn to scale. It is not done by experts but by the local people. The local people are considered to have an in-depth knowledge of the surroundings where they have survived for a long time. Hence the resource map social map drawn by the local people is considered to be accurate and detailed. Resource maps have been used for depicting of various aspects related to the natural resources management of a locality including:

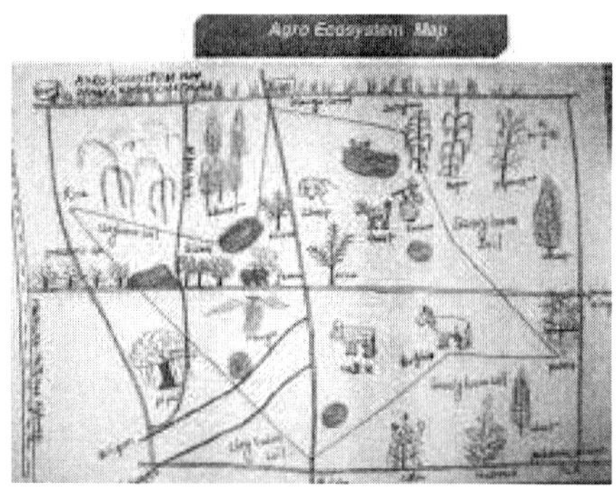

- Topography, terrain and slopes
- Forest, vegetation and tree species
- Soil-type, fertility, erosion and depth
- Land and land use, command area, tenure, boundaries and ownership
- Water, water bodies, irrigation sources, rivers and drainage.
- Watershed development, various soil and water conservation measures, denuded areas, etc.
- Agricultural development, cropping pattern, livestock rearing, productivity, etc.

Key questions asked to elicit the information about resources

1. What resources are abundant?
2. What resources are scarce?
3. Does everyone have equal access to land?
4. Do women have access to land?
5. Do the poor have access to land?
6. Who makes decision on land allocation?
7. Where do people go to collect water?
8. Who collects water?
9. Where do people go to collect firewood?
10. Who collects firewood?
11. Where do people go graze livestock?
12. What kind of development activities do you carry out as a whole community? Where?
13. Which resource do you have the most problem with?

2. Transect walks

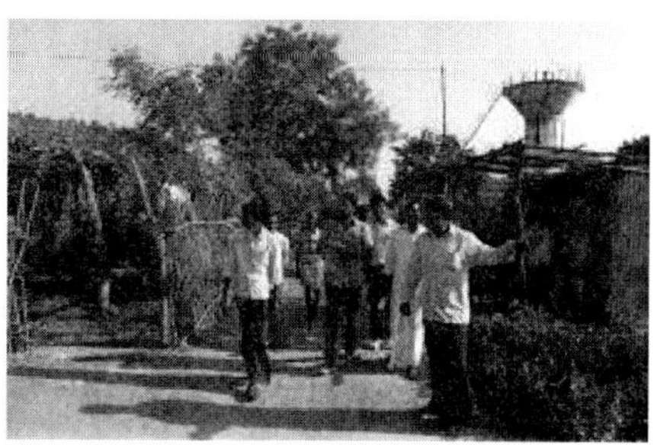

Transect walks are a participatory exercise, where members of the community, planners and others walk through the village with key informants, interviewing passers-by and drawing a map with observations of characteristics, risks and existing solutions after the walk. These walks are typically applied in villages to obtain first-hand information about the resources available in the village. A transect walk is a systematic walk along a defined path (transect) across the community/project area together with the local people to study the different conditions of the village by observing, asking, listening, looking and producing a transect diagram. An important part of the method is discussion and active listening, identification of problems and their solutions. The main objective of the transect walk is to understand and study the major land uses, cultivation pattern, livestock rearing practice, topography, water resources, natural vegetation and different ecological zones by observing, interacting and discussing with the key informants , while walking in the deciding direction.

Mobility Map

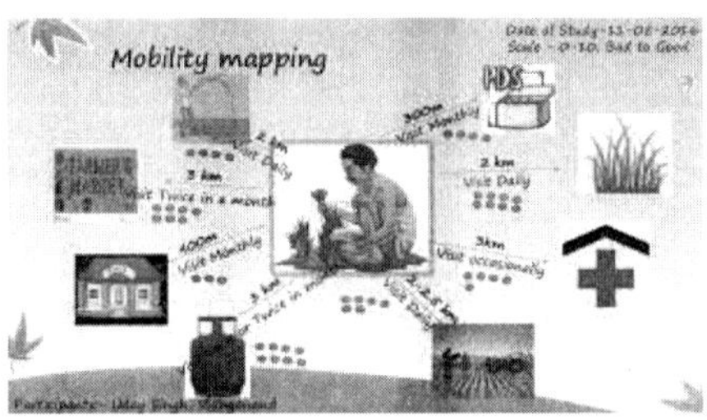

Mobility map is a PRA method used to explore the movement pattern of an individual, a group, or the community to outside of their village for various purposes like purchasing fodder, inputs, family needs, selling of milk, medical needs, educational needs, etc. The focus is on where people go and for what. Other aspects, like the frequency of visits, distance, and the importance of the place visited, may also be studied and depicted. It reflects the people's perception of movement patterns and the reasons there of.

Time Line

Time lines establish well known past events and provide a framework for discussing changes that have taken place. It is an important PRA method which captures the chronology of events as recalled by local people. It is drawn as a sequential aggregate of past events. It thus provides the historical landmarks of a community individual or institution. The important point to note here is that it is not history as much the events of the past as perceived and recalled by the people themselves.

Objectives

- To learn from the community what they considered to be important past events.
- To understand from the community the historical perspective on current issues.

- To generate discussions on changes with respect to issues you are interested in e.g. education, health, food security, gender relations, economic conditions, etc.
- To develop a rapport with the villagers, since a discussion about the past of the village can be a good non-threatening and enjoyable starting point.

Trend Analysis

It captures and trends related to certain variables over different spans of time. It is, thus, people's account of the past and of how things have changed and hence also provides a historical perspective. The local people have a good understanding of the present situation and the changes that have taken place over the years. Trend analysis can provide a good idea of the quantitative changes over time in different aspects of village life, such as yields, population, livestock population, the number of trees, area under cultivation, rainfall, etc., it helps to understand increases and decreases in the variables under study over a period of time.

Livelihood Analysis

Livelihood analysis refers to finding out the degrees to which the pattern of life differs from one social class to another social class in term of family size, annual income, landholding size, type of house, income from different sources, expenditure pattern, crisis management pattern, indebtedness etc. Studies have brought out clearly that livestock rearing helps the resource poor people to reduce the intensity of poverty as the livestock offer livelihood options, security in the event of financial crisis to the families.

Stakeholder analysis

Stakeholders are those who are either directly or indirectly effected by the programmes or policies of the government. The stakeholder's analysis would identify who are going to be benefitted by the programme. For an example, a deworming programme in a village may benefit the dairy farmers, medicine supplier, Self Help Groups, Milk Cooperative Societies, veterinary department, etc.

Seasonal Diagram

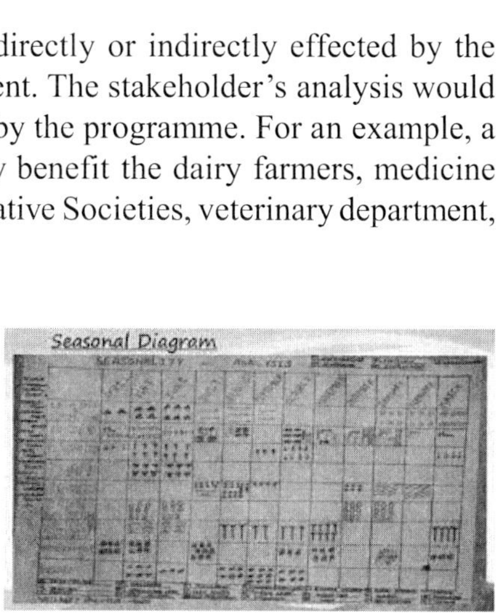

Season diagram is also called seasonal calendar, seasonal activity, profile and seasonal analysis. Seasonal diagram is one of the popular PRA methods that have been used for temporal analysis across annual cycles, with months or seasons as the basic unit of analysis. It reflects the perceptions of the local people regarding seasonal variations on a wide range of items. Seasonal diagram, however, are not based on statistics, but they may be triangulated against secondary or primary data in order to verify the information generated. One of the examples is availability of different types of fodder for livestock in a village.

Cause -Effect Diagram (Problem Tree)

Cause effect diagram is a popular PRA method which falls under the family of flow and linkage diagram methods. Also known as fishbone or Ishikawa diagram, it focuses on the causal factors of a phenomenon, activity, or problem, and the effects thereof. The cause effect diagram presents visually the causes, effects and their interlinkage, which help in arriving at an in-depth understanding of a particular topic, and provide scope for analysis and subsequent action by the local people.

Well-being ranking methods/Wealth Ranking

Wealth ranking is an ingenious and simple method of eliciting relative wealth or wellbeing in a community. It is PRA method commonly used for ranking and grouping household and communities on the basis of income, wealth, and other perceivable well-being criteria. Well-being ranking is based on the perception of the local people. It helps to understand the local people's perception of wealth, well–being and their views on socio-economic disparities between households. Wealth ranking is based on the assumption that the community members have a good sense about fellow villagers in their own village and are able to categorize themselves. Wealth ranking helps the extension workers, developmental staff, researchers and others concerned with rural and livestock development to find out the inequalities and differences in wealth in every farmer and which in turn lead to overall understanding of socio-economic conditions of entire village community and develop extension interventions accordingly. This also will help in selecting the right type of beneficiaries for various programmes.

Venn Diagram

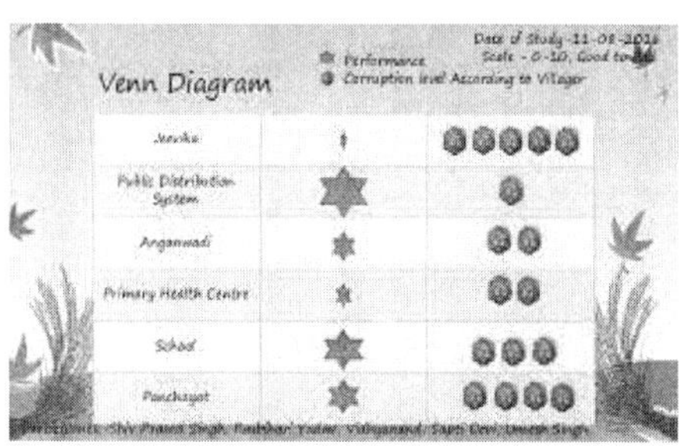

Venn diagram is one of the commonly used methods in PRA to study institutional relationship and is sometimes also referred to as institutional diagram. It is however, popularly known as Chapati diagram (Chapati means 'round bread' in Hindi) as the method uses circles of various sizes to represent institutions or individuals. The bigger the circle, the more important is the institution or individual. The distance between circles represents, for example, the degree of influence or contact between institutions or individuals. Overlapping circles indicate interactions and the extent of overlap can indicate the level of interaction.

Objectives

- To study and understand local people's perceptions about local institutions, individuals, programmes, etc.
- The method provides valuable insights into and analyses of the power structure, the decision- making process, etc., the need to strengthen the community's institutions can also be ascertained.
- The relative importance of services and programmes has also been studied using the Venn diagram.

Venn diagram is particularly useful when you want to study and analyse

- Various institutions and individuals and their influence on the local people.
- Various groups and individuals in the locality and their influence.
- The main actors in the community and their conspicuous and inconspicuous influence.

The following information is elicited in Venn diagram

a. relative importance of various institutions in the village
b. relationship among them,
c. linkages among them
d. weaknesses with respect to decision making process
e. development of the village by institutions
f. duplication of efforts among institutions
g. gap identification between institutions
h. objectives and felt needs of farmers
i. concentration of power within villages

Disadvantages of PRA Methods

Although PRA techniques have a potentially wide application in the field of project development and research, it is important that they are applied appropriately, with sufficient resources and should not be conducted hastily.

The process of carrying out PRA methods requires mutual respect and trust between external facilitators and village participants, this takes time, and requires an understanding of the local culture. Hence, the general messages to consider are to avoid being dogmatic, be flexible in field study design without losing direction, be sensitive to the context of the field study and adjust the approach accordingly.

The following is a list summarising lessons learnt from existing PRA surveys:

- A common mistake is; projects do not contact local government officials from the start hence no local government support which is a prerequisite for success.
- The step from problem identification with participatory PRA methods to follow up project definition is often poorly prepared.
- Project Officers should leave any class and gender biases they may carry at home!
- There should be continual analysis of the qualitative data whilst in the field.
- PRA methods require that the researcher knows the context and participates.
- Dialogue between the target group and Project Officers will be of benefit to both parties. The researcher must be able to listen but also to establish dialogue and share own experience.
- Very few project results are shared with the people who most need them. The filters are too many and too closed.
- Participants are introduced to a 'code of conduct':
- Time suitable to the villagers
- Cultural protocol
- Avoid raising expectations
- Avoid lecturing - listen and learn
- Stay in the village throughout the training session.

Suggested Readings and References

1. Dasgupta (1989). *Diffusion of Agricultural Innovations in village India*, Wiley Eastern Limited, New Delhi.
2. Rogers E.M., Shoemaker F.F. (1971). *Communication of Innovations*, The Free Press, New York.
3. Swanson B.E. (1984). Agricultural Extension - A Reference Manual, Second Edition, FAO, Rome, Oxford and IBH Publishing Co. Pvt. Ltd., New Delhi.

4. Domains Czech Conroy And Alistair Sutherland Network Paper No. 133 January (2004). Agricultural Research & Extension Network, Participatory Technology Development with Resource- Poor Farmers: Maximising Impact Through The Use Of Recommendation.

5. Gonsalves, J., T. Becker, A. Braun, D. Campilan, H. De Chavez, E. Fajber, M. Kapiriri, J. Rivaca-Caminade and R. Vernooy (eds), (2005). Participatory Research and Development for Sustainable Agriculture and Natural Resource Management: A Sourcebook. Volume 1: Understanding Participatory Research and Development. International Potato Center-Users' Perspectives With Agricultural Research and Development, Laguna, Philippines and International Development Research Centre, Ottawa, Canada.

6. Salas Maruja, Jianchu Xu & Tillmann Timmi, July, (2002). Field Manual Participatory Technology Development – Linking Indigenous Knowledge and Bio-diversity for Sustainable Livelihood, Yunnan Science and Technology Press, Kunming,

7. Chambers, R; Arnold Pacey and Lori Ann Thrupp (eds.), (1989). Farmer First – Farmer Innovation and Agricultural Research. Intermediate Technology Publications, London, UK.

8. Kumar, B. and Hansra, B.S. (2000). Extension Education for Human Resource Development, Concept Publishing Company, New Delhi. Leagans, J.P. (1961), India s Experience with Training

9. Baxter M, Slade Roger and Howell John (1989). Aid and Agricultural Extension-Evidence from the World Bank and Other Donors, World Bank Technical Paper Number 87, Washington, D.C. 20433, U.S.A.

10. Kelsey, L.D., and Hearne, G.C. (1963). Cooperative Extension Work, Comstock Publishing Associates, New York.

8

Rural Sociology

1. What is Sociology?
2. What is Rural Sociology?
3. Impotance and significance of Rural Sociology in Animal Husbandry Extension
4. Relationship between Sociology and Livestock Extension
5. Society, Community, Association and Institution
6. What is Society?
7. Attributes of Society
8. What is Community?
9. What is Association?
10. Characteristics of Rural Society
11. Comparison between Rural, Tribal and Urban Societies
12. Livestock Production Practices in Rural, Urban and Tribal Societies
13. Social control
    - a) Social Norms
    - b) Folkways
    - c) Mores
    - d) Custom
    - e) Religion
    - f) Family
    - g) Neighbourhood
    - h) Laws
    - i) Education
    - j) State
14. Social stratification
15. Caste and Class System in India
16. Institutions in Rural Society
    1. Social Institutions
        - a) Marriage
        - b) Family
        - c) Kinship
    2. Economic Institution

Rural Sociology

Significant proportion of Indian population lives in village and derives their livelihood from villages. India is a land of agriculture and its customs, traditions, social structure, etc. are unique in the world. Understanding of rural society is must for successful implementation of developmental programmes. The understanding of rural people requires study of rural sociology. Rural sociology, as indicated by its name, studies rural society, rural social structures and institutions. The rural society is primarily depending on agriculture and hence rural sociology also concerns itself on the peasant society. There is a stark difference between the social structure, processes, social dynamics and social control in rural society and urban society. Thus, rural sociology has been specially designed to study the rural phenomena and it is a systematic study of the varied aspects of the rural society. It is the study of the rural social networks and how they operate for the smooth functioning of the society. The rural society is generally rooted in the villages, and rural sociology studies the facets of the villages, the way it functions, the various problems it faces and the how it tackles to face the imminent challenges. Rural sociology offers viable solutions and ways of mitigating the problems that hound over the villages.

What is Sociology ?

> August Comte:
> Father of Sociology
> Socio-Society
> Logos: Scientific Study

The term sociology was coined by **Auguste Comte** (1789-1857) who is often referred as the father of Sociology. It comprises two words: In Latin, *Socio* means companion, friend, association but in a broader sense group or society. In Greek, *logos* mean scientific study. Thus, the literal or etymological meaning of sociology is called as 'Science of Society'. Comte wished to establish a science of society that would help to reveal social laws which control development and change. Sociology is a simple way of study of people. Sociologist wants to know why people behave the way they do, why they form groups, why they worship, why they practice certain things, etc., all such things happen when people interact with one another. Sociology is the scientific study of man's behaviour in relationship to other individuals with whom he interacts. The sociologists define sociology in different ways and some of them are:

According to Rogers, sociology is defined as a study of ways in which social experiences function in developing, maturing, refreshing human beings through interpersonal stimulation.

According to Chitamber, sociology is the study of human beings in their group relations. It studies the interaction within and between groups of people.

According to Max Weber, sociology as a science which interprets social behaviour with the aim of arriving at causal explanation of human behaviour.

According to L.T. Hobhouse , sociology is comprehensive science of society which aimed at the interpretation of social life.

According to Morris Ginsberg, sociology as the study of the conditions and consequences of human interactions and interrelations.

According to Park and Bugess, sociology is the science of collective behaviour.

According to Emile Durkheim, sociology is the study of social phenomena.

From these definitions, we may conclude that the sociology is the study of human society and social behaviour as well as study of social relationships and its forms.

What is Rural Sociology ?

Rural sociology is a field of sociology that is connected with the study of social life in rural areas. The sociologists define rural sociology in different ways and some of them are:

According to Sanderson, "Rural sociology is the sociology of rural life in the rural environment".

According to Bertand, "Rural sociology is that study of human relationships in rural environment".

According to T.L. Smith, "Such sociological facts and principles as are derived from the study of rural social relationships may be referred to as rural sociology".

According to F.S Chapin, "The sociology of rural life is a study of rural population, rural social organization, and the rural social processes operative in rural society".

According to A.R Desai rural sociology is, "the science of the laws governing the specific Indian rural and social organisation has still to be created. Such a science is, however, the basic premise for the renovation of the Indian rural society, as indispensable for the renovation of the Indian society as a whole".

The above definitions clearly justify that rural sociology studies the social interactions, institutions and activities and social changes that take place in the rural society.

Thus,

- Sociology is the study of human relationships. Rural sociology involves the study of human relationships in rural situations.
- It is the study of man in relation to groups with whom he or she interacts. It is the study of human behaviour that too in groups.

- Human relationships and human interactions are the central core of the field of sociology. Around them are built social groups, organizations, institutions and other components of the structure of society.
- Man lives and interacts within human groups both in his immediate environment and outside of it. Sociology studies man in his group relations.

Major components of society

1. A group of people
2. Lived together long enough to become organized
3. Sharing common interests and values (likeness)
4. Sharing common culture
5. Inter-dependence and
6. Co-operation

Importance and Significance of Rural Sociology in Animal Husbandry Extension

Rural sociology holds immense significance in a county like India that is predominantly agrarian and majority of its population resides in villages. Dependence on agriculture and allied sectors forms the fundamental base of the Indian rural life and it also acts as a backbone for the rural population. It hasnot only an economic role to play but also helps in shaping the moral, psychological and ideological life of the rural people. The major aim of animal husbandry extension is to develop the rural society through a variety of extension programmes. However, the success of the programmes depends on rural population's support, co-operation and participation in these programmes. The knowledge on structure, culture, customs, laws, beliefs of the rural society is very important on the part of the extension workers because these factor affect the attitude, approach behaviour etc. of the rural people. The understanding of rural sociology is very important in animal husbandry extension for the following reasons:

- The basic purpose of animal husbandry extension is changing the behaviour of livestock farmers as desired. Therefore, knowledge and understanding of rural people (livestock farmers) is essential. It is the rural sociology which provides this knowledge and understanding about the farmer vis-à-vis rural social system in which he lives.
- It helps in devising an animal husbandry extension plans for farmers.
- It helps in identifying the groups, individuals, organisations and leaders. Besides this, the interrelationship between animal husbandry extension and rural sociology also highlights the importance or rural sociology in animal husbandry extension.

Relationship between Sociology and Livestock Extension

Livestock extension and rural sociology are extremely close to each other. Both fields are greatly concerned with the study of rural life. However, following are the major points which clearly indicate the relationship.

Rural Sociology	Livestock Extension
Rural sociology is the scientific study of rural man's behaviour in relationship to other groups and individuals with whom he interacts.	Livestock extension is a non-formal education for livestock farmers (rural people) with a view to develop rural society on desirable lines
Rural sociology studies the attitude and behaviour of rural people	Livestock extension seeks to modify or change the attitude and behaviour of farmers
Rural sociology studies the needs and interests of rural society	Livestock extension helps farmers to discover their needs and problems and build educational programmes based on these needs and wants.
Rural sociology analyses rural social relationship or group or organisation and leaders in rural areas.	Livestock extension utilises the knowledge pertaining to groups, organisations and leaders to achieve the objective or livestock development.
Rural sociology studies social situation s and collects social facts of rural society	Livestock extension makes uses of such social data as basis for building up extension programmes for farmers.
Rural sociology investigates the social, cultural, political and religious problems of rural society	Livestock extension also studies these problems with special reference to their impact on agricultural extension work in the village

From the above interrelationship between the rural sociology and livestock extension, one could understand that rural sociology will help the extension agent to identify problems of livestock farmers and develop an extension programme to help in solving the problems. Thus, it can be concluded that both sciences are closely related and benefited with each other by sharing the knowledge of each other.

Society, Community, Association and Institution

Rural sociology is a science of rural society which focuses on certain basic units like society, community, association and institution to understand how human beings live and carry out their activities.

What is Society ?

We, common people, understand society is an aggregation or collection of individuals. But in sociology, it is not only congregation of individuals but the sum total of the relationship between them. Society is a web of social relationships and is always changing. A society is a network of social relationship and individuals in the society are related to each other through the ties of kinship, marriage, religions, groups, etc. Therefore, the sociologists define society as the pattern of social relationships formed through interactions of its members.

Attributes of Society

The main attributes of society are:

a) Likeness and differentiation

b) Inter-dependence

c) Co-operation and conflict

Members of the family and kin group, person belonging to the same group, village, occupation and members of the same caste generally have feeling of likeness.

Members of the society differ from one another in terms of caste, class, occupation, income, education, etc., Even in a family, the members differ from one another in terms of gender, age, personality, outlook and preferences. These differences complement each other in such a way that family stability is maintained.

The members of society depend on one another for its smooth functioning. In a village, you might have seen that washer man, carpenter, cobbler, sweeper, religious leader is doing their own task yet depending upon each other. No individual can perform all functions on one's own. Therefore, individuals depend on each other to live smoothly in society.

The existence of society will be difficult, if the members do not cooperate with each other. Cooperation is obtained at every level in the society like between husband and wife, between neighbours, between group members, etc. Like cooperation, there exist conflict in the society. We may enter in to conflict, if our interests are not met.

What is Community ?

According to sociologists, 'whenever the members of any group, small or large, live together in such a way that they share the basic conditions of a common life, we call that group a community. Thus, community refers to a group of individuals living in a geographical area. Society is an abstract notion, idea or thought whereas community is a concrete entity.

Society-
Abstract notion
Community-
Concrete entity

Characteristics of Community

a) Community refers to an aggregate of individuals

b) Community members have strong community sentiments or sense of belongingness.

c) Community is established over a long period of life

d) community serves wider purposes than the group

What is Association ?

Associations are functional groups that are brought into existence for various but well defined purpose by collective action and functioning. Association is a group of people expressly organised around a particular interest. When a group of people organise itself for the pursuit of some common interests, an association is born. e.g.: Dairy Farmers association for the purpose of sale of milk and milk products, cricket club, farmers' club, Mahila mondal in our neighbourhood.etc.

Characteristics of Association

a) It consists of group of individuals

b) The people are organised

c) There are rules and regulations for governance of the association

d) The members carry out activities to meet the objectives of the association.

Characteristics of Rural Society

Rural society in India has some distinct characteristics. The technological advancement has eroded some of its characteristics, still many of these characteristics are significant. Some of these basic characteristics are listed below:

1. **Occupation:** A sizable number of rural people are engaged in agriculture, which is the mainstay of their lives. In addition, a rural society has several other groups, engaged in various other occupations of arts and crafts, usually known as artisans and craftsmen, who regularly supply their services to agriculturalists in exchange for grains and cereals.
2. **Size of Community :** Usually small scale agriculture demands a higher land to man ratio than industries.
3. **Density of population**: Density of the rural population is low and it may be clustered according to the criteria of social status. The low density brings greater intimacy among the members.
4. **Homogeneity of population**: Rural population is homogenous in terms of occupations, culture, customs etc.

5. **Social differentiation and stratification**: Low degree of social differentiation and stratification due to their homogenous nature.
6. **Social mobility:** Low levels of social mobility in village
7. **Social interaction**: Low levels of interaction (fewer contacts) due to low density of population but rural masses have more primary contacts (informal)
8. **Social control**: High degree of social control. Strict punishments like ostracism for deviation.
9. **Social Solidarity**: More pronounced in rural areas.
10. **Leadership pattern:** Usually traditional and based on known personal qualities of the individual or sometimes hereditary.
11. **Standard of living:** Normally low
12. **Governance:** Rural societies are generally governed by certain regional and local traditions.
13. **Social Institutions** Less enacted social institutions and more informal institutions.

Comparison between Rural, Tribal and Urban Societies

Human beings live in rural and urban societies. There are differences in social life in both the cases. two different environments of rural and urban. Since, there is difference in social life in both environments it is of interest to know the differences. Further, extension workers are concerned themselves to rural environment, they must be in a position to differentiate the rural from urban environment. While comparing and contrasting it has to be kept in mind that both the societies are the part of one human society. As a result of development one particular society assumes the name of rural society while the other becomes urban society. The two societies are basically the same. The difference that exists between the two is of theoretical and academic than the real. A comparison between rural, urban and tribal societies will help us to understand the nature of rural and tribal societies and how they differ from the urban societies.

S.No.	Criteria	Rural Society	Tribal Society	Urban Society
1	Occupation	Predominantly agriculture and allied occupations and artisans Similar type of occupation	Forest and agriculture based operation. Similar type of occupation	Non-agriculture like manufacturing, trade, commerce, professionals, etc. Varied occupation
2	Environment	Direct relationship with nature	Very close to nature	Greater isolation from nature; predominance of man – made environment

3	Heterogeneity and Homogeneity of population	More homogeneity in respect of socio-psychological and other aspects like behaviour, belief, language etc.	Highly homogenous	More heterogeneity
4	Size of community	Small	Very small	Usually larger
5.	Density of population (No. of people/sq. km)	Low	Very low	Very High
6.	Rate of literacy	Medium to high	very low	High
7.	Culture	Conservative and tradition bound Guided by customs and superstitions	Very Conservative and tradition bound Guided by customs, superstitions and blind beliefs	Free from conservation and tradition Free from superstition and customs Influenced by scientific invention which bring about changes in everyday life
8.	Social stratification	Low and follows traditional systems; status determined by birth. It changes with changes in values. Poor becomes rich and thus changes occur in status.	Very low and follow traditional system.	High; stratification on the basis of economic, social, political, educational and other features. Wider gap
9.	Social mobility	Lack of social mobility. People normally do not change their place, occupation, religion, political view etc.	Lack of social mobility and people do not change their settlement	High level of Social mobility.
10.	Systems of interaction	Less contact Narrow area of interaction. More of primary contacts. Predominance of personal contacts.	Very l ess contact Narrow area of interaction. More of primary contacts. Predominance of personal contacts.	Numerous contacts. Wider area of interaction. Predominance of secondary contacts. Impersonal, formal and short- lived relations.
11.	Social control	Informal due to smaller size of community. It is the primary institutions like	Informal due to smaller size of community. Very harsh	More formal because of more laws. Besides primary institutions,

		family and neighbourhood that control life and the society		secondary institutions like economic and other institutions control social life.
12	Social change	Takes place at a very slow rate due to little competition	Takes place at a very slow rate due to little competition	Fast because of stiff competition
13.	Social tolerance and family domination	More due to cultural uniformity, lack of varieties (different castes/religion etc.) and people do not face the new situation	More due to cultural uniformity	Low because people often face new situation, varieties in culture and other aspects.
14.	Family type	Joint	Joint	Mostly nuclear
15.	Status of women	Low, inferior to men, role confined to house, live with serious restrictions	Low, inferior to men	Not so low. Free to take part in outdoor activities. Enjoy a good deal of freedom.
16.	Standard of living	Low to medium	Very low	High
17.	Neighbourhood environment.	Important because rural society's strength is based on co-operation and mutual good will. Generally consists of same caste and economic status.	Generally consists of same caste	No institution like neighbourhood is built. Belong to different castes and economic status.
18.	Leaders	Based on personal qualities	Hereditary	More impersonal leaders.
19.	Solidarity	Stronger, informal	Very strong relationship with the members	Not stronger
20.	Caste	More predominant	Highly predominant. Mostly same type of caste in each settlement	Less predominant
21.	Income	Less	Very less	More
22.	Sense of belonging ness	More	Very high	Less
23.	Migration	People migrate from rural to urban areas	Nomadic or no migration	Low migration
24.	Infrastructure facilities	Poor infrastructure facilities	Very poor infrastructure facilities	Good infrastructure facilities
25.	Level of industrial pollution	Low	Very low	High

Livestock Production Practices in Rural, Urban and Tribal Societies

Differences exist between rural, urban and tribal areas in the animal rearing patterns. These differences stem from the purpose for which the animals are being reared. The table below exhibits the differences in livestock production practices among rural, urban and tribal communities. These differences form the basis for the extension agent to develop suitable programmes which address differential needs of the societies

S.No	Particulars	Rural	Urban	Tribal
1	Purpose	Economic as well as social / religious	Primarily economic	Way of life
2	Number of animals / household	Less (2 to 3)	More (>5)	Less (<3)
3	Quality of animals	Predominantly indigenous	Predominantly cross bred	Indigenous / non-descript
4	Productivity of animals	Low to medium	Medium to high	Very low
5	Dry and wet ratio	High	Low	High
6	Animal sheds	Open yard	Mostly pucca	Open yard
7	Feeding	Mostly grazing	Mostly stall feeding	Grazing
8	Type of feeds	Dry, green fodder with little or no concentrate	Dry fodder with little or no green fodder, concentrate feeding common	Green grasses
9	Management	Less scientific	To a greater extent scientific	Not scientific
10	Adoption of technologies to improve productivity of animals	Low level	Early adoption	No adoption of scientific practices. Adopt traditional practices
11	Cost of production / kg. of milk / meat	Low	High	Meagre
12	Occupation	Traditional	Entrepreneurial	Traditional
13	Profit / unit of milk / meat sold	Marginal or nil	High	Marginal or nil
14	Sentimental attachment with animals	Very much present	Not to that extent as in rural areas	Very much present
15	Person involved in the maintenance of animals	All members of the family / part time	Specific person as full time job	All members of the family
16	Marketing	Own use / vendor / co-operative	Private	Own use. At times do not milk the animas

Social Control

For smooth functioning of any society, it is essential that its members conduct themselves in a manner that is acceptable to other members of the society. Our behaviour is controlled by the norms and customs of the society. Social control is the method of regulating the behaviour of an individual in the society. It is the pattern of influence the society exerts on individuals and groups to maintain order and establish rules in the society. Social control includes those laws by which an individual behaves in concurrence with the mores of the group. It is by the social control that every particular group and individual member outcomes tensions and conflicts. Mannheim has defined social control as," the sum of those methods by which a society tries to influence human behaviour to maintain a given order. The aim of the social control is to bring about conformity in a particular group or society.

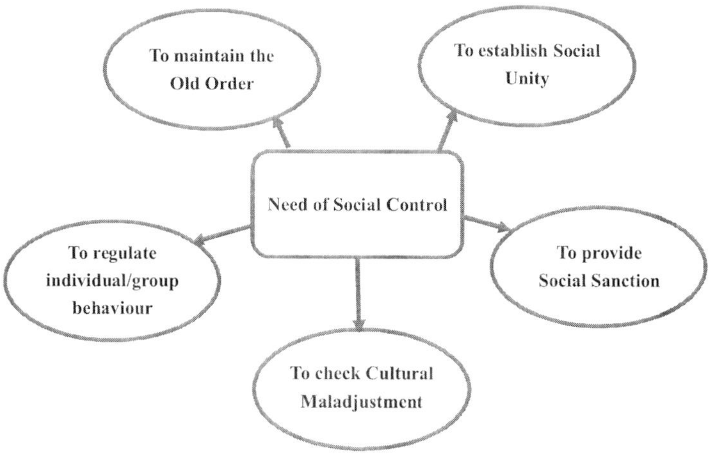

Many eminent sociologists have classified social control mainly as two types.

a. **Informal means of social control (Internal social control)**: These are personal, unofficial and uncodified. It lies within the individual and it is developed during socialisation. This type of social control is maintained by informal mechanisms, i.e. customs, traditions, folkways and religion. These are adopted by means of informal groups.

b. **Formal Social Control (External Social Control) :** This types of social controls are codified, systematic, and with written set of rules. External social controls are formal mechanism enforced by state, government, legitimate institutions to prevent chaos in society. They apply coercion in case of deviance. For instance, a person stolen some one's property may be sentenced to imprisonment. The institutions of the state exercise the legal power to control the behaviour of the individual.

Formal means of Social Controls	Informal means of Social Controls
• Law • Education • Coercion or Physical force	• Social norms • folkways • mores • values • customs • religion • family • peer-group • public Opinion

i) Social Norms

Norms are established behaviour patterns for the members of a social system. It is expected that the members of a society shall follow the norms. A person who deviates from the norm is generally regarded as a deviant by the other members of the system.

Folkways

Folkways are socially acceptable ways of behaviour to which individual conform. It is customary to do so. e.g. Good Manners. Folkways are customary ways of behaviour in society in which society exerts force for conformity. It is not enforced by law or any other agencies of the society. Persons who do not conform may subject to criticism or to be considered strange, but would not necessarily penalised. Folkways are manifested in matters of dress, food, rituals, worships, greetings, etc., For example, in north Indian villages people are expected to enter home only after the removal of shoes.

Mores

Mores are socially acceptable ways of behaviour that do involve moral standards, violation may result in severe social action such as ostracism; e.g., inter-dining of an orthodox high caste Brahmin with an outcaste Hindu Harijan. Mores are the pattern of behaviour considered essential by society. They are rigidly enforced, and if not followed, the individual incurs severe penalty from society. They influence the value system of a society and are in the form of social regulations which aim to maintain social order. Of course, clear lines of distinction between mores and folkways are not often distinguishable, and borderline cases certainly occur.

Custom

Customs are long established practices of people which regulate social life and bind the people. In primitive societies, customs were powerful , means of social control but in modern times, they have weakened due to rise in the force of individualism and diversity.It is a social phenomenon. It refers primarily to practices that have been repeated by a multitude of generations, practices that tend to be followed simply because they have been followed in the past. In a day to day talk custom is used as synonymous with habit, but here are vital differences between the two. Habit is a personal phenomenon while custom is a social phenomenon. Custom is an important mean of controlling social behaviour. They are so powerful that no one can escape their range. There is no country or community wherein customs are not found. In some communities they are regarded so sacred that their violation cannot be even thought of. The society wishes us to follow them. These are socially prescribed forms of behaviour transmitted by tradition and enforced by social disapproval of their violation. In other words, the socially accredited ways of acting are the customs of society. eg. Ways of taking bath, washing, cutting hair, eating, drinking and fasting.

Religion

Religion is the unified system of beliefs and practices related to sacred things. Religion occupies a significant place in the life of an individual and fulfils the spiritual, social and psychological needs of an individual.

Family

Family is the most important institution for social control. Every member learns from its environment, which is first provided by the family. The family socialise the members in to norms, values, traditions and customs of the group.

Neighbourhood

Neighbourhood in the villages comprises people normally belonging to the same kin group or caste. Hence, relationship that exists are intimate and informal. The village neighbourhood is an enthusiastic participant in many daily activities of a family. It thereby fulfils its role as a medium of social control. It ensures conformity and corrects deviant behaviour. For an example, a village neighbours would subject a son not looking after his aging parents to sharp disapproval and even sarcasm.

Laws

Formalized norms with legal and / or political enforcement such as acts, statutes etc. e.g: Laws to prevent cruelty to animals.

Education

Along with law, education has been an important agency od social control. It prepares the individual for social living and teaches him the values of discipline, cooperation, tolerance and integration.

State

State has a vital role in administering social control. State enact different laws and enforce them for wellbeing of its members.

Social Stratification

Social stratification is the division of society into a series of levels indicating positions of individuals and groups in the value system existing in that society. The social groups or individuals are categorised in the societies higher or lower to one another in terms of their relative position on the scale of wealth, power, prestige, privileges. etc., Position in the stratification level denotes 'Status' of the group or individual. Factors influencing social stratification are caste, religion, income, number of family members, land size, animal herd size etc. The societies could be classified into rich and poor; landless, marginal, small and large farmers and the like. Social stratification is a type of social inequality. It refers to the presence of social groups which are ranked one above other, usually with respect to the amount of power, wealth, prestige and status their members possess. Those who belong to a stratum usually share a set of common thoughts and interests. Generally, they also share a similar style of life that distinguishes them from the members located in other strata.

There are three major organizing principles of social stratification. These are. status, wealth and power. Status in the language of social stratification means ranking of groups in a society on the basis of their relative position in terms of honour or respect. Honour is a qualitative attribute which members in a status group enjoy by birth. Any such attribute which is inherited by birth is ascribed and cannot be acquired by effort. Ascribed statuses are given to the individual because of the facts related to his/her birth. In our country, caste is a very appropriate example of status groups. The position which are achieved due to competition is known as achieved status. If a person gets through the Civil Service Examination and becomes a civil servant, then we would say that he has achieved the status.

The groups which had greater control over the economic resources and wealth or which possessed more wealth were ranked higher in society than groups which controlled less of it, or groups which had little or negligible access to wealth (for example, landless workers or industrial workers). Wealth refers to material possessions-such as property, livestock, land, building, jewellery, money, etc., -that are regarded as valuable in most societies. The social stratification based on class is its prime example.

The principles of power in social stratification means having authority by an individual or group or institution in exercising their will on citizen of the society. A relative example could be power of political party, power of state administration, power of individual in different positions, etc.

Caste and Class System in India

Caste and class are principles of social stratification which illustrate respectively the role of status and wealth in the ranking of groups in societies. Caste is a prime example of a status group. Class, on the other hand, is based on the principle where groups are ranked on their access to wealth or their relative ability to have a control upon the wealth resources in society. Caste is different from class. A class is defined in economic terms, whereas caste is understood as a hereditary unit, defined as a way of life. An individual is borne in a class but he always has a chance to improve upon it. Whereas the position of an individual in the caste system is fixed forever. Caste system is close system and class system is open system. In a class system, an individual may work hard, try newer avenues of improving upon his economic condition and move up from lower to middle class and so on. Caste system in India derives its legitimacy from religion. Some of the salient characteristics of caste are mentioned below:

1. Caste system is based on the ideas of purity and pollution
2. Each caste has its own style of living, besides occupation.
3. Each cast has its own complex of gods and goddess, ritual and folklore.
4. Each caste follows certain defined rules of marriage system.

Institutions in Rural Society

We normally mean organisation like hospital, school, panchayat, etc., are institutions. But, in sociology, the meaning of institution is different. In sociology, the institutions refer to established codes of conduct for carrying out group activities. They refer to a set of rules and procedures which provide guidelines for human activities. We consciously or unconsciously imbibe codes of conduct to perform worship, marriage functions, education, etc., in the society. We conduct such a way in the society which is acceptable. We attain a school and learn what to do and what not to do in a society. Institutions are basic constituents of any society and found in all culture and in all societies. There are six primary institutions found in all societies. They are:

a) Social institutions (e.g. family, marriage and kinship)
b) Political institutions
c) Educational institution
d) Economic institutions (e.g. agriculture, livestock, industry or any other)
e) Religion, and
f) Expressive institutions such as music, dance, fine arts, literature, etc.

Social Institutions

a) Marriage

Marriage is a social institution to satisfy physical, psychological, social, cultural and economic needs of men and women. It permits men and women to establish a stable relationship with each other in order to form a family and authorise husband and wife to produce children and engage in many other socioeconomic activities together.

Functions of Marriage

i) Satisfaction of sex: Marriage regularises sexual relations
ii) Procreation and nurturing of children: Procreation and nurturing of children is done in a family set-up, where both the husband and wife together look after their children so that they can survive and become physically and mentally strong.
iii) Economic co-operation and security: The husband and wife look after the economic activities of each other. Together, they take care of their children's economic requirements such as food, clothing, shelter, education, medical and recreational needs and so on.
iv) Companionship and emotional support: Marriage provides a constant companion, a life-partner in the form of husband and wife. They help each other socially, economically and emotionally, in joy and sorrow and develop a better understanding of each other's perspective in managing the family.

b) Family

Every individual in this world is a part of one family or the other. All of us are born and brought up in a family. The family is often the focal point, the centre around which our whole life revolves. Family is the basic unit of society. In its minimal form, family may consist of a husband, wife and children. An adult person is part of two types of families. The family in which one is born is called the family of orientation. A person is identified as son or daughter in this type of family. Such family exerts formative influence on his life and personality.

The family which a person sets up after marriage is called the family of procreation. It is the family in which a married couple gives birth to children and brings them up. The family is the most multifunctional of all institutions in the society and is a system of organised relationships involving workable and dependable ways of meeting basic social needs.

Characteristics of Family

i) Universality: In all society, family is found. It performs biological, economic, social and psychological functions efficiently and simultaneously that it has become indispensable for everyone.

ii) Emotional Basis: Family members are emotionally bound to each other and provide love, care and protection to each other.

iii) Limited Size: A family is basically made up of a husband, wife and their unmarried children.

iv) Nuclear Position in social structure: Family is regarded as basic, nuclear or fundamental to all social groupings.

v) Social Regulations: Family is run according to social norms.

Specifically, family fulfils the following tasks in society.

1. Sex regulation
2. Reproduction and perpetuation of the family and human race.
3. Socialization.
4. Provision of economic maintenance and livelihood.
5. Provision of love, affection and security to the individual and
6. Provision of class status to the individual of the family into which he / she has been born.

Secondary Institutions

1. Engagement,
2. Marriage,
3. Courtship and
4. Relationship with the family into which marriage has taken place.

c) Kinship

Man is social by nature. He establishes many types of relationship with a number of persons. The most important of these relationships is known as kinship. A normal adult male is a son, a brother, a nephew, an uncle and so on. Similarly, a female is a daughter s sister, a wife, a mother and aunt, etc. Such relationships based either on marriage or blood-ties re known as kinship relations.

Economic Institution

Economy is concerned with production, exchange, distribution and consumption of good and services. None of the activities are performed in isolation. For the production of goods, human beings enter in to relations with other human beings.

Political Institution

In each social relationship, there are some who exercise power over others. Polity is concerned with the distribution of power in the society. Power is the ability to take decision for oneself and others, and to see that others abide by the decisions taken on their behalf. Power is central to every group and institution. For example, the principal exercises his or her power, which he or she has by virtue of the head of the institution. But, this power is different from political power. The political power has wider application. It is not confined to a group or institution rather it embraces all of them. Political power is closely connected with governance. It administers the regulatory functions of law and order and maintains security in society.

Religion

In each society, religion is concerned with a set of relations people have with what they regard as 'superior' to them. This superiority entity is not human. It is beyond the world of human beings. That is way the terms used for conveying the superior entities are 'super natural', 'extramundane', and 'spiritual'. These entities are revered, they are worshiped and their favour is sought. People believe in the existence of these powers, which control human affairs. They think that if these powers are worshiped through certain acts such as rites and rituals, etc. Happiness and peace will follow, and their life will be fulfilled. In brief, we may define religion as a set of beliefs and practices dealing with the objects and ideas that people regard as super natural and worthy of worship. The function of religion is to provide means where man can face the crisis with strength and fortitude. Most religions of the world have the following elements:

1. A set of beliefs regarding the ultimate power in the universe.
2. A set of beliefs regarding the ideal and proper pattern of behaviour.
3. A set of ceremonial way of expressing these beliefs.

Secondary institutions of religion - forms of worship and organised groups for propagating religion.

Educational Institution

Educational institutions are those which seek to socialise individuals in society or introduce them in formal ways in to their social and cultural world. Education as an institution in various parts of the world seeks to fulfil its functions of transmission of cultural heritage, social integration of society by moulding the individual to conform with norms, socialisation and personal development in various forms and in various ways that are socially acceptable and culturally defined. Every new generation must be prepared and trained to play a role in society. This process referred as the process of socialisation, commences informally at home and then formally in the institution of education.

Social Change

Human society has always been undergoing change. We have experienced changes not only in our life but also in the family and community. The changes may be social, political, economic, technological and so on. Change can be described as "transformation in the organisation of society and in patterns of thought and behaviour over time" (Macionis, 1987).

Characteristics of Social Change

a) Social Change is Universal

Everything in nature is subject to laws of change. All societies experience change, but each society experiences change at different rates and in different ways. Some societies do not experience many changes, because of conscious effort and/or compulsion of circumstances. The rate of change is believed to be much more rapid in societies which are technologically advanced. Each new major invention, as you might have noticed, brings in major changes.

b) Social Changes are both Unplanned and Planned

Planned changes are brought in the society with deliberate tempts by different agencies, institutions or groups. For example, the planned changes by implementing different developmental programmes in the society by Government. Some changes are unplanned. The industrialisation of a particular area may change the life style of the adjacent community.

Social Change and its Consequences

Whether change is sought or unplanned, all social change involves consequences which may be positive or negative. For example, the introduction of High Yielding Variety programme yielded Green Revolution in the country as positive or anticipated consequence of social change whereas it also produced negative or undesired social consequence like regional disparity in food grain production leading to social unrest.

Social Groups

> **Groups**
>
> Unit of two or more persons in the reciprocal interaction

Human beings live in society and can not lead an isolated life. They need to have people around them with whom they can share their problems, happiness, ideas, experiences, etc. They look for company. Therefore, human beings are social animals. Every human being from birth until he dies is associated with one or other group, by one or the other ways. These groups directly or indirectly have impact on the psychology of an individual. These groups influence the attitudes, thinking and behaviour of the people throughout the life period. These groups deeply influence the development of the personality and play a role in the socialisation. Every individual is born in the family. Afterwards, other groups outside the family interact with various ways. From birth period and from family he interacts with neighbourhood, school, community and outer society. These groups contact, expands outward as individual develop and assumes various roles as a member of the society.

What is a Group ?

A social group is a unit of two or more persons in the reciprocal interaction or communication with each other. It establishes social relationships among the members. We live in a groups such as family; we belong to groups like caste, clan, profession, etc. Persons in all socities are involved in several forms of interaction.

Characteristics of a Social Group

a. **Number of person:** A group always consists of at least two or more persons.

b. **Membership Consciousness:** Each member is conscious of his or her membership in his or her group.

c. **Communication:** Each group must have a communication and interaction among its members. The communication among the members should be always two ways. One-way communication does not constitute the group interaction, which should influence each other. The duration of the group exists only as long as there is reciprocal psychological interaction. Continuity of a culture from one generation to other helps for the formation of a group.

d. **Organised Structure:** Every group is structurally organised

e. **Common goals and interest:** Common interests, shared values and norms may be important constituents of a group.

f. **Nomenclature:** Each group is normally known by a name

g. **Group Norms:** Each group has its own rules and norms, which the members are expected to follow,

h. **Belongingness:** The formation of group is affected by many forces i.e. blood, marriage, religion, caste, common possessions, common areas, common interacts, responsibilities and occupation etc.

i. **Reciprocal Relations:** The members of the group are reciprocally related to each other.

Types of Groups

Based on the presence or absence of formal rules, groups could be classified as formal group or informal group. For an example, family is an informal group while school as formal group. However, social groups are classified as primary, secondary and tertiary group based on the nature of contacts. Social groups are classified on the basis of their structure and functions. The nature and characteristics of the different groups are discussed below.

a) Primary and Secondary Groups

The persons in the primary group have face to face relationships, such as family and playgroup. A secondary group is one where the relationships are indirect. The members of secondary group have little personal affection and their relationships are governed by the fulfilment of some objectives. The specific characteristics of primary and secondary groups are compared here

S.No	Primary groups	Secondary groups
1.	Small, mostly less than 20 to 30 persons are members	Larger in size
2.	Personal and intimate relationships among the members	Impersonal relationships with little personal affection
3.	Face to face interactions	Contact through mostly other communication media
4.	Mostly permanent membership	Temporary membership
5.	Relations among the members mostly informal	The relation is mostly formal
6	Physical proximity of the memebrs is more close	Physical proximity of the members is less close
7	Diffused interest	Specific interest
8.	Rural society	Urban society

b) Tertiary Group

These groups comprise of many groups having similar character and the contact or interaction is only notional in character. For an example, Federation of SHG groups, Federation of labour unions.

c) Formal and Informal Groups

This classification is based on mode of organisation and functions of group.

i) **Formal:** These groups have a name, title, written purposes and place. There are definite rules and procedures, awards and punishments and standard discipline is followed here. For example, Self Help Group, Poultry Group, etc.

ii) **Informal:** Informal groups like friends, neighbours, community members do not have such characteristics. There is no organization, rules etc. and no definite mode of functions is followed here.

d) Reference group

This is a group of persons whom an individual consult before taking an important decision. Here the members may be form primary, secondary, formal and informal groups. Sometime an individual may not have reference group, but may be consulting some experienced person in a society to seek the advice.

e) Cultural Interest Group

These groups are created for the development of special interest like economic, religious, political, educational, or recreational interest etc.

f) Temporary and Permanent Groups

Group for short period is called temporary group i.e. Crowd. The groupings living in a common geographic area for longer period are called as permanent group i.e. Village, State, Religion, Tribe etc.

g) Classification on the basis of the structure of the Groups

i) **Horizontal Group:** Horizontal group is that type of group who interacts among each other without giving significance to hierarchy. For example, a group of friends or peer groups

ii) **Vertical Group:** Vertical group refers to that organised aggregate of individuals who interacts among each other with a conscious sense of hierarchy. For example, class, cast and bureaucracy.

iii) **In-groups and out-groups:** In-groups refers to that aggregate of members who interact with a sense of intra-group solidarity. These member possess prejudices and superiority-inferiority complex towards several other groups, which are called 'outgroups'. For example, in a village upper caste and lower caste are 'in groups' in themselves but for one another each becomes an out-group. In general sense, in groups are called 'we-group' and out-groups are called 'they-groups'. These two groups differ on the basis of feelings.

iv) **Ephemeral group or chance group and Enduring group:** These are the groups based on duration. For example, farmers meet in exhibition ground is an ephemeral group. The enduring group is one, which continues for a longer period of time. For example, goat producers' group.

v) **Open Group and Closed Group:** Open groups are those where membership is voluntary and mobility of members is possible. For an example, football club.

In closed groups, membership is restricted and mobility is relatively difficult. For an example, caste group.

Difference between Group and Society

Group	Society
A collection of human beings	A system of social relationship
an artificial creation	A spontaneous and natural growth
Group is organised	Society is loose collection of groups
Group may be temporary	Society is permanent
Group is concrete aggregation	Society is an abstract concept of peple
Group is marked by 'we feeling'	A sense of belongingness

Difference between Group and Community

Group	Community
It is created	It grows naturally and is also created
Comparatively temporary	Comparatively permanent
Group is a part of community	Community consists of many groups

Socialization

Socialization is a process by which people acquire the attitudes, values and actions appropriate to individuals as members of a particular society. Society forms and instils the rules and regulations of the society to which he / she belong. For an example, we show our respect to elders by touching their feet, greet them with folded hands and simply bowing down our heads before them. These behaviours we learn from the society in the process of socialisation. Socialization occurs through human interaction. We learn a great deal from our family members, best friends, teachers and all those for whom we nurture affection and respect other. We also learn, though to a limited extent, from the people on the street, characters, portrayals, and depictions of characters in films and magazines and other sources. By interacting with people, as well as, through our own observations, we learn how to behave 'properly' and what to expect from others if we follow (or challenge) society's norms and values.

It involves the development of

- Personality
- Attitudes
- Habits
- Expected social roles

Social Process

Social processes are the ways in which individuals and groups interact, adjust and readjust and establish relationships and pattern of behaviour which are again modified through social interactions. The meaning of social interaction is that as man is a social animal, it is difficult for him to live in isolation. They always live in groups. As members of these groups they act in a certain manner. Their behaviour is mutually affected. This interaction or mutual activity is the essence of social life. Social life is not possible without interactions. The four basic forms of social processes are:

1. Cooperation

Cooperation is one of fundamental processes of social life. It is a form of social process in which two or more individuals or groups work together jointly to achieve common goals. Cooperation is the form of social interaction in which all participants benefit by attaining their goals. The term 'cooperation' has been derived from two Latin words – 'Co' meaning 'together and Operation meaning 'to work'. Hence, cooperation means working together for the achievement of a common goal or goals. When two or more persons work together to gain common goal, it is called cooperation.

2. Accommodation

Adjustment is the way of life. It can take place in two ways such as adaptation and accommodation. Adaptation refers to the process of biological adjustment. Accommodation, on the other hand, implies the process of social adjustment. "Accommodation is the achievement of adjustment between people that permits harmonious acting together in social situation. It is achieved by an individual through the acquisition of behaviour patterns, habits and attitudes which are transmitted to him socially. It is a process through which individuals or groups make adjustment to the changed situation to overcome difficulties faced by them. Sometimes new conditions and circumstances arise in the society. Individuals have learned to make adjustment to the new situation. Thus, accommodation means adjusting oneself to the new environment.

3. Competition

Competition is one of the dissociative from of social processes. It is actually the most fundamental form of social struggle. It occurs whenever there is an insufficient supply of anything that human beings desire, in sufficient in the sense that all cannot have as much of it as they wish. Competition is considered to be very healthy and a necessary social process. It is indispensable in social life. It has played a major role in the survival of human beings. It is the basic law of life. It is extremely dynamic. It performs both positive and negative functions. They are mentioned below:

Positive functions

a) Assignment of right individual to proper place
b) Source of motivation
c) Conducive to progress

Negative functions

a) Competition may lead to frustration
b) Competition may lead to monopoly
c) Competition may lead to conflict

4. Conflict

Conflict is one of the dissociative or disintegrative social processes. It is a universal and fundamental social process in human relations. Conflict arises only when the attention of the competitors is diverted from the object of competition to themselves. As a process, it is the anti-thesis of cooperation. It is a process of seeking to obtain rewards by eliminating or weakening the competitors. It is a deliberate attempt to oppose, resist or coerce the will of another or others. Conflict is a competition in its occasional, personal and hostile forms. Conflict is also goal oriented. But unlike cooperation and competition, it seeks to capture its goal by making ineffective the others who also seek them.

Type of Conflict

Conflict expresses itself in thousands of ways and various degrees and over every range of human contact. There are two fundamental types of conflict. Direct and Indirect conflict.

i) Direct Conflict

When a person or a group injures, thwarts or destroys the opponent in order to secure a goal or reward, direct conflict occurs; such as litigation, revolution and war.

ii) Indirect Conflict

In indirect conflict, attempts are made by individuals or groups to frustrate the efforts of their opponents in an indirect manner. For example, when two manufacturers go on lowering the prices of their commodities till both of them are declared insolvent, indirect conflict in that case take place.

Culture

Concept of Culture

Culture is an integral part of our existence. Yet, it is different from people to people. We can understand culture better with the following example: whenever we meet our elders, we offer respect by touching elders' feet. When we meet our friend we greet him with folded hands. Shaking hands, hugging and kissing are different ways of greeting friends and relatives in the western world. Our culture makes us Indian and distinguishes us from the American or the German. Thus, culture is the distinguishing element of the society or group. Culture is a way of life that is common to a group of people. It includes a collection beliefs and attitudes, shared understandings and patterns of behaviour. Culture is one of the most important constituent as well as tool of the study of sociology. Our society is continuously changing, new ideas and experiences are acquired by the units of the society. These experiences or learned behaviour are shared by the members in the society. The culture is the sum total of the thought and behaviour, leading to total way of life of people in society. Therefore, culture may be defined as, "socially standardized ways of feeling, thinking and acting, which an individual acquires as a member of the society". It is the continually changing patterns of learned behaviour and the products of learned behaviour (including attitudes, values, knowledge and material objects), which are shared by and transmitted among the members of society." [Cuber, 1968]. It is not merely customs, though customs are a part of culture. In other words, "culture is that complex whole which includes knowledge, beliefs, arts, morals, laws, customs an any other capabilities and habits acquired by man as a member of society".

Characteristics of Culture

i. It is dynamic in nature: continuously changing.

ii. It is a learned behaviour. An individual learns the various ways of thinking, values and attitudes from the family itself.

iii. It is an organization of phenomena of acts (pattern of behaviour), objects (tools, things made with tools), ideas and sentiments. Because of this character, culture is easily and readily transmitted from one human organism to another.

iv. It satisfies ones biological and socio-cultural needs, not only for food, shelter and clothing but various relationships.

v. It is integrative in nature. Some forces may sometime tend to pull it in different directions, even there is a general tendency towards integration, so that the society is held together.

vi. It is adaptive to various external forces. It must try to maintain its structure and functions in spite of all external forces.

vii. It builds certain norms, rules and actions for creating harmony among various members of a particular group or society. As it provides common interests and needs. It helps the individual to come closer in touch to share their various day to day interests.

viii. Culture is reality of human beings; it produces informal attachments with other members of the same group.

ix. Only human being possess the culture, other animals do not possess it. Man has created the culture during the process of controlling himself, others and nature.

x. All the societies in the world have culture but each society has a different culture from one another. Indian culture – African culture – Western culture.

xi. Culture is learned or acquired after birth and through life consciously or unconsciously through agents influencing directly or indirectly on individuals. It is not innate.

xii. Culture is a social and not individual heritage of man. One has to learn the tradition, customs as the society in which he is living.

xiii. Culture is transmitted from one generation to another generation during the process of socialization and is disseminated among members of society.

xiv. Culture is adoptive – It must adjust itself to external forces of various kinds.

xv. Culture is integrative – culture has general tendency towards consistency and integration so as to held society together.

xvi. Culture is idealistic – it stands for ideal norms of human behaviour toward which persons are expected to strive.

xvii. Culture is shared – Learned behavior and products of learned behavior is nor exclusive property of a single individual or group but belong to all members of society and are shared by a large proportion of the.

xviii. Culture is gratifying. It satisfies the man's bio-logical and socio-culture needs- foods, clothing, shelter and for various relationship with other individuals and group.

xix. Culture is accumulating. It goes on increasing in size, act to the funds of his knowledge, regarding the science or literature in each generation. This knowledge is preserved in the form of books, films and pictures.

Functions of Culture

1. Culture provides us with design for living. It is always learned and acquired.
2. Culture provides a series of pattern by which biological and socio-cultural demands of group members are met e.g. food, shelter, and reproduction and relationship with group and individuals.
3. Culture provides a set of rules to ensure co-operation of the individuals of a group in adjusting environmental situation.
4. Culture provides individual a set of ready-made definition of situation.
5. Culture helps in understanding and predicting the human behavior and also it provides channels of interaction for individuals within the group.
6. Culture provides us a guidepost or kind of map for all our life activities. It defines the pattern of behavior for individuals so that he acts according to the behavior pattern prescribed and defined by culture.
7. Culture acts as a means of social control through norms, folkway, and moves laws.

Thus, culture functions to deeply influence control and direct behaviour and life of the individual and of group. All these functions are controlled through norms or rules made in society. These norms may be governed by sanctions or punishment, so the study of norms, mores, folkways, laws etc. is necessary for knowing the culture of society.

Terms associated with Culture

a) Culture area

Geographic area within which culture exists.

b) Culture trait

Simplest functional unit into which culture may be divided and is defined as a 'reportedly irreducible unit of learned behaviour pattern or material product thereof'. e.g., a dhothi, a sari, a bamboo pen are examples of material culture trait whereas bowing slightly in respectful greeting to an elder is a non-material trait.

c) Culture complex

Organization of culture traits around one dominant trait. It is a group or cluster of related traits. eg.' the sacred thread ceremony in a Hindu Brahmin home involving a large number of related culture traits.

d) Culture pattern

It is a group of culture complexes, formed in the same way to form a complex culture.

e) Culture lag

The term cultural lag refers to a situation when ideas, values and norms and beliefs used to regulate social life do not keep pace with changes in the technology of society. Time difference between some technological change and the resulting change in culture is termed as cultural lag.

f) Material Culture

Material culture refers to the tangible aspects of culture, those things that can be seen or touched; e.g. temples, bridges, furniture etc.

g) Non-material culture

Non material culture consists of the abstract aspects of culture, which cannot be directly seen or touched; e.g. values, folkways, ways of thinking and feeling etc.

h) Cultural Integration

Cultural integration is the blending of two or more different cultures that happens without one of the cultures sacrificing the characteristics that make it unique. The exchanges include a culture's popular beliefs, rituals and practices.Cultural integration is considered to be a positive thing. This is because it doesn't involve taking anything away from one culture. This type of integration lets people from different cultures blend their beliefs and their rituals into a cohesive new unit without giving up anything. Times to find cultural integration in practice include when people from one culture move into a culturally different community, when people from different cultures marry or when people from different cultures work together. The times when cultural integration is seen as negative include times when it is a forced situation.

i) Ethos

The term 'ethos' is used to signify those traits that are characteristic of, or peculiar to a particular culture, which may be used to differentiate one culture from another. eg. In USA- Mechanization and mass production. In India- handicrafts and cottage industries, production by masses.

j) Ethnocentrism

This term means the preferential feeling we have for the way we do things in our culture. It is the tendency of man to consider his own culture of high value and superior to all others, and to judge other cultures in terms of standards and values that exist in one's own culture. We assume that ours is the best of all cultures, and the way we do things is the right way to do them. This is common characteristic found among peoples of all cultures.

k) Taboo

Taboo refers to anything (food, place, activity) which is prohibited and forbidden. The observance of a taboo has the social sequence of binding a social group together behind common rituals and sentiments. The taboo is a symbol of group membership.

l) Ritual

Ritual is any formal action, following a set pattern, which express through symbol in public or shared. Rituals are typically the practical aspects of a religious system and they express sacred values rather than seek to achieve some utilitarian end. For example, ritual is often used to refer to any regular pattern of interaction – 'how do you do?' As a routine method of starting conservation it could be regarded as ritual of everyday interaction.

m) Conventions

Conventions are customs regulating more significant social behaviour. e.g. Being polite to others. Conventions are violated less often than folkways on usages and the sanctions are more severe.

n) Tradition

Tradition refers to any human practice, belief, in-situation or artifact which is handed down from generation to the next. While the content of tradition is highly variable, it typically refers to some element of culture regarded as part of the common inheritance of a social group. Tradition is often regarded as a source of social stability and legitimacy. But, appeal to tradition may also provide basis for changing the present.

Role of Cultural Concepts in Livestock Extension

Cultural concepts are important tools for understanding and analyzing society. Before starting any development programme, extension worker analyze the situation, where programme has to be executed. Cultural concepts have practical implications for programmes of promoted change such as rural community development. In this way cultural concepts play a role in livestock extension and extension worker cannot ignore their importance and role in their developmental programmes. Most of the livestock farm practices are inherited from past. We have to understand the importance of old practices in the context of rural culture and try to find out the compatibility methods to improve the practices for better income of the farming communities.

Social Value and Attitudes

The function of extension education is to bring about desirable changes in the behaviour ofpeople. The overt behaviour or what we call as action is based on attitude. Unlike action,attitude cannot be seen. They can only be inferred by way of tendency to act or react positively or negatively to some stimuli. These tendencies or attitudes in turn are based upon individual's values. Social values are ideas which help an individual to discriminate whether a particularobject or behaviour is good or bad, desirable or undesirable. There are at times rules whichgovern the action which is known as "Norms". People are expected to behave in accordancewith the values held by the individual and in the expected behaviour which is known as "normative behaviour". Social values constitute what is right and important in society. Those feelings which constitute assumption of what is right and important are abstract and often unconscious. The sharing of feeling or attitudes is of vital importance to the operation and functioning of society. Attitudes held by society that define what society considers correct and of relative importance are referred to as social values.

Values

> **VALUES**
> Abstract, hierarchical and dynamic concepts that essentially describe what we desire or seek to achieve.

Values are the basis for our behaviour and motivation. Values are abstract, hierarchical and dynamic concepts that essentially describe what we desire or seek to achieve. We may hold values such as "loyalty", "truthfulness", "charity", "service" and many others. When we say we hold a value, what we are really saying is that we aspire to something, or we feel that value is worth something to us. So if we say that we hold "charity" as a value we are saying that we aspire to be charitable, even at personal cost. However, values are an abstract concept. You may have a very good idea of what it means to be charitable. But the idea of charity hold from another person may be very different than yours. Everyone has an internalized system of beliefs and values that they have developed throughout their lives. These may stem from religion or may develop separately to religion.

In summary, it can be said that beliefs and values are different concepts. Values represent our aims, desires, and goals. They are usually abstract, and are further defined by criteria. Beliefs are judgments that connect our values and criteria to our experiences, in other words are convictions that we generally hold to be true, usually without actual proof or evidence. They give our experiences meaning, and provide context for our values. Both values and beliefs shape the way we view ourselves and the world around us. They act as filters for our perceptions, and actually create our maps of reality. They literally make our reality, and make us who we are. For this reason:

1. Beliefs are concepts that we hold to be true.
2. Beliefs may come religion, but not always.
3. Values are ideas that we hold to be important.
4. Values govern the way we behave, communicate and interact with others
5. Beliefs and values determine our attitudes and opinions.

Social values have been defined in various ways by sociologists.

According to Rogers, "abstract and often unconscious assumption of what is right and wrong.

Social values are attitudes, held by individuals, groups or society as a whole, as to whether material or non-material objects are good, bad, desirable or undesirable.

Type of Values

Value may be classified in different ways. **Fraenkel** (1976) classified as:

Moral Value : Deciding particular alternative as better than other because of its just or humane

Real Value : Deciding based on real worth in terms of legal, aesthetic, etc.

Market Value : Based on how much can be paid- value in terms of price

Personal Value : Based on ones likes and preferences over things of similar nature

Instrumental Value : Based on some standards that help us to achieve or acquire other values

Spranger classsified value as like:

Theoretical value : Expressed in the urge for discovery of truth

Economic value: Based on the criteria of usefulness

Aesthetic Value: Based around form and harmony

Social Value : Referring to interest of people on others

Political Value : Centre round power

Religious Value : Meaning therby a mystic sense of utility

Types of Social Values

Ultimate Values

These are often referred to as dominant values. These values constitute the core of society's value system. Ultimate values express the general views of society and found most easily in social institutions such as family, religion and government. These are abstract and often not attainable.

Intermediate Values

Intermediate values are derived from ultimate values and can be categorised into more reasonably attainable category e.g. freedom of speech, religious freedom, free public education, non-discrimination, housing etc. in framework of social institutions such as religion, government and education.

Specific Values

The sub-division of in values are called specific values and are almost unlimited in members. Specific values must be in conformity with the total value system of which they form the smallest unit.

Socio-psychological determinants of values

People will be eager to change and many times they accept changes, when changesgive prestige to them and/or increase their socio-economic changes. Though change iscommon every idividual will not accept changes. Only some individuals accept the changes.

An analysis of factors that influences the changes were studied by Reddy (1987). They arecaste of the individual, age, possession of land and type of tenure, wealth and economicposition, hard work and physical stamina, personal characteristics like truthfulness, honesty,reliability etc. These factors have obvious implications in the introduction of improvedpractices.

Major values prevailing

1. **Importance of described status :** Status of individual in a group is decided by the group to which he belongs. There is an established order of hierarchy of casts in Indian society.

2. **Recognition of inequality :** Still exists on caste basis
3. **Patrilineal tendency :** Eldest male member of the family has supreme power and tends to act automatically
4. **Status of women :** Though there is tendency to give greater respect they are still inferior to men.
5. **Charity :** There is religious significance and approval for giving of alms. A person with a charitable disposition is respected.
6. **Tendency of non-violence :**Killing of animals except for the purpose of food is considered to be immoral. It sometimes brings conflict.
7. **Respect to old age and elders :** They are generally given respect and recognition.
8. **Religious attitude :** People in rural areas are religious.

Role of Values in Livestock Extension

We have already seen that culture of the people is changing and it is dynamic. The development workers or extension workers are the major strongest forces to bring changes in the culture of rural India. In fact, community development programmes are the promotion of cultural changes among rural people towards desired goals. Accepted on that irrespective of the involvement of extension workers the changes happen. But the desired changes in the direction deemed desirable by the government in the rural society only when extension workers are involved the change agents. Scientific understanding of culture of people among whom extension work operate helps the effective functioning by these workers. This is particularly significant in countries like India. For instance, piggery is not introduced in Muslim areas, poultry farming in Brahmin areas, and the like. Thus, the study on caste structure would reveal certain types of improvements of change. Religious festivals and other local functions form important part of village life. Extension workers can look upon these festivals and melas as potentially useful for technology transfer through exhibition, demonstration, etc. It is generalised that greater success may be anticipated when a new improved practice is introduced in familiar terms something that is already present in the culture. Change is more likely to occur where there is lack of adjustment. For example, when poultry birds are wiped out due to Ranikhet Disease outbreak, that would be an opportunity for the livestock extension worker to introduce the concept of vaccination. There would be less resistance to the introduction. Recently coloured birds are becoming popular in village due its colour liked by the buyers. These are good examples of how the value factor changes due to the influence of extension activities.

Attitude

Attitude is of feeling of like, dislike, attraction, repulsion, interest or apathy toward other persons, objects, situation or ideas. Attitudes are essentially acquired and learned. Learning or acquisition or attitudes may be conscious or unconscious. Attitudes involve some knowledge of a situation. However, the essential aspect of the attitude is found in the fact that some characteristic feeling or emotion is experienced and, as we would accordingly expect, some definite tendency to action is associated. Subjectively, then, the important factor is the feeling or emotion. Objectively, it is the response, or at least the tendency to respond. Attitudes are important determinants of behaviour. If we are to change them, we must change the emotional components. Attitude as a mental and neutral state of readiness organized through experience, exerting a directive or dynamic influence upon the individual's response to all objects with which it is related .A farmer may vote for a particular political party because he has been brought up to believe that it is "right" party. In the course of experience, he may learn something about the policies of that party. In that case his attitude will probably change. As a result, he may be expected to vote in a different way. Knowledge, attitude and behaviour are then very closely linked.

Attitude change

Well established attitudes tend to be resistant to change, but others may be more amenable to change. Attitudes can be changed by a variety of ways. Some of the ways of attitude change are as follows:

1. By obtaining new information from other people and mass media, resulting in changes in cognitive component of a person's attitudes.
2. Attitudes may change through direct experience.
3. Attitudes may change through legislation.
4. Since person's attitudes are anchored in his membership group and reference groups, one way to change the attitude is to modify one or the other.
5. Attitude change differs with reference to the situation also.

Suggested Readings and References

1. A.R. Desai: Rural Sociology; Popular Prakashan, Mumbai.
2. Gough, Kathleen (1981). Rural Society in South India. Cambridge: Cambridge University Press.
3. Mukherjee, Ramkrishna (1979). Sociology of Indian Sociology. Allied Publishers, Bombay.

4. Sharma K.C. (1997). Rural Sociology in India; Rural Publication; New Delhi
5. Vasant Desai: *A* Study of rural economics; Himalaya Publishing Company; New Delhi.
6. Srinivas M. N.: Social Change in Modern India; Orient Black Swan, New Delhi.
7. David G Mandelbaum: Society in India; Popular Prakashan, Mumbai.
8. P. Gisbert: Fundamentals of Sociology; Orient Black Swan Pvt. Ltd., New Delhi.
9. Breman, J., P. Kloos, and A. Saith. (eds.), (1997). The Village in Asia Revisited. Delhi: Oxford University Press.
10. Madan, Vandana (ed.), (2002). The Village in India. Oxford University Press: New Delhi.
11. Beteille, Andre (1986). Studies in Agrarian Social Structure. Oxford University Press: Delhi.
12. Anderson, M. (ed.) (1980), [1971]. Sociology of the Family. Penguin Books: Harmondsworth.
13. Chakravorty, C., and A.K. Singh (1991). Household Structures in India. Census of India, occasional Peper 1. Census of India: New Delhi.
14. Dube, L. (1974). Sociology of Kinship. Popular Prakashan: Bombay.
15. Karve, Irawati (1953). Kinship Organization in India. Deccan College Monograph Series: Poona.
16. Jha, Hetukar (1991). Social Structure of Indian Villages: A Study of Rural Bihar. New Delhi: sage Publications.
17. Sharma, K.L. (ed.), (2001). Social Inequality in India. Jaipur and New Delhi: Rawat Publications
18. Srinivas, M.N. (1996). Village, Caste, Gender and Method. Delhi: Oxford University Press.
19. Baradwaj, A.N. (1985). Problems of Scheduled Castes and Scheduled Tribes in India. New Delhi: Light and Life Publications.
20. Rath, R. (1995). Reservation and Social Transformation Among Scheduled Castes and Scheduled Tribes. New Delhi: InterIndia Publications.
21. Dube, L. (1974). Sociology of Kinship. Popular Prakashan: Bombay.
22. Singh, S. (1987). Scheduled Castes of India, Dimensions of Social change. Delhi: Gian Publishing House.

9

Diffusion and Adoption of Livestock Innovation

1. Diffusion and Adoption process
2. Diffusion
3. Diffusion process
4. What is an Innovation ?
5. Diffusion of Innovations
6. Elements of Diffusion of Innovation and their Functions
    a. Innovation
    b. Attributes of Innovation
        i. Relative Advantage
        ii. Compatibility
        iii. Complexity
        iv. Trialability
        v. Observability
        vi. Predictability
    c. Communication Channels
    d. Time
        i. Innovation – Decision Process
        ii. Innovativeness
        iii. Innovation's Rate of Adoption
    e. Social System
7. System norms
8. Reinvention:
9. Forced discontinuance
10. Consequences of Innovation
    a. Desirable versus undesirable consequences
    b. Direct versus indirect consequences
    c. Anticipated versus unanticipated consequences

11. Adoption process
12. Stages in Adoption Process
    a) Awareness Stage
    b) Interest Stage
    c) Evaluation Stage
    d) Trial Stage
    e) Adoption Stage
13. Other Models of Adoption Process
14. Skipped Stages of Adoption
15. Adoption Period
16. Innovation – Decision Process

a. Knowledge stage
b. Persuasion Stage
c. Decision Stage
d. Implementation Stage
e. Confirmation Stage

17. Dissonance
18. Discontinuance
19. Over adoption
20. Innovation – Decision Period
21. Sources of information (communication media) in adoption process
22. Sources of information in Innovation-Decision Process
23. Innovativeness and Adopter Categories
    a. Innovativeness
    b. The S-shaped Curve of Adoption and Normality
24. Classification of adopter categories
    a. Innovators: Venturesome
    b. Early Adopter: Respectable
    c. Early Majority: Deliberate (Local Adoption Leaders)
    d. Late Majority: Skeptical
    e. Laggards: Traditional
25. Factors influencing in adoption of improved AH Practices
26. Opinion Leadership and Change Agents
27. Suggested Readings and References

Diffusion and Adoption of Livestock Innovations

One of the important functions of livestock extension worker is communication. This communication is not mearly informing the livestock owners about the improved technologies and practices, but to ensure the application of technologies for their benefits. Livestock extension worker's efficency are always judged and measured (a) by the speed or quickness with which the gap between what is known and what is done by the livestock farmers is bridged, (b) by the number of new practices adopted; and (c) also by the number of livestock farmers and communities that adopt the new practices. While discharging the technology dissemination function, livestock extension worker often faces with some of the difficult questions:

1. Why there is lag between what is known and what is done by most farmers?
2. Where do most farmers get their new ideas?
3. Why some farmers accept new ideas and put them into practice faster than others?
4. Why some new ideas and practices are accepted quickly and with little apparent efforts, while others are accepted only after years of effort put forth by extension agencies?
5. Why, in spite of best efforts, all the livestock farmers do not acept the technologies?
6. Why some of ideas are more popular and ready accepted by the livestock farmers, while some other ideas are not accepted ?

Diffusion and Adoption Process

Diffusion of Innovations is a theory that seeks to explain how, why, and at what rate new developmental ideas, practices and technology spread through the social system. The concept was first studied by the French sociologist Gabriel Tarde (1890) and by German and Austrian anthropologists such as Friedrich Ratzel and Leo Frobenius. In 1962 Everett Rogers, a professor of rural sociology published 'Diffusion of Innovations'. In this book, Rogers synthesized research from over 508 diffusion studies and produced a theory for the adoption of innovations among individuals and organizations.

Diffusion

Diffusion is the process by which an innovation is communicated through certain channels over time among the members of a social system.It is a special type of communication, in that the messages are concerned with new ideas. It is this 'newness' of the idea in the message content of communication that gives diffusion its special character. The diffusion of innovations is essentially a social process in which subjectively perceived information about a new idea is communicated.

Diffusion Process

Diffusion of innovations refers to the spread of those innovations through a population, and is simply the result of a host of individual adoption decisions. If individual adoption decisions are, to an extent, predictable, then the larger diffusion process is also predictable. It follows a pattern, and that element of predictability has substantial implications. Therefore, the diffusion process can be explained with the terms given by Rogers as "the spread of a new idea from its source of invention or creation to its ultimate use of adopters". The diffusion of innovations is essentially a social process in which subjectively perceived information about a new idea is communicated.

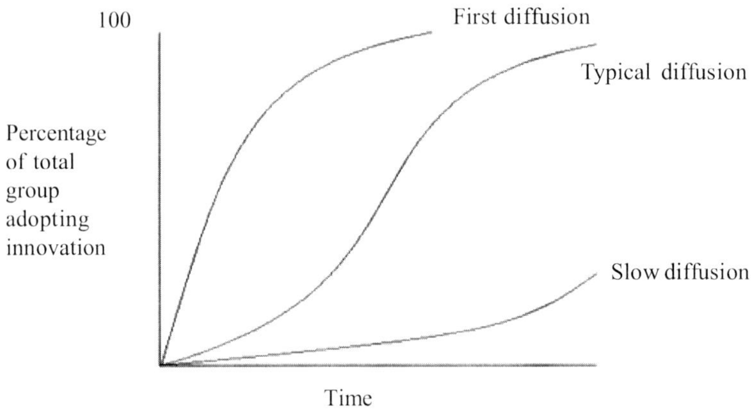

The Diffusion process

What is an Innovation ?

An innovation is an idea, practice or object that is perceived as new by an individual or other unit of adoption. Perception is an activity through which an individual becomes aware of objects around oneself and of events taking place. The technologies, practices developed through research are innovations. These may be new breeds of livestock, new medicines, new technique of doing things etc.Farmers themselves may develop some new practices, which are also innovations. Irrespective of the time period the idea or practice was originally developed, when a person first become aware of it, it is an innovation to that person.

> **Innovation**
>
> Idea, practice or object that is perceived as new by an individual or other unit of adoption.

Diffusion of Innovations

The process by which an innovation spreads within a social system is called "diffusion". An innovation, however, diffuse within a social system through its "adoption" by individual and groups.Diffusion and adoption are thus closely interrelated even though they are conceptually distinct.It takes time for an innovation to diffuse throughout a social system. There is variation among the memebrs of the social system in the way they respond to the new idea or practice.

Elements in the Diffusion of Innovations and their Functions

The diffusion is the process by which an innovation is communicated through certain channels over time among the members of a social system. There are four main elements that influnces the spread of new idea are :

1. Innovation
2. Communication channels
3. Time
4. Social System

Types of Innovations

There are three main types of innovations that are diffused in different ways:

a) Continuous Innovation

This type of innovation is a simple changing or improving of an already existing product where the adopter still uses the product in the same fashion as they had before. An example of a continuous innovation is now seen in the dairy implements industry as it continues to change and develop.

b) Dynamically Continuous Innovation

Here the innovation can either be a creation of a new product or a radical change to an existing one. Here the consumption patterns of people are altered some. An example of this type of innovation would be android mobile.

c) Discontinuous Innovation

This is a totally new product in the market. This is the big idea innovation. In this situation, because the product has never been seen before, there are total changes to consumers buying and using patterns.

1. Innovation

Rogers defined an innovation is an idea, practice, or object that is perceived as new or an improvement over the existing one by the individual or members of a social system. The 'idea' constitutes the central element of an innovation which often manifests itself in a material or behavioural form.

Examples for Material Form : Improved cattle feed, Milking machine, New deworming medicine, etc.

Examples for Behavioural Form: Improved animal husbandry practices.

An innovation do not diffuse at the same rate. An innovation which represents only a slight modification of an existing idea or practice will obviously diffuse at a faster rate than the one which represents a significant departure from it.

Important attributes of an innovation which influence the rate of adoption are:

Attributes of Innovation

i) Relative advantage
ii) Compatibility
iii) Complexity
iv) Trialability and
v) Observability
vi) Predictability

Key Elements in Diffusion Process

Element	Meaning
Innovation	Idea, practice or objects that is perceived as new or an improvement over the existing one by the individual or members of a social system
Communication channel	A communication channel is the means by which messages get from one individual to another
Time	The innovation-decision period is the length oftime required to pass through the innovation decision process.
Social system	A social system is defined as a set of interrelatedunits that are engaged in joint problem solvingto accomplish a common goal.

a) Relative Advantages

The degree to which an innovation is perceived as better than the idea it supersedes. The relative advantage may have number of dimensions. For example, if a new technology or practice gives more yield or income or saves time, labour and cost: or has less risk than the existing one; it has more relative advantage.

Relative Advantage

The degree to which an innovation is perceived as better than the idea it supersedes

Multiple use of an innovation may be a form of relative advantage. For example, an equipment or material, which may be used for a number of activities, has more advantage than an equipment or material that can be used for a single purpose. Location specific enterprises in specific areas mayprovide some relative advantage. For example, Pashmina goat rearing in Jammu and Kashmir having more favourable climate for pashmina goat rearing.

Factors of Relative Advantage

Economic Factors: One of the most important factors deciding the rapid rate of adoption.

Example: When android mobile hand set cost was reduced, lot of individual purchased the hand set.

Social Factors: In some cases, social prestige, status and social approval are important factors for adoption of technologies.

Example: Even when there is huge subsidy from Government for pig farming, majority of the Brahmin community would not go for pig farming

The sub- factors / dimensions of relative advantage include:

i) Degree of economic profitability
ii) Low initial cost
iii) Decrease in discomfort
iv) Social prestige
v) Savings in time and effort, and
vi) Immediacy of the reward.

b) Compatibility

Compatibility is the degree to which an innovation is perceived consistent with the existing values, past experiences and needs of the receivers. Compatibility ensures great security and less risk to the receiver and makes the new idea more meaningful.

An innovation may be compatible with :

1. Socio-cultural values and beliefs
2. Previously introduced ideas
3. Client needs for innovations

> **Compatibility**
>
> The degree to which an innovation is perceived consistent with the existing values, past experiences and needs of the receivers.

Physical and Cultural Compatibility

Physical compatibility refers to the degree to which a new idea or practice is consistent with existing practices relating to economic activities.

Example : Rearing of crossbred cow in the tribal community is found to be physically incompatible with their farming situation because they do not have AI facilities in their areas.

Cultural compatibility refers to the degree to which an innovation is consistent with the existing values, beliefs, habits and tradition in a social system.

Example: The lack of cultural compatibility contributed to the failure of piggery farming in many villages.

Compatibility with Previously Introduced Ideas/Names

Compatibility of an innovation with a preceding idea can either speed up or retard its rate of adoption. Old ideas are the main mental tools that individuals utilize to assess new ideas and give them meaning. Farmers cannot deal with an innovation except on the basis of familiarity. Previous practice provides a standard against which an innovation can be interpreted thus decreasing its uncertainty.

Example: Application of the cow dung in the fodder field is a common practice in the village. If we promote, the preparation and application of vermi-compost as a new innovation, the dairy farmers may adopt the same as they are familiar with the similar type of practices.

Compatibility with Felt Needs

Livestock extension worker must determine the needs of their clients and then recommends innovations that fulfill these needs. The one dimension of compatibility is the degree to which an innovation is perceived as meeting the needs of the client system. When felt needs are met, a faster rate of adoption usually occurs.

Indigenous Knowledge System

The basic notion of the compatibility attribute is that a new idea is perceived in relationship to existing practices that are already familiar to the individual change agent and others who introduce an innovation often commit an "empty vessels fallacy" by assuming that potential adopters are blank slates who lack any relevant experience with which to associate the new idea. The empty vessels fallacy denies that compatibility is important.

c) Complexity

Complexity is the degree to which an innovation is perceived as relatively difficult to understand and use. Any new idea may be classified on the complexity – simplicity continuum. Some innovations are clear in their meaning to potential adopters others are not. The complexity of an

> **Complexity**
>
> The degree to which an innovation is perceived as relatively difficult to understand and use.

innovation, as perceived by members of a social system, is negatively related to its rate of adoption. Diffusion of an innovation which is too complex to communicate and to apply, is slow. As has been described, the relative simplicity of F 1 vaccination practice in chicks has diffused rapidly in the commercial poultry farm whereas due to relative complexity of the practice of R_2 B vaccination, it has not diffused so well.

Generally speaking, the more complex a practice and the more change it requires in the existing operations, the more slowly it will be adopted.

The following classification of practices in the form of their complexity, roughly represents the decreasing order of speed with which acceptance may be expected to occur.

a) *A simple change*: A change in materials and equipment only, without a change in techniques or operations. Example: New variety of fodder seed.
b) *Improved practice*: Change in existing operation with or without a change in materials or equipment. Example. Clean Milk Production
c) *Innovation:* Change involving new technique or operations. Example: Artificial Insemination
d) *Change in total enterprise*: Eg. Dairy farming to Poultry farming

d) Trialability

Trialability (divisibility) is the degree to which an innovation may be experimented with on a limited basis before deciding to adopt. The feeling of insecurity associated with the adoption of something new and previously unknown is greatly minimized if it can be tried out on a small scale. The result of the trial, if successful, not only minimizes the risk and insecurity, it also gives the farmer on opportunity to evaluate the innovation in terms of its feasibility and applicability to his own situation. An innovation that is trialable represents less uncertainty to the individual who is considering it for adoption, as it is possible to learn by doing.

> **Trialibility**
> The degree to which an innovation is perceived as relatively difficult to understand and use.

Example: Adoption of feeding of balanced cattle feed is more, compared to purchase of a new Crossbred animal for dairy farming, simply because balanced cattle feed can be purchased in small units and can be tried. Whereas, CB animal, requires large investment and cannot be tried in parts.

e) Observability

Observability is the degree to which the results of an innovation are visible/observable, demonstrable and communicable to farmers.

Example: The result of feeding of balanced ration to a milch cow is clearly visible to dairy famrers in terms of increase in milk production. The farmer will adopt the recommendation of feeding balanced ration than the feeding of traditional ration as the result is observable. But, the result of clean milk productionis not obvious to the farmer. That is why recommendation like clean milk production has been less adopted. The problem of lack of observability may, however, be overcome by strengthening extension efforts like training, communication etc. that can enlarge one's vision and reasoning. Observability is sometimes referred as communicability. The observability of an innovation is positively related to its rate of adoption. The visible impact of an innovation facilitates its diffusion in the social system.

Obervability

The degree to which the results of an innovation are visible/observable, demonstrable and communicable to farmers.

f) Predictability

Predictability has also been perceived as an attribute of innovations. Predictability refers to the degree of certainty of receiving expected benefits from the adoption of an innovation. Subsistence farmers are often very cautious when making adoption decisions, because crop failure or substantial reduction in output due to failure of agricultural innovations to achieve expected production goals, can result farmers are reluctant to adopt any technology or technique which introduces a higher level of uncertainty into the operation of the farm enterprise.

Predictability

The degree of certainty of receiving expected benefits from the adoption of an innovation

2. Communication Channels

A communication channel is the means by which messages get from one individual to another. The following classification of channels would help the communicator to use them appropriately:

i) **Interpersonal channels -** It refers to those which are used for face to face communication between two or more individuals.

ii) **Mass media channels -** These enable the messages to reach a larger, diverse audience simultaneously in a relatively shorter time. e.g.: Radio and T.V.

iii) **Localite channels -** They originate within the social system of the receiver. eg: neighbours, relatives, opinion leaders etc.

iv) **Cosmopolite channels -** They originate outside a particular social system. eg: Extension worker, sales personnel etc.

More effective communication occurs when two or more individuals belong to the same groups, live or work near each other, and share the same interests (homophilous). More effective ommunication occurs in homophilous condition. When they share common meanings, a mutual sub cultural language, and are alike in personal and social characteristics, the communication of new ideas is likely to have greater effects in terms of knowledge gain, attitude formation and change, and overt behaviour change. When homophily is present, communication is therefore likely to be rewarding to both participants in the process. One of the most distinctive problems in the diffusion of innovations is that the participants are usually quite heterophilous. A livestock extension officer, for instance, is more technically competent draw his or her farmers. This difference frequently leads to ineffective communication as the participants do not talk the same language. In fact, when two individuals are identical regarding their technical grasp of an innovation, no diffusion can occur as there is no new information to exchange. The very nature of diffusion demands that at least some degree of heterophily be present between two participants.

Heterophily and Homophily vis-a-vis Communication Channels

Homophily is the degree to which pairs of individuals who interact are similar in certain attributes, such as beliefs, education, social status, and the like. When given the choice, individuals usually choose to interact with someone similar to him or herself. Furthermore, homophilous individuals engage in more effective communication because their similarities lead to greater knowledge gain as well as attitude or behaviour change. However, most participants in the diffusion of innovations are heterophilous, meaning they speak different languages, so to speak. The problem is that diffusion requires a certain degree of heterophily; if two individuals are identical, no diffusion occurs because no new information can be exchanged. Therefore, an ideal situation would involve two individuals who are homophilous in every way, except in knowledge of the innovation.

3. Time

The third elelment of diffusion process is time.The time is involved in diffusion in :

1. Innovation decision process
2. Innovativeness and
3. Innovation's rate of adoption.

1. Innovation – Decision Process

The innovation – decision process is the mental process through which as individual or other decision making unit passes from first knowledge of an innovation to forming an attitude towards the innovation, to a decision to adopt or reject, to implementation of the new idea, and to confirmation of this decision. This process consists of a series of choices and actions over time through which an individual or a system evaluates a new idea and decides whether or not to incorporate the innovation into ongoing practice. We conceptualize five steps in this process

1. Knowledge,
2. Persuasion,
3. Decision,
4. Implementation, and
5. Confirmation

Types of Innovation-Decisions

Two factors determine what type a particular decision is :

i) Whether the decision is made freely and implemented voluntarily,
ii) Who makes the decision.

Based on these considerations, three types of innovation-decisions have been identified within diffusion of innovations.

Type	Meaning
Optional Innovation-Decision:	This decision is made by an individual who is in some way distinguished from others in a social system
Collective Innovation-Decision:	This decision is made collectively by all individuals of a social system.
Authority Innovation-Decision:	This decision is made for the entire social system by few individuals in positions of influence or power.

An individual seeks information at various stages in the innovation – decision process in orderto decrease uncertainty about innovation's expected consequences. The decision stage leads to adoption, a decision to make full use of an innovation as the best course of action available, or (2) to rejection, a decision not to adopt an innovation.

2. Innovativeness

Innovativeness is the degree to which an individual or other unit of adoption is relatively earlier in adopting new ideas than other members of a social system. Based on innovativeness, the adopters can be classified into five categories viz.,

1. Innovators
2. Early adopters

3. Early majority
4. Late majority and
5. Laggards

3. Innovation's Rate of Adoption

Rate of adoption is the relative speed with which an innovation is adopted by members of a social system. The rate of adoption is usually measured by the length of time required for a certain percentage of the members of a system to adopt an innovation. It is a system perspective rather than an individual as a unit of analysis. There are differences in the rate of adoption for the same innovation in different social system.

4. Social System

A social system is defined as a set of interrelated units that are engaged in joint problem solving to accomplish a common goal. The members or units can be individuals, informal groups, organizations, or sub systems. The sharing of common objective binds the system together. Diffusion occurs within a social system. The social structure of the system influence how and what information is disseminated. Knowledge of social structure is important to consider while studying diffusion. A village as a social system is made up of a variety of individuals and groups with distinctive statuses, roles, norms and goals all of which, at least in ideal terms, functionally relate to each other to attain its major goals and objectives. The structure of a social system constitutes a set of boundaries within which innovation diffuse. The differences in the adoption of livestock innovations at the village level can often to explained in terms of their differences in structural characteristics. The degree to which a village is structurally homogeneous or heterogeneous, unitary or highly stratified, affects the rate of diffusion of agricultural innovations within its boundaries.

System Norms

Norms are the established behaviour patterns for the members of a social system. They define a range of tolerable behaviour and serve as a guide or a standard for the members' behaviour in asocial system. The norms of a system tell an individual what is expected behaviour. A system's normscan be a barrier to change. In our country, for example, sacred cows roam the country side while millions of people are malnourished. Pork is not consumed by Muslims. Polished rice is eaten inmost of our Asian countries even though the whole rice is nutritious. These are examples of cultural and religions norms. Norms can operate at the level of nation, a religious community, an organization,or a local system like a village.

Diffusion of a Medical Drug Among Doctors

According to Rogers, the diffusion theory became more widely accepted after Coleman et al. (1966) conducted a study on the diffusion of tetracycline, a new medical drug, in 1966. The Pfizer drug company invented this successful new drug and wanted to investigate the effectiveness of their tetracycline advertisements, which were placed in medical journals. The company asked three professors at Columbia University to find out how physicians adopted the new innovation and how mass communication influenced this adoption process. They conducted a survey to gather accurate and reliable data. Different with previous diffusion research that relied on respondents' recall of how they adopted new technology, this study gathered data both from physicians' responses and pharmacies' prescription. In addition to this, Coleman et al. (1966) asked their respondents to list their interpersonal connections in order to investigate the effect of interpersonal network links with the new drug adoption. The result shows that the percentage of adoption of the new drug followed an S-shaped curve, but that the rate of tetracycline adoption was faster than the rate of other innovations adoption. The researchers also found that doctors who are cosmopolite were likely to adopt the new drug. One of the most important findings was that doctors who had more interpersonal networks adopted the new medical drug more quickly than those that did not. This meant that interpersonal communication channels with peers had a strong influence on the adoption process. Rogers noted that this Columbia University study is "one of the most influential diffusion studies in showing that the diffusion of an innovation is essentially a social process that occurs through interpersonal networks". In fact, Rogers mentioned that the Columbia University Drug Study made a contribution to identify the importance of social networks in the diffusion process.

Re-invention

Re-invention is the degree to which a technology is changed or modified by auser in the process of its adoption and implementation. Re-invention is beneficial to adopters. Flexibilityon the process of adopting technology may reduce mistakes and encourage customization of the technology to fit it more appropriately to local and / or changing conditions. Reinvention may occur because the technology advocate influences the clients to modify or adopt a technology.

Re-invention occurs due to the following reasons

1. Technologies that are relatively more complex and difficult to understand
2. Re-invention can occur only to adopter's lack of selected knowledge about the technology such as when there is relatively little direct contrast between the adopters and the change agent or the previous adopter

3. A technology that is a general concept or that is a tool with many possible applications is more likely to be re-invented.
4. When a technology is implemented in order to strive a wide range of user's problems re-invention is more likely to occur.

Forced Discontinuance

Sometimes the technology itself is banned due to several reasons. For example, DDT and BHC were banned by the Government due to their deleterious effects.

Consequences of Innovation

Consequences are the changes that occur to an individual or to a social system as a result ofthe adoption or rejection of an innovation. Consequences are not uni-dimensional. They can take many forms and are expressed in various ways. We find it useful to analyze three dimensions of consequences:

1. Desirable versus undesirable consequences
2. Direct versus indirect consequences
3. Anticipated versus unanticipated consequences.

Desirable versus Undesirable Consequences

Desirable consequences are the functional effects of an innovation for an individual or for a social system. Undesirable consequences are the dysfunctional effects of an innovation to an individual or to a social system. The determination of whether consequences are functional or dysfunctional depends on how the innovation affects the adopters. An innovation can cause consequences for individuals other than its adopters. For instance, rejecters of a new idea may be affected because an innovation benefits the other members of the system who adopt it, widening the socio-economic gap between adopters and rejecters. Everyone in a system usually is touched by the consequences of a technological innovation, whether they are adopters or rejecters. For example, the adoption of Artificial Insemination in cattle and buffalo led to White Revolution in India. The white revolution led to increase milk production resulting higher income for the farmers those adopted the technology. The white revolution also led to decrease in animal population, migration of traditional dairy farmers to other sector, increased unemployment in the villages. Although, many livestock farmers were benefited, the white revolution created unequal conditions for the system as a whole. So whether the consequences are desirable or undesirable depends on whether one takes certain individuals, or the entire system, as a point of reference. We may conclude with generalization that the effects of an innovation usually cannot be managed so as to separate the desirable from the undesirable consequences.

Windfall Profits / Loss

By being the first in the field, innovators frequently secure a kind of economic gain called **windfall profits.** Windfall profits are a special advantage earned by the first adopters of a new idea in a system. Their unit costs are usually lower, and their additions to total production have little effect on the selling price of the product. But when all members of a system adopt a new idea, total production increases, and the price of the product or service eventually drops. An innovator must take risks in order to earn windfall profits. Not all new ideas turn out successfully, and occasionally the innovator gets his or her fingers burned. Adoption of a non-economic or unsuccessful innovation can result in **"windfall losses"** for the first individuals to adopt. An example of windfall losses occurred in the diffusion of mobile hand set. The first model of hand set sold in India was approximately Rs.20,000/-. Within 3-4 years, the price was dropped to Rs.400-5000/-, and after decade it became Rs,500. In this case, later adopters gained a windfall benefit by waiting to adopt.

Direct versus Indirect Consequences

A change in one part of a system often initiates a chain reaction of indirect consequences stemming from the direct consequences of an innovation. Direct consequences are the changes to an individual or a social system that occur in immediate response to adoption of an innovation. Indirect consequences are the changes to an individual or a social system that occur as a result of the direct consequences of an innovation. These are the consequences of consequences.

Anticipated versus Unanticipated Consequences

Anticipated consequences are changes due to an innovation that are recognized and intended by the members of a social system. Unanticipated consequences are changes due to an innovation that are neither intended nor recognized by the members of a social system. No innovation comes without strings attached. The more technologically advanced an innovation, the more likely its introduction will produce many consequences, both anticipated and latent. Unanticipated consequences represent a lack of understanding of how an innovation functions, and of the internal and external forces at work in a social system. For example, introduction of HYV seeds in India led to Green revolution there by increasing the food grain production. This increase of food grain production was anticipated consequence. The unanticipated consequences of Green Revolution in the country were regional imbalance, social disharmony, degradation of soil quality, unemployment, etc.

Adoption Process

An innovation diffuses within a social system through its adoption by individuals and groups.The decision to adopt an innovation, however, "is not normally a single, instantaneous act", it involves as a process. The "adoption process" is a decision-making process goes through a number of mental stages before making a final decision to adopt an innovation. First the livestock farmer comes to know the idea, then collect information and form an attitude and finally take decision to adopt or reject. Some times it so happens, farmer may reject even after taking the decision to adopt due to some conflicting messages. At all the stages of adoption, communication sources actively help the farmer to take appropriate decision. Adoption is essentially as Decision – Making process. Johnson and Haver (1955), decision-making involves the following steps.

i) Observing the problems
ii) Making analysis of it
iii) Deciding the available courses of action
iv) Taking one course and
v) Accepting the consequence of the decision

Stages in Adoption Process

Ryan and Gross (1943) first drew attention to the existence of a sequence of stages in the process of adoption viz.,

i) 'Awareness' of the existence of an innovation
ii) 'Conviction' of usefulness
iii) 'Acceptance' in the sense of willingness to try the innovation, and
iv) 'Complete adoption'

According to Wilkening (1953) adoption of an innovation is a process composed of learning, deciding, and acting over a period of time. That means the adoption of specific practices is not the result of a single decision to act but series of actions and thought decisions. He identified four adoption stages:

i) Awareness
ii) Obtaining information
iii) Conviction and trial, and
iv) Adoption

It indicates that initial knowledge of a practice, its mental acceptance as a "good idea", its use on a trial basis and finally its full adoption. Wilkening's first two stages were later extended into three and the resulting five stages identified by the North Central Rural Sociology Sub Committee for the study of Diffusion of

Farm practices (1955) are widely accepted and received world wide attention. The five stages of adoption process are:

1. Awareness
2. Interest
3. Evaluation
4. Trial
5. Adoption

Stages	
Awareness - the individual is exposed to the innovation but lacks complete information about it	Awareness ↓
Interest - the individual becomes interested in the new idea and seeks additional information about it	Interest ↓
Evaluation - individual mentally applies the innovation to his present and anticipated future situation, and then decides whether or not to try it	Evaluation ↓
Trial - the individual makes full use of the innovation	Trial ↓
Adoption - the individual decides to continue the full use of the innovation	Adoption

1. Awareness Stage

This is the starting stage wherein the farmer comes to know the existence of the new idea but he doesn't have full information about the idea.For instance, the farmers may know Machine Milking only and may not know what it is, what it will do and how it will work ?

2. Interest Stage

The farmer develops interest in the innovation and seeks additional information about it either from extension officer or from fellow farmers or from any source, which he feels credible. That means the farmer at the interest stage acquires more information about an innovation or idea. Farmer wants to know, what the innovation/idea is, how it works and what its potentialities are.

3. Evaluation Stage

The farmer here makes mental application of the new idea in the present and anticipated future situations and decides whether or not to try it. The farmer at this stage judges the utility of the innovation. He/she makes an assessment whether the idea is applicable to own situation and if applied what would be the result. The dairy farmers after acquring more information about machine milking at the intest stage, mentally judge contribution of machine towards milking.

5. Trial Stage

The farmer actually applies the new idea on a small scale in order to determine its utility or feasibility & applicability in own situation. Even though, the farmer takes a decision to try the idea by virtue of its plus points or merits, generally the effectiveness of the idea is tested taking this as small scale trials in their own field standards, even though farmers has thought about it for long time and gathered information concerning it.

6. Adoption Stage

Being satisfied with the performance of the new idea tested on small scale in his own situation, the farmer uses the new idea continuously on a full scale. Trial may be considered as the practical evaluation of an innovation. The innovation becomes a part of his normal farming activity. It provides the advantage of the innovation and hence the farmer takes final decision and applies the innovation in a scale appropriate to own situation on a continued basis.

Other Models of Adoption Process

According to Singh (1965) the stages of adoption are dynamic and not static. The same fivestages do not occur with all the adopters and all the practices sequence is not always the same. Sometimes one stage appears more than once.Singh andPink have developed a seven-stage model of the adoption process. Need, awareness, interest,deliberation, trial, evaluation and adoption.

1. **Need**: Need is nothing but the difference between what is and what ought to be. Here at this stage, farmer himself wishes to change his existing practice inorder to get more yield/income.
2. **Awareness**: The farmer just comes to know about an innovation without knowing the details of it.
3. **Interest**: Farmer makes an attempt to know more about the innovation.
4. **Deliberation**: Farmer at this stage look for possibility of application of the innovation under own conditions. Seeks advice of opinion leaders observe the performance at different places and discusses with the members of family. The farmer then takes a decision to try out & reject the idea.
5. **Trial**: Puts the practice on a limited scale to observe the performance under own conditions.

6. **Evaluation**: The farmer observes performance of the innovation on various dimensions. He/she collects data on the performance of the innovation on others situation. Compares performance of the new with the old one and figures out other changes which will be necessary if the innovation isadopted. Calculates input – output, risks, uncertainties etc.
7. **Adoption**: In this stage the farmer takes the decision to extend the use of the innovation on a continued basis.

Skipped stages of Adoption

Not all farmers go through each stage of the adoption process before making a final decision about the adoption of an innovation. A farmer may decide to adopt or reject an innovation at any stage of the adoption process or may skip one or several stages. For example, a farmer may skip the evaluation and trial stages and proceed directly from awareness to the trial stage, skipping interest and evaluation stages. The skipping of stages appears to be more common among later rather than earlier adopters, for they can learn from the experience of their friends, relatives, or neighbours who adopted the practice before them. It should be emphasized, however, that although there are instances of skipped stages, they are the exceptions rather than the rule. The majority of farmers appear to pass through all stages of the adoption process.

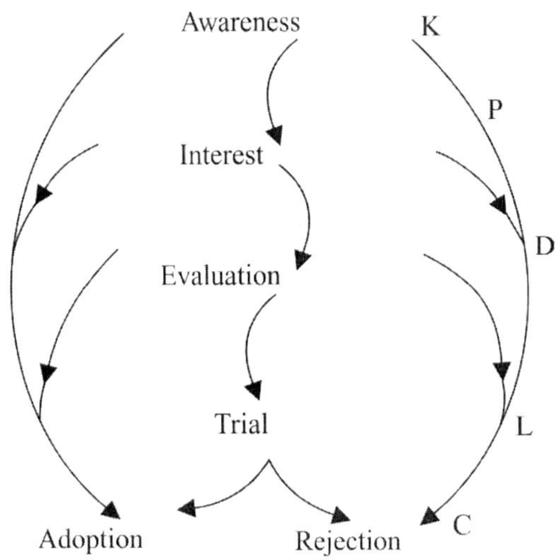

Skipped stages in the Adoption Process

Adoption Period

The time taken to pass from the awareness of an innovation to its adoption is called the "adoption period". The major aim of agricultural extension workers is to shorten the length of the adoption period of individual farmers so that an innovation will diffuse rapidly within a social system. The livestock extension worker try to attain this goal by making farmers aware of the innovation as quickly as possible and persuading them to move rapidly through the stages of the adoption process and adopt the innovations.

Innovation - Decision Process

Meaning of Innovation Decision Process

According to Rogers (198),the Innovation - Decision process is the process through an individual (or other decision making unit) passes from first knowledge of an innovation, to forming an attitude toward the innovation, to a decision to adopt or reject, to implementation of the new idea, and to confirmation of this decision. This process should be distinguished from the diffusion process by which new ideas are communicated to the members of a social system. The major difference between the two processes is that diffusion occurs among the units in a social system, whereas innovation-decision making takes place within the mind of an individual. The adoption or rejection of an innovation is a decision by an individual. If he adopts, he begins using a new idea, practice, or object and ceases using the idea that the innovation replaces. The innovation-decision is a special type of decision-making; it has certain characteristics not found in other kinds of decision-making situations. In the case of the adoption of an innovation, an individual must choose a new alternative over those previously in existence.THe Innovation-Decision process consists of a series of actions and choices over time through which an individual or an organization evaluates a new idea and decides whether or not to incorporate the new idea into the ongoing system. This behaviour consists essentially of dealing with the uncertainty that is inherently involved in deciding about a new alternative to those previously in existence. The perceived newness is a distinctive aspect of innovation-decision making, compared to other types of decision-making.

Stages of Innovation Decision Process

Innovation-decision is a process that occurs over time and is conceptualized to have five stages and they are :

1. Knowledge
2. Persuasion
3. Decision
4. Implementation
5. Confirmation

The model contains three major divisions viz.,

i) Antecedents
ii) Process
iii) Consequences

Antecedents are those variables present in the situation prior to the introduction of an innovation which consist of:

i) Personality characteristics of individuals, like general attitude toward change
ii) Social characteristics of individuals, like cosmopoliteness
iii) Strength of individual's perceived need for the innovation.

Communication sources and channels provide stimuli to the individual during the innovation-decision process. The typical individual gains initial knowledge of the innovation mainly from cosmopolite and mass media channels. At the persuasion function, the individual forms his perception the innovation from more localite and interpersonal channels. An innovation may be adopted at the decision stage in the process and be used continuously or rejected at a later date (a discontinuation).

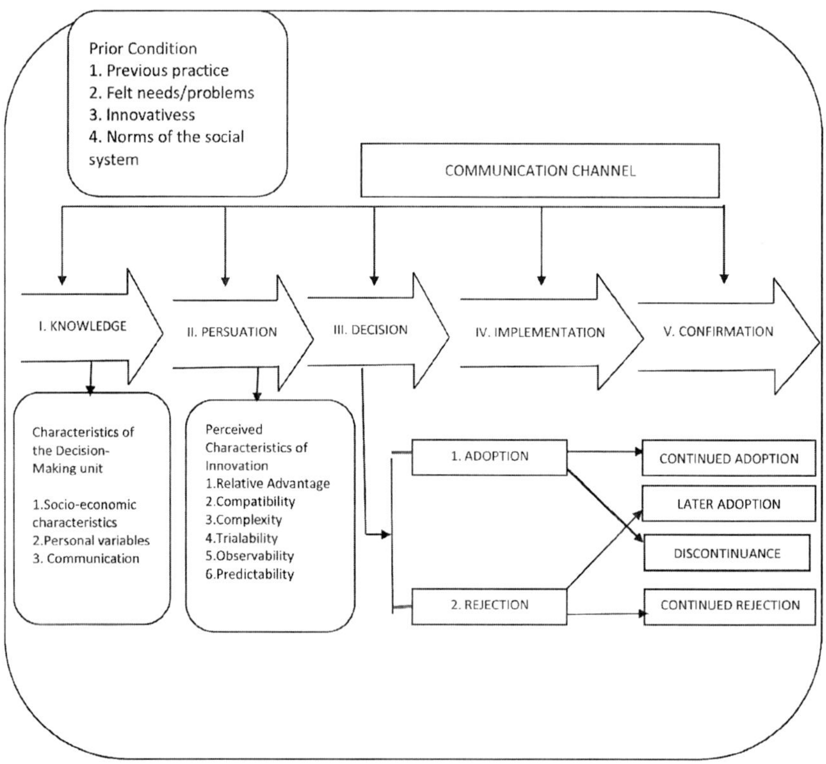

Innovation-Decision Process Model with Five Stages (Source : Rogers, 1983)

Discontinuance may be due to the innovation's replacement by an improved idea or to disenchantment (disappointment) with the innovation. The new idea may be rejected at the end of the process but adopted at a later date due to changes in how the individual perceives the innovation. Continued information seeking often occurs throughout the confirmation function, because the individual seeks to reinforce his decision. Sometimes, however, contradictory (to the innovation- decision) messages reach the individual, and this leads to discontinuance or later adoption.

1. Knowledge stage

Innovation-decision process begins with knowledge stage, which commences when the farmer is exposed to the innovation's existence and gains some understanding of how it functions. Knowledge function is mainly cognitive or knowing. Knowledge seeking is initiated by an individual and is greatly influenced by one's predispositions. Generally, individuals tend to expose themselves to chose ideas which are in accord with their interests, needs, or existing attitudes. An individual may develop a need when he learnt that an improved method, an innovation, exists. Therefore, innovations can lead to needs, as well as vice versa. Some change agents use this approach to change by creating needs among their clients through pointing out the desirable consequences of new idea. Thus, knowledge of innovations can create motivation for their adoption.

Selective Exposure vs. Selective Perception

Individuals tend to expose themselves to ideas which are in accord with their interests, needs, or existing attitudes. The tendency is called 'selective exposure'. Hassinger (1959) argues that individuals will seldom expose themselves to messages about an innovation unless they first feel a need for the innovation, and that even if such individuals are exposed to such innovation messages, there will be little effect of such exposures unless the individual perceives the innovation as relevant to his needs and as consistent with his existing attitudes and beliefs. This tendency is called 'selective perception'.

Example: We are all exposed daily to hundreds of mass media messages about new products. But few of these only register on our minds.

Example: A dairy farmer is used to feed his animal locally prepared feed to his dairy animals for years. After hearing to the balanced ration for dairy animals having high potentiality from the KVK scientist the dairy farmer would feel it as a need for his situation to adopt it.

A need can motivate an individual to seek information about an innovation and the knowledge of an innovation may develop the need.

Types of Knowledge

There are three types of knowledge related to innovation viz.,

i) Awareness-knowledge

ii) How-to-knowledge

iii) Principles' knowledge

Awareness-knowledge: Awareness-knowledge - is information that an innovation exists which motivates an individual to seek 'how-to-knowledge and 'principles' knowledge. This type of information-seeking is concentrated at the knowledge stage, but it may also occur at the persuasion and decision stages.

How-to-knowledge: How-to knowledge consists of information necessary to use an innovation properly. The adopter must understand what quantity of an innovation to secure, how to use it correctly, and so on. In the case of innovations that are relatively more complex, the amount of how-to knowledge needed for proper adoption is much greater than in the case of less complex ideas. When an adequate level of how-to knowledge is not obtained prior to the trial and adoption of an innovation, rejection and discontinuance are likely to result.

Principles' knowledge: Principles-knowledge consists of information dealing with the functioning principles underlying how the innovation works.

Examples: Functioning of vaccinations; Functioning of deworming medicine.

Knowledge about Innovation vs. Use

Having knowledge about an innovation is quite different from using the idea.

Most of the dairy farmers know about the importance of milking machine, but many of them do not use. Why they do not use? Possible reasons could be the machine may not be useful to his situation.

Knowing about new idea does not mean using the idea. One must seek sufficient knowledge to become adequately informed so that can entre to persuasion stage of adoption.

Knowledge Stage – Cognitive (Knowing)

Persuasion Stage- Affective (feeling)

Psychologically involved

Actively seek information

2. Persuasion Stage

At the persuasion stage in the innovation-decision process ,the individual forms a favourable or unfavourable attitude towards the innovation. Whereas the mental activity at the knowledge function was mainly cognitive (or knowing), the main type of thinking at the persuasion function is affective (or feeling). Until the individual knows about a new idea, of course, he cannot begin to form an attitude toward it. At the persuasion stage the individual becomes more psychologically involved with the innovation and actively seeks information about the idea. His personality as well as the norms of his social system affects information seeking behaviour and interepretation. Thus, selective perception is important in determining the receiver's communication behaviour at the attitude formation stage. At the persuasion stage, a general perception of the innovation is developed. Such perceived attributes of an innovation as its relative advantage, compatibility, and complexity are especially important at this stage. In developing a favourable or unfavourable attitude toward the innovation, the individual may mentally apply the new idea to present or anticipated future situation before deciding whether or not to try it.

Attitude vs. Action

A dairy farmer may have a positive attitude towards fodder cultivation, but may be giving concentrate feed to his animals.

Positive attitude does not lead to always to Action.

3. Decision Stage

At the decision stage in innovation-decision process, the individual or some other decision making unit engage in activities which lead to a choice to adopt or reject the innovation. This decision involves consideration of whether or not to try the innovation. Most of the livestock farmers will not adopt an innovation without trying it first on a pilot basis to determine its utility in their own situation. The small-scale trial is often part of the decision to adopt, and is important as a means to decrease the perceived risk of the innovation for the adopter. In some cases, innovation cannot be divided for trial, and so it must be adopted or rejected in total. Innovations, which can be divided for trial use, are generally adopted more rapidly. If the innovation has a certain degree of relative advantage in the trial stage, then individual move to an adoption decision.

4. Implementation Stage

Implementation occurs when an individual or other decision making unit puts an innovation into use. At this stage the individual is generally concerned with where to get the innovation, how to use it and what operational problems will be faced and how these could be solved. Implementation may involve changes in management of the enterprise and/or modification in the innovation, to suit more closely to the specific needs of the particular person who adopts it.

Re-invention

The degree to which an innovation is changed or modified by a user in the process of its adoption and implementation.

Re-invention often occurs at the implementation stage. Re-invention is defined as the degree to which an innovation is changed or modified by a user in the process of its adoption and implementation. Re-invention often is beneficial to the adopters of an innovation. Flexibility in the process of adopting an innovation may reduce mistakes and encourage customization of the innovation to fit it more appropriately to local situations or changing conditions. As a result of re-invention, an innovation may be more appropriate in matching an adopter's pre-existing problems and more responsive to new problems that arise during the innovation-decision process.

> **Rejection of an Innovation**
>
> Rejection is decision not to adopt an innovation.
>
> **Active rejection**
>
> When an individual rejects after adopting the innovation including even its trial, is called active rejection
>
> **Passive rejection**
>
> A simple non- adoption is called passive rejection.

5. Confirmation Stage

At the confirmation function the individual seeks reinforcement for the innovation-decision he has made, but he may reverse his previous decision if exposed to conflicting message about the innovation. If the individual perceives that the innovation is consistently giving satisfactory or unsatisfactory results the person may continue to adopt or reject the innovation as the case may be. The confirmation stage continues after the decision to adopt or reject for an indefinite period in time.Throughout the confirmation function the individual seeks to avoid a state of internal disequilibrium or dissonance or to reduce it if it occurs. Farmer seeks to accomplish it by changing his knowledge, attitude or actions.

Rejection is decision not to adopt an innovation. This may be of two types Active rejection and Passive rejection.

When a farmer rejects after adopting the innovation including even its trial is called Active rejection and simply non- adoption is called Passive Rejection.

Dissonance

Human behaviour change is motivated in part by a state of internal disequilibrium or dissonance,an uncomfortable state of mind that the individual seeks to reduce or eliminate. When an individualfeels dissonant, he will ordinarily be motivated to reduce this condition by changing his knowledge,attitude, or actions.

In the case of innovative behaviour, this may occur in the following three methods of dissonance reduction:

i) When the individual becomes aware of a felt need or problem and seeks information about some means such as an innovation to meet this need. Hence, a receiver's knowledge of a need for innovation can motivate information-seeking activity about the innovation. This occurs at the knowledge stage in the innovation-decision process.

ii) When individual becomes aware of a new idea for which he has a favourable regard, then the individual is motivated to adopt the innovation by the dissonance between what he believes and what he is doing. This behaviour occurs at the decision stage in the innovation-decision process.

iii) After the innovation-decision to adoption, the individual may secure further information which persuades him that he should not have adopted. This dissonance may be reduced by discontinuing the innovation. Or if he originally decided to reject the innovation, the individual may become exposed to pro-innovation messages, causing a state of dissonance which can be reduced by adoption. These types of behaviour (discontinuance or later adoption) occur during the confirmation function in the innovation decision process.

These three methods of dissonance reduction consist of changing behaviour so that attitudes and actions are more in line.

Discontinuance

Discontinuance is a decision to reject as innovation after having previously adopted it. Discontinuance also may take three forms.

i) Replacement discontinuance is a decision to reject an idea in order to adopt a better idea that supersedes. Eg. Artificial Insemination over Natural Insemination

ii) Disenchantment discontinuance is a decision to reject an idea as a result of dissatisfaction with the performance. Eg. Rearing of indegenous birds are repalced by Vanaraja birds by a farmer due to dissatisfaction of poultry farmer with the performance of indegenous birds.

iii) Forced Discontinuance Farmers are forced to discontinue the existing practices because of Government Policies. For example, Government has banned the use of Oxytocin for milk production.

Over Adoption

The continuation of adoption, even vigourously, when experts (Scientists or extension officers) feel that it should not be done is known as over adoption. Over adoption produces negative effect and may cause distortion or deterioration of the related systems. In sufficient knowledge about an innovation and inability to predict its consequences generally leads to over adoption. As a livestock extension worker, your role is to prevent the excessive adoption of the innovation by providing adequate knowledge about the innovation through training and communication.

Innovation - Decision Period

The innovation – decision period is the length of time required to pass through the innovation – decision process. The time elapsing from awareness-knowledge of an innovation to decision for an individual is measured in days, months, or years. This period is thus a gestation period in which a new idea is fermenting in the individual's mind.

Sources of Information (Communication Media) In Adoption Process

An integral part of the adoption process is the communication of information at the stages of adoption and innovation-decision processes. The research indicates that people use different sources of information at the various stages in this process. The communication channels are classified as follows

1. Mass media – newspapers, radio, magazines etc.
2. Government agencies – extension workers etc
3. Neighbours and friends
4. Salesman and commercial dealers

Based on the research conducted in U.S.A, the information sources were given in ranking order at each of the stages of the process in the table below.

Active Adoption

It is the process by which the individual who takes up an innovation influences others to do so.

Example: A livestock farmer not only adopts deworming practices for his calf but also influences other farmers to do the same.

Passive Adoption

If the livestock farmer who adopts the practice do not influence the other farmers to do the practice, the innovation is confined to the individual farmer who has adopted.

In the active adoption, diffusion effect is more compared to passive adoption.

Rank order of Information sources in USA (By stages of Adoption)

Awareness Knows about it; lacks detail	**Interest** Gathers more information and fats	**Evaluation** Mental trial, application to personal situation Can I do it ?	**Trial** Small scale experimental use. How to do it?	**Adoption** Large scale continued use; satisfaction
1. Mass Media 2. Neighbours and friends 3. Govt. agencies 4. Salesmen and dealers	1. Mass Media 2. Neighbours and friends 3. Govt. agencies 4. Salesmen and dealers	1. Neighbours and friends 2. Govt. agencies 3. Salesmen and dealers 4. Mass Media	1. Neighbours and friends 2. Govt. agencies 3. Salesmen and dealers 4. Mass Media	1. Neighbours and friends 2. Govt. agencies 3. Salesmen and dealers 4. Mass Media

It is very clear from the Table that when people are making a decision to adopt an idea, they apparently rely on sources which they consider to be objective. Neighbours and friends, and government agencies evidently rank high as valid sources of information. Farmers seem to suspect mass media, and salesmen and dealers of pushing an idea mainly for the purpose of selling a product.

Table below gives the details of the seven-stage-adoption model and the relative importance of different information sources or media based on a number of studies in India.

S.No	Adoption Stage	Important media source
1	Need	Village level change agent and to some extent mass media
2	Awareness	Village level change agent, mass media and other farmers
3	Interest	Formal sources as extension agency and other farmers
4	Deliberation	Informal personal sources including family members
5	Trial	No communication for simple substitute practice. For complex or new practices, change agent and fellow farmers
6	Education	Fellow farmers and neighbours
7	Adoption	Self-experience gained at the trial stage

Note: In all stages of the adoption process, the complexity of the idea is related to the choice of information sources. The more complex the idea, the greater is the tendency to rely on government agencies (change agents)

Sources of Information in Innovation-Decision Process

Communication channels were categorized as (1) interpersonal or mass media in nature, and (2) originating from localite or cosmopolite sources.

Mass media channels are all those means of transmitting messages that involve a mass medium, such as radio, television, newspapers, and so on, which enables a source to reach an audience of many. The formation and change of strongly held attitudes, however, is best accomplished by interpersonal channels. Interpersonal channels involve a face-to-face exchange between two or more individuals.

Localite sources of information belong to the same social system as that of the receivers. Their knowledge about objects and events are restricted, generally confined to the local system. Examples, relatives, friends, neighbours etc. On the other hand, cosmopolite sources of information are from outside the social system of the receivers. Their knowledge about objects and events are wider, and as such, they can bring new ideas to the receivers. Examples, extension agents (personal cosmopolite), mass media (impersonal cosmopolite) etc.

Dey (1976) studied the channels of communication used by the farmers in different stages of the innovation-decision process. For this purpose, he selected high and low urbanized villages in West Bengal and found out the channels of communication used by the farmers of these two types of villages in each stage of the innovation-decision process. The categories of channels of communication have been arranged according to importance as perceived by the farmers in each stage of the innovation decision process. A similar situation may be found in progressive and non-progressive villages.

High urbanised villages	Low urbanised villages
Knowledge (Awareness) stage	
1. Personal cosmopolite	1. Personal cosmopolite
2. Impersonal cosmopolite	2. Impersonal cosmopolite
3. Personal localite	3. Personal localite
Persuasion stage	
1. Personal cosmopolite	1. Personal cosmopolite
2. Impersonal cosmopolite	2. Impersonal cosmopolite
3. Personal localite	3. Personal localite
Decision stage	
1. Personal cosmopolite	1. Personal cosmopolite
2. Impersonal cosmopolite	2. Impersonal cosmopolite
3. Personal localite	3. Personal localite

The findings indicated that in all stages of the innovation-decision process, personal cosmopolite channels like extension agents are most important for high urbanized villages and personal localite channels like other farmers are most important for the low urbanized villages. In low urbanized villages, after getting initial information about the innovation from other farmers (who belong to the local social system), for going ahead with the adoption of new technologies, the farmers seek technical and scientific guidance about the innovation from the extension agents, who are perceived as competent. It has been further observed that personal channels are more important than impersonal channels like radio and other mass media in all types of villages and in all stages of the innovation-decision process, except knowledge stage in the high urbanized villages. Further he found that while taking more information about the innovation (persuasion stage) and putting it into trial (decision stage), the chief concern of the farmers is the 'method' i.e. 'how to' information. The next important information the farmers would like to have is about 'yield potentiality' or 'increase in yield' in the persuasion stage and 'availability of inputs' in the decision stage.

In this context, Rogers (1995) made the following generalizations –

1. Mass media channels are relatively more important at the knowledge stage, and interpersonal channels are relatively more important at the persuasion stage in the innovation-decision process

2. Cosmopolite channels are relatively more important at the knowledge stage, and localite channels are relatively more important at the persuasion stage in the innovative-decision process.

For successful livestock technology transfer programme, the livestock extension workers have to plan their communication strategy based on the actual information needs of the client system.

Innovativeness and Adopter Categories

When an innovation is introduced in the social system, all farmers do not adopt at atime. Some of them adopt immediately and put in to practice, others may take long time to adopt it. There is variation among farmers in adoption of innovation. According to the rate of adoption, the farmers are categorised in to different categories. Some times it happens also that an innovation is readily accepted by the farmers, and some of the innovations are not easily accepted by the farmers and take considerable time for adoption. This is due to certain attributes of the innovation. All individuals in a social system do not adopt an innovation at the same time. Rather, they adopt in an ordered time sequence, and they may be classified into adopter categories on the basis of their innovativeness.

Innovativeness

Innovativeness is the degree to which an individual or other unit of adoption is relatively earlier in adopting new ideas than other members of a system.

Innovativeness is a relative dimension, in that an individual has more or less of this variable than others in a system. Innovativeness is a continuous variable, and partitioning it into discrete categories is a conceptual device, much like dividing the continuum of social status into upper, middle, and lower classes. Such classification is a simplification that aids the understanding of human behavior, although it loses some information as a result of grouping individuals.

The S-shaped Curve of Adoption and Normality

The adoption of an innovation over time follows a normal, bell-shaped curve when plotted over time on frequency basis. If the cumulative number of adopters is plotted, it results in an S-shaped curve. The S-shaped curve rises slowly at first when there are few adopters in a time period. Then the curve accelerate to a maximum when about half of the individuals in the system have adopted and then increases at a gradually slower rate as the few remaining individuals finally adopt .Then it decreases at a gradually slower rate as fewer and fewer remaining individuals adopt the innovation. The S-shaped curve is like that of a 'learning curve' as propounded by the psychologists. Each adoption in the social system is in a sense equivalent to a learning trial by an individual.

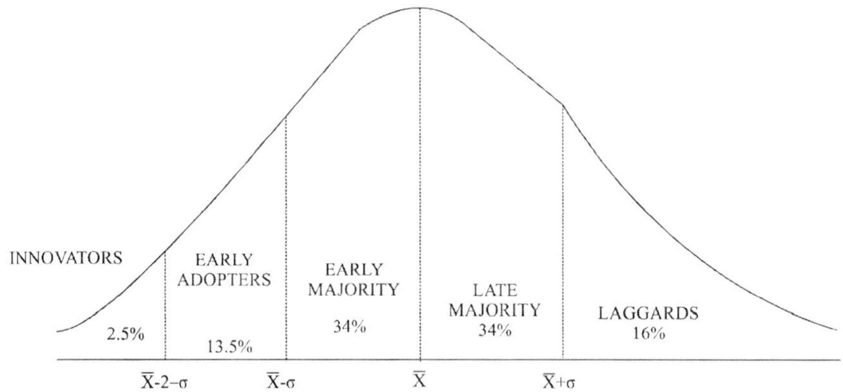

Adopters distribution follow a bell shaped curve over time and approaches normality. The normal frequency distribution has several characteristics that are useful in classifying adopters. One characteristic or parameter is the mean or average, of the individuals in the system. Another parameter of distribution is its standard deviation, a measure of variation or dispersion about the mean. The standard deviation indicates the average amount of variance from the mean for sample individuals. These two statistics, the mean (**x**)and the standard deviation (**ó**), are used to divide a normal adopter distribution into five categories. Vertical lines are drawn to mark off the standard deviations on either side of the mean so that the normal curve is divided and categorized with a standardized percentage of respondents in each category. Figure below shows the normal frequency distribution divided into five adopter categories. The area lying to the left of the mean time of adoption (of an innovation) minus two standard deviations includes 2.5 per cent of the individuals who are the first to adopt an innovation and are known as innovators. The next 13.5 per cent between the mean minus one standard deviation and the mean minus two standard deviations to adopt the new idea are called as early adopters. The next 34 per cent laying between mean and mean minus one standard devaition are known as early majority. Between the mean and onestandard deviation to the right of the mean are located the next 34 per cent to adopter who are known as the late majority. The last 16 per cent to the right of mean plus one standard deviation are the last to adopt the innovation who are known as laggards in the social system.

Classification of Adopter Categories

There are different categories of farmers. According to Rogers (1971), the farmers based on their innovativeness can be classified as

1. Innovators (Venturesome)
2. Early adopters (Respectable)
3. Early majority (Deliberate)
4. Late majority (Skeptical)
5. Laggards (Traditional)

Innovators: Venturesome

These are the first people to adopt a new idea, much ahead of other people. They are very few in numbers, probably not more than one or two in a community. They are eager to try new ideas. This interest leads them out of a local circle of peers and into more cosmopolite social relationships. Communication patterns and friendships among a clique of innovators are common, even though the geographical distance between the innovators may be great. Being an innovator has several prerequisites. These include control of substantial financial resources to absorb, understand and apply complex technical knowledge. The salient value of the innovator is venturesome-ness, due to a desire for the rash, the daring, and the risky.

Characteristics

a) Have larger farms
b) High net worth and risk capital.
c) Willing to take risks.
d) Usually not past middle age
e) Generally well educated
f) Have respect and prestige in progressive communities but not in conservative type of communities.
g) Mentally alert and actively seeking new ideas.
h) Their sphere of influence and activity often goes beyond the community boundaries.
i) They have many formal and informal contacts outside the immediate locality.
j) They often by-pass the local extension worker in getting information from the originating sources, and may learn about new things even before he does. They sometimes manage to get samples of seeds or chemicals even before they are released for public use.
k) They subscribe to many farm magazines and specialised publications.
l) Other farmers may watch the innovators and know what they are doing but the innovators are not generally named by other farmers as "neighbours and friends" to whom they go for information.

Early Adopter: Respectable

Early adopters are a more integrated part of the local Social system than the innovators. Whereas innovators are cosmopolites, early adopters are localities. This adopter's ategory, more than any other, has the greatest degree of opinion leadership in most social systems. Potential adopters look to early adopters for advice and information about the innovation. The early adopter is considered by many in the community as "the man to check with" before using a new idea.

Characteristics

a) Have large farms.

b) High income.

c) Higher education than those who adopt more slowly.

d) Respected by his or her peers

e) Younger than those who have a slower adoption rate, but not necessarily younger than the innovators

f) They are not the persons who test the untried ideas but they are quickest to use tried ideas in their own situations.

g) They are sought by the extension worker for spreading the difussion process

h) They participate more in the social activities of the community.

i) They also participate more in government programmes.

j) This group usually furnishes a disproportionate amount of the formal leadership (elected positions) in the community.

k) They read papers and farm journals and receive more bulletins than people who adopt later.

l) They are be regarded as community adoption leaders.

Early Majority: Deliberate (Local Adoption Leaders)

The early majority adopt new ideas just before the average member of a social system. The early majority interact frequently with their peers, but leadership position; are rarely held by them.The early majority's unique position; between the very early and relatively late to adopt make them an important link in the diffusion process. The early majority are one of the most numerous adopter categories, making up one third of all member of a system.

Characteristics

a) Slightly above average in age, education and farming experience.

b) They take a few more farm journals and bulletins than the average.

c) They have medium high social and economic status.

d) Less active in formal groups than early adopters, but more active than those adopting later.

e) In many cases, they are not formal leaders in the association

f) They also attend extension meetings and farm demonstrations.

g) They are most likely to be informal resources than early adopters and innovators, and so cannot afford to make hasty or poor decisions.

h) They associate mainly with people of their own community.

i) They value highly the opinions their neighbours and friends hold about them; for this is their main source of status and prestige.

j) They are mostly mentioned as "neighbours and friends" from whom the majority of farmers seek information.

Late Majority: Skeptical

The late majority adopt new ideas just after the average member of a social system. Adoption may be both an economic necessity and the answer to increasing social pressures. Innovations are approached with a skeptical and the late majority do not adopt until most other in their social system have done so. Like the early majority, the late majority make up one third of the members of a system.

Characteristics

a) Those in this group have less education and are older than the early majority.

b) They form the major part of formal organisational membership, although they participate less in such formal groups.

c) They take fewer leadership roles than the earlier adopters.

d) They take and read fewer papers, magazines and bulletins, than the early majority.

e) They do not participate in as many activities outside the community as do people that adopt earlier.

Laggards: Traditional

Laggards are the last in the social system to adopt an innovation. They possess almost no opinion leadership. They are the most localite in their outlook of all adopter categories, many are near solates. The point of reference for the laggard is the past. Decisions are often made in terms of what has been done previously and these individuals interact primarily with others who also have relatively traditional values. Laggards tend to be suspicious of innovations and of change agents. Their innovation-decision process is relatively lengthy, with adoption and use lagging far behind awarenessknowledge of a new idea. Resistance to innovations on the part of laggards may be entirely rational from the laggards' viewpoint, as their resources are limited and they must be certain that a new idea will not fail before they can adopt. The laggard's precarious economic position forces the individual to be extremely cautious in adopting innovations.

Characteristics

a) Least education.
b) Oldest.
c) Participate least in formal organisations, cooperatives and government programmes.
d) They hardly read farm magazines and bulletins.

Factors Infulencing in Adoption of Improved Animal Husbandry Practices

The factors influencing the adoption of innovations can be discussed under the following subheads.

I. Personal

1. **Age:** Elderly farmers seem to be somewhat less inclined to adopt new practices than younger ones. (However, the findings of several Indian studies do not support the existence of a negative relationship between the age and adoption)
2. **Education:** More than eight years schooling is almost always associated with higher adoption rates than lesser amounts.
3. Psychological characteristics:
    a) Exposure to reliable sources of farm information may create a state of rationality which in turn predisposes an individual to the adoption of new practices
    b) A mentally flexible person has higher adoption rates than one with mental rigidity.
    c) Some people are found to be more prone to change than others
4. Values and attitudes (cultural characteristics)
    a) Values found to be positively related to farm practice adoption rates are: a desire by farmers to provide a high school or college education

for their children, a high emphasis on science and material comfort, and also wide contacts within and beyond the community.

b) A high emphasis on traditionalism, isolationism, and security (e.g., owning farm free of debt) has been found to be negatively associated with adoption of improved practices.

Situational

Reasons why farmers adopt farm practices more quickly at one time than another relate to the situation in which they find themselves when alternative course of action becomes known.

1. **The nature of the practice:** The speed with which adoption will take place is partly dependent on the nature of practice itself. The more complex a practice and the more change it requires in the existing operations, the more slowly it will be adopted. Less costly inputs seem to be adopted more rapidly than those, which are more expensive. Similarly, practices which yield the greatest marginal returns per rupee invested, and in the shortest time seem to be adopted most readily.
2. **Farm income:** High farm income nearly always is associated with high adoption level.
3. **Size of farm:** Size of farm is nearly always positively related to the adoption of new farm practices
4. **Tenure status**: Adoption scores are usually higher for owner cultivators than for tenant cultivators.
5. **Sources of farm information used:** The number of sources used or the number of contacts with information sources is positively related to adoption rates. A high positive correlation is particularly evident with the use of such sources as Government agencies. High dependence on relatives and friends as sources of information is usually negatively associated with the adoption of new farm practice.
6. **Level of living:** Since successful farm practice adoption is instrument in providing the means for supporting a higher level of living, a positive correlation between the two would be expected and is generally found.

Social

Community standards and social relationships provide the general framework wherein the process of change occurs, and they account for the differences between one community (or group) and another.

Social values: The value, norms, culture, belief, progressiveness, etc of a society put grate pressure towards the adoption of new technologies. Society which value material gains, more income, prestige, status, etc., would adopt faster than the society which are closed and not open to the new ideas.

Opinion Leadership and Change Agents

Opinion leadership is thedegree to which an individual is able to influence other individuals' attitudes or overt behaviourinformally in a desired way with relative frequency. This informal leadership is not a function of theindividual's final position or status in the system. Leadership is earned and maintained by individuals'technical competence, social accessibility, and conformity to the system's norms. By their close conformity to the system's norms, opinion leaders serve as an opt model for the innovation behavioursof their followers. Opinion leaders thus exemplify and express system's structure. Opinion leaders have more exposure to external communication, higher social status greater mass media exposure,greater change agent contact, greater social participation, more cosmopoliteness and moreinnovativeness. It is important to remember, however, that social power, educational attainment, and public are not absolute requirements for opinion leadership. Despite the existence of opinion leaders, it is not always easy to distinguish them from the other members of groups. This is because opinion leadership is not a trait, but rather a role taken by some individuals under certain circumstances. In other words, anyone can be an opinion leader at any given time. Such leadership changes from time to time and from issue to issue. Opinion leaders also play important roles in movements of social change. Opinion leaders can bring legitimacy to a social movement. Known as "legitimizers," these social opinion leaders are judges, politicians, business executives, clergy members, sports figures and entertainers. Such people help "legitimize" a cause in the eyes of the public by marching in demonstrations, appearing at rallies, donating money, speaking in favour of the cause, and so forth.

Suggested Readings and References

1. Rogers, E.M. (1995). Diffusion of Innovations (4th ed.). New York: Free Press.
2. Dasgupta (1989). Diffusion of Agricultural Innovations in village India, Wiley Eastern Limited, New Delhi.
3. Swanson B.E. (1984). Agricultural Extension - A Reference Manual, Second Edition, FAO, Rome, Oxford and IBH Publishing Co. Pvt. Ltd., New Delhi.
4. Rogers, E.M., and Shoemaker, F.F. (1971). Communication of Innovations, Free Press, New York.
5. Reddy, A.A. (1987). Extension Education, Sree Lakshmi Press, Bapatla
6. Ray G.L. (2005). Extension Communication and Management, Kalyani Publishers, New Delhi.

7. Coleman, J.S., Katz, E., & Mentzel, H. (1966). Medical innovation: Diffusion of a medical drug among doctors. Indianapolis, MN: Bobbs-Merrill.

8. Rogers, E.M. (1976). New product adoption and diffusion. Journal of Consumer Research, 2: 290–301.

9. Wejnert, B. (2002). Integrating Models of Diffusion of Innovations: A Conceptual Framework, Annual Review of Sociology (Annual Reviews) 28: 297–306.

10. Supe, S.V. (1994). An Introduction to Extension Education, Oxford and IBH Publishing Co. Ltd. New Delhi.

11. Sandhu, A.S. (1993). Textbook on Agricultural Communication: Process and Method, Oxford and IBH Publishing Co Pvt. Ltd. New Delhi.

10

Extension Programme: Planning Monitoring and Evaluation

1. Programme
2. Assumptions on Extension Planning
3. Extension Programme Planning
4. Objectives of Programme Planning
5. Need identification in Programme Planning
6. Principles of Programme Planning
7. Programme Planning Process
8. Steps in Extension Programme Planning
9. Extension Programme Planning Model Proposed By Sandhu
10. Extension Programme Monitoring and Evaluation
    a. Monitoring
        i. Meaning of monitoring
        ii. Basic concepts and elements in monitoring
        iii. Types of monitoring
        iv. Tools and techniques of monitoring
        v. Indicators of monitoring
    b. Evaluation
        i. Definitions of evaluation
        ii. Nature of Monitoring and Evaluation
        iii. Features of Evaluation
        iv. Difference between Appraisal, Monitoring and Evaluation
        v. Types of evaluation
        vi. Extension evaluation process
        vii. Various Aspects Of Evaluation
11. Suggested Readings and References

Extension Programme: Planning and Evaluation

The first step to promote any extension programme is to prepare useful programme based on community need. Extension Programme planning is a blueprint or plan to an extension worker for effective execution. It is a procedure of working with people in an effort to identify and recognise the unsatisfactory situations or problems and to determine the possible solutions. To understand the extension programme planning process, certain basic concepts of an extension programme, planning and extension planning need to be understood.

Programme

The word 'programme' has several distinct meanings in the dictionary. It means a proclamation, a prospectus, a list of events, a plan of procedure, a course of action prepared or announced beforehand, a logical sequence of operations to be performed in solving a problem. This is a written statement which describes the extension activities proposed, the problems they address, the premises on which they are based, the objectives they seek to attain, the actions and the resources they require.

Programme

It is a written statement which contains the following four elements:

Objectives which the extension worker expects to be achieved in the area within a specified period of time. This will often be a one-year period, to enable the agent to review the programme at the start of each farming year.

Means of achieving these objectives.

Resources that are needed to fulfil the programme

Work plan indicating the schedule of extension activities that will lead to the fulfilment of the programme objectives.

According to Kelsey and Hearne (1949), an "extension programme" is a statement of situation, objectives, problems and solutions'.

According to the USDA (1956), an "extension programme" is arrived at co-operatively by the local people and the extension staff and includes a statement of:

- The situation in which the people are located;
- The problems that are a part of the local situation;
- The objectives and goals of the local people in relation to these problems; and
- The recommendations or solutions to reach these objectives on a long-time basis (may be several years) or on a short-time basis (may be one year or less).

Leagans (1961) says that an "extension programme" is a set of clearly defined, consciously conceived objectives or ends, derived from an adequate analysis of the situation, which are to be achieved through extension teaching activity. Lawrence (1962) says that an "extension programme" is the sum total of all the activities and undertakings of a county extension services. It includes: (i) programme planning process; (ii) written programme statement; (iii) plan of work; (iv) programme execution; (v) results; and (vi) evaluation.

- From the above definitions, it is clear that an extension programme:
- Is a written statement;
- Is the end product of extension programme planning;
- Includes a statement of situation, objectives, problems and solutions;
- Is relatively permanent but requires constant revision;
- May include long-term as well as short-term programme objectives;
- Forms the basis of extension teaching plans;
- Has been drawn up in advance; and
- Has been built on the basis of content.

Plan or Plan of work

Plan is schedule of development work outlining different activities in a specific period. It answers the questions like what, why, how, and when as well as by whom and where the work is to be done.

Planning

Planning is a designing courses of action to achieve ends. It is a progressive step by step process. It is never completed.

Social Planning

Social Planning has been defined as a conscious, collaborative, interactional process combining investigation, discussion, agreement and action in order to achieve the conditions, relationship and values regarded as desirable.

Programme Planning

Programme planning is the process of making decisions about the direction and intensity of extension education efforts to bring about desirable changes among people/community.

Extension Programme

Extension programme is a statement of situation, objectives, problems, strategies and solutions to developmental problem and issues. This is a very simple and comprehensive definition of extension programme which is widely accepted by the extension professionals.

Situation

Situation is a statement of affairs that includes the cultural, social, economic and physical conditions in which a particular group of people find themselves at a given period of time. The situation which constitutes the environment is continuously changing. The changing environment aspects that are relevant to extension and development work are:

- Changes in technology.
- Changes in Government policy.
- Changes in overall economic activity including prices, employment of labour, raw material etc. Changes in social norms and attitudes of people towards development.

Aims are generalised and broad statement. It is a very generalised statement of direction and may have several objectives.

Example: Improvement of standard of living condition of dairy farmers of India.

Objective

Objectives are expression of ends towards which our efforts are directed. The dictionary meaning of objective is 'something that one's efforts or actions are intended to attain or accomplish'.

Example: Increase the yield of milk production by 20 per cent.

Goal: Goal is the distance in any given direction one expects to go during a given period of time. Example: Increase the average yield of milk production from 5 litres to 5.5 litters per day per animal in the current year by introducing scientific feed management practices.

Problem

Problem is an unsatisfactory situation. It is an issue or obstacle which makes it difficult to achieve a desired goal, objective or purpose. It refers to a situation, condition, or issue that is not yet resolved. In a broad sense, a problem exists when an individual becomes aware of a significant difference between what actually is and what is desired. It is a situation that causes concern and its solution is not known.

Example: A farmer may notice low milk yield of cow due to mastitis but may not know how to control it.

Need

It is a problem situation, the solution for which is also known. But the ability to make the use of the solution is presently not there.

Example: A farmer may want a milking machine to milk more animals but may not know how to get it.

Solution

Solution is a course of proposed action to change an unsatisfactory condition to one that is more satisfying.

Example: Increase in milk yields of cow by providing treatment facilities of mastitis to animals

Calendar of work: It is a time schedule of work arranged chronologically, according to the time period. It indicates, for any given point of time, the kind of activities to be pursued.

Example: Clean milk production awareness programme on first Sunday of every month during the year 2020.

Project: This pertains to one selected component of the extension programme. Thus, when extension programme is a composite plan of action, extending over a period of years, and extension plan is an annual plan of work, extension project refers to the plan of solving a single problem. A project is a specification of work to be done or procedures to be followed in order to accomplish a particular objective.

Project Management

It is the process of managing and directing the appropriate use of resources such as people, materials, money and time to complete a particular project according to the objectives set forth.

Extension Planning

The concept of extension planning is based on a number of assumptions. Boyle (1965) has listed the following assumptions in this regard:

- Planning change is a necessary prerequisite to effective social progress for people and communities.
- The most desirable change is predetermined and democratically achieved.
- Extension education programmes, if properly planned and implemented, can make a significant contribution to planned change.
- It is possible to select, organize and administer a programme that will contribute to the social and economic progress of people.

- People and communities need the guidance, leadership and help of extension educators to solve their problems in a planned and systematic way.

Assumptions on Extension Planning

According to Kelsey and Hearne (1967), the objectives of having a programme are as follows:

1. To ensure careful consideration of what is to be done and why
2. To furnish a guide against which to judge all new proposal
3. To establish objectives toward which progress can be measured and evaluated
4. To have means of choosing the important (deep rooted) from incidental (minor, less important) problems and the permanent from temporary changes
5. To develop a common understanding about the means and ends between various functionaries and organisations.
6. To ensure continuity during changes in personnel
7. To help develop leadership
8. To avoid waste of time and money and promote efficiency.
9. To justify expenditure and to ensure flow of funds.
10. To have available on written form a statement for public use.

Extension Programme Planning

Extension programme planning is viewed as a process through which representatives of the people are intensively involved with extension personnel and other professional people in four activities (Boyle, 1965) and they are :

i) Studying facts and trends
ii) Identifying problems and opportunities based on these facts and trends.
iii) Making decisions about the problems and opportunities that should be given priority and
iv) Establishing objectives and recommendations for future economic and social development of a community through educational programmes.

Objectives of Programme Planning

Properly planned programme gives many benefits. Objectives of any extension programme is to influence people to make changes in their life and making a living. The postulation is that there is need for change and people are not aware. It is necessary to make them aware about their problems and develop their needs. Important objectives of having a programme planning as per Kelsey and Hearne (1966) are as follows;

i) To ensure careful consideration of what is to be done and why.
ii) To furnish a guide against which to judge all new proposals
iii) To establish objectives toward which progress can be measured and evaluated.
iv) To have a means of choosing the important/deep rooted from incidental/ minor/less important problems and the permanent from the temporary changes.
v) To develop a common understanding about the means and ends between various functionaries and organisations.
vi) To ensure continuity during changes in personnel.
vii) To help develop leadership.
viii) Avoid wastage of resources, money and promote efficiency.
ix) To justify expenditure and ensure flow of fund.
x) To have available in written form a statement for public use.

Need Identification in Programme Planning

Successful programme planning is one of identifying accurately what people want, think they need, and actually getting these items converted into a realistic well organized and concerted series of forceful developmental activities. Effective programmes to promote change are developed through finding people's needs and arranging action that helps meet them. Hence, a clear understanding of the nature and role of people's needs in programmes is essential to a livestock extension worker. In development programmes, people participate only when they think that the programme is valuable to them in meeting personal, family, group or community needs which they themselves recognize. The element of need and need identification therefore, should be the fundamental concern in extension programmes.

Principle of Programme Planning

Planning of extension programme is to be done on the basis of certain well recognised principles which should be clearly understood and followed by extension workers. The main principles are:

1. Extension programme planning should be based on analysis of the factual situation

It is important to take into account the conditions that exist at a particular time. This implies that factors such as land, crops, economic trends, social structure, economic status of the people, their habits, traditions and culture, in fact, everything about the area in which the job is to be done and its people, may be considered while planning an extension programme. The present situation is to be analysed and interpreted on the basis of past experiences.

2. Extension programme planning selects problems based on people's interests and needs

Sound programme building selects problems based on people's needs. I t is necessary to select these problems which are most urgent and of widest concern. Choice of problems must be from among those highlighted by an analysis of the facts regarding what are felt as unfelt needs. To be effective, extension work must begin with the interests of the families. It must meet interest and use them as a spring-board for developing further interests. It is common knowledge that people join together because of mutual interests and needs.

3. Extension programme planning determines definite objectives and solutions which offer satisfaction

In order to hold interest, we must set working objectives and offer solutions which are within reach and which will give satisfaction on achievement. This is related to motivation for action. People must see how they or their communities are going to benefit from the proposed solutions. Very often the simplicity or dramatic effect of the practice recommended is the most potent factor in its wide adoption. Further, if there is to be progress and not more evolution in the development of man, the objectives must be periodically revised in view of the progress made. In other words, as changes occur, objectives need to be re determined to allow for even further progress to be realized.

4. Extension programme planning has permanence with flexibility

Any good programme must be forward looking and permanent. Permanence means anticipating years of related and well organized effort. Along with this lower process, which both follow and makes a long-term trend, experience has shown that particular items will need to be changed to meet unforeseen contingencies or emergencies. Without flexibility, the programme may not, in fact, meet the needs of the people. A programme should be prepared well in advance of its execution but not too far ahead of time. Ordinary events may subject it to change in part though not in total. It is obvious that an extension programme must be kept flexible to meet the changing needs and interests of the people.

5. Extension programme planning has both balance and emphasis

A good programme should cover the majority of people's important interests. It must be comprehensive enough to embrace all groups, creeds and races at all levels and community, block, state, national and international problems. It is futile to deal with only one phase of life in a community as an end in itself. At the same time, a few of the most important or timely problems should be chosen for emphasis. To avoid scattered effort, something must stand out. Decisions must be made as to which of the needs are most urgent. The next consideration in choosing items for emphasis is to promote efficiency by permitting a good distribution of time and effort throughout the year. Too many things carried out simultaneously will divide either the worker's or the people's attention.

6. Extension programme planning has a definite plan of work

No matter how well a programme is thought through, it is of no use unless carried out. This implies good organization and careful planning for action. A plan of work is an outline of procedure so arranged as to enable efficient execution of the entire programme. It is the answer to what, where, when and how the job will be done. In carrying out programme plans, different leaders and groups may work on various phases, i.e., the women in the community may work on one segment, the men on a second segment and youth-club members on a third. Organization should be used as a tool to accomplish these purposes, never as an end in itself.

7. Extension programme planning is an educational process

The people who do the planning may participate in local surveys and neighbourhood observations. This provides an opportunity for them to learn more about their own community and area and increases their interest. The extension worker has the responsibilities of providing local leaders with the knowledge, skills and attitudes they must have if they are to help in educationally serving the people. Essentially, learning takes place through the experiences the learner has and the responses he makes to the stimuli of his environment. The experience gained in finding facts, analyzing situations, recognizing problems, stating objectives and thinking of possible solutions and alternatives should make for a better and more effective learning environment. The extension personnel should remember this fact and provide opportunities for the effective participation of local people in programme planning.

8. Extension programme planning is a continuous process

Since programme planning is viewed as an educational process and since education is seen as a continuous process, therefore it logically holds that extension programme planning is a continuous process. There is no question of exhausting new knowledge, either in the subject matter with which we deal or in the methods of teaching.

9. Extension programme planning is a co-ordinating process

Extension programme planning finds the most important problems and seeks agreement on definite objectives. It coordinates the efforts of all interested leaders, groups and agencies and considers the use of resources. It obtains the interest and co-operation of many people by showing them why things need to be done. This is important in working with people. Within the extension organization, the block staff may work together on an integrated programme.

10. Extension programme planning involves local people and their institutions

Involvement of local people and their institutions is very essential for the success of any programme for their development. People become interested and give better support to the programme when they are involved in the planning process. So, extension programmes should be planned and implemented with the people.

11. Extension programme planning provides for evaluation of results

Since extension programme planning involves decision-making procedures, so evaluation is important in order to make intelligent decisions aimed at achieving the stated objectives. Matthews (1962) pointed out that extension programme planning and evaluation go together.

Effective evaluation will, of course, depend on clear objectives, knowing which people we are trying to teach and having records of the results in terms that reflect changes in their action. Starting a programme with the intention of engaging in a careful evaluation at the close of a specific period has a salutary effect on all the intermediate processes. However, provision has to be made both for concurrent and ex-post facto types of evaluation.

Programme Planning Process

Three phases involved in programme planning process are :

i) Programme Formulation
ii) Programme Execution
iii) Programme Evaluation

Steps in Extension Programme Planning

There are eight steps which form a continuous cycle of programme planning process under three distinct phases mentioned above. These steps are:

1. Collection of facts
2. Analysis of situation
3. Identification of problems
4. Programme Formulation visible
5. Developing plan of work and calendar of operations
6. Implementation of activities
7. Evaluation of programme
8. Reconsideration and revision of the programme

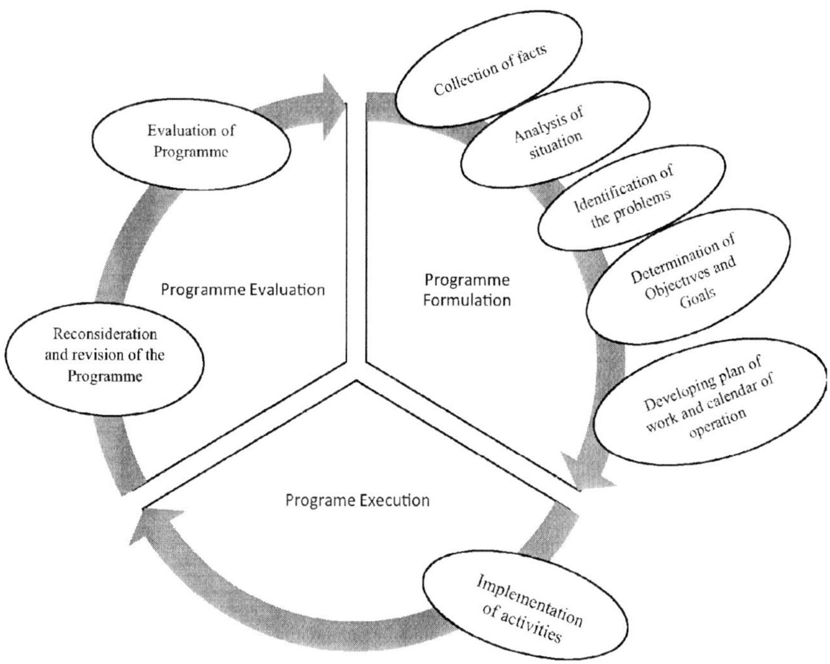

Development Programme Planning Process

Suppose you want to start an extension programme in a block to reduce the mortality level of backyard poultry farming. Now, you have only perceived that there is mortality in backyard poultry in a particular block. To address that problem, we need an extension programme. To develop, design and implement the programme, we have to follow the following steps.

1. **Collection of facts:** It is the starting point of a programme planning process. We need facts related to poultry rearing practices prevailing in the area, mortality rate in poultry, provision of veterinary services in the area, socio-

economic status of the poultry farmers, etc. All these related facts, we may get from the records available at veterinary dispensary or LAC, or we may survey the area or we may get the required facts from other sources like panchayats, cooperatives, etc. to develop a programme.

2. **Analysis of situation:** Facts do not yield much information. The data collected from various sources are then analysed with the help of poultry farmers, suppliers and experts like veterinary doctors and para-veterinary workers of that area. If we analyse the situation, we may get the answer like that there is poultry mortality due to non-vaccination of birds or poor management of the backyard poultry by the farmers. We may also get conflicting information from different sources, and must judge which one is reliable. This helps us in understanding the local situations in a proper perspective.

3. **Identification of the problems:** A proper analysis and interpretation of data related to poultry farming shall help in correctly identifying the problems related to poultry mortality. Here, our technical knowledge on the subject would be much helpful. There may be many problems, but only the urgent and significant ones which may be solved with the available resources and within the limits of time, should be selected. We should not rely too much only on our expertise and experience in identification of local problems, rather we should involve the farmers in identification of problems.

4. **Determination of Objectives and Goals:** Once the situation analysis is done correctly and problems are identified, it would be easier to take decision about what to do to address the problems faced by the farmers. The key questions would be how the problems of poultry mortality be checked. The solutions to check poultry mortality require clear, real and attainable objectives. We should express objectives of the extension programme in terms of amount and numbers rather than general statements. Instead of stating to "reduce the poultry mortality" as objective we may state to "reduce poultry mortality to 10 percent in the project area within 05 years". Once objective is set, the goals to achieve the objective may be stated. For an example to the objective of reducing poultry mortality to 10 percent within 05 years, the goals may be to (i) reduce poultry mortality from 50 percent to 30 percent in the first year, (ii) to train 50 percent of the poultry farmers of the project villages on prevention and control of Ranikhet and Fowl pox in poultry in the first year, (iii) to aware 50 percent of poultry farmers of project villages on good poultry management practices in the first year, etc.

5. **Developing plan of work and calendar of operations :** Once programme objectives and goals are set clearly, we have to develop schedule of activities indicating who should do what job. We have to decide what knowledge and skills the farmers need; what type of technical information required from specialist; what extension methods should be used; resources and support required from the user and Department of Veterinary and Animal Husbandry. The plan of work should have all the essential details to implement the activities in the field. The calendar of operations should have dimensions of 'when', 'where', 'how' and by 'whom'. The calendar of activities should indicate clearly when to start the activities and to finish it preferable mentioning the year, month, date and time. In 'where' aspect, it must be clearly stated where the activities to be performed. The 'how' aspect covers what are the methods used to perform the activities like by conducting meeting, training, demonstration, etc. besides how much quantity of different inputs are required for the programme. The calendar of works should also mention by whom- veterinary doctor, livestock inspector, para-veterinary workers, etc. the activities are going to be done.

6. **Implementation of activities :** Based on the plan of work and calendar of activities, the implementation of activities is the next step in programme implementation. For effective implementation, advance preparation is essential to ensure that the activities are done as per planning. We have to make all arrangements for teaching aids and inputs. The persons who are responsible to perform the activities require to take up the activities in right time to complete the work in schedule time as per the project plan. If there is any problem in performing the activities, necessary rescheduling may be done.

7. **Evaluation of programme :** Evaluation is the process by which the effectiveness of programme is assessed. It is done to measure the degree of success of the programme in terms of the objective set forth. Every extension programme should have inbuilt system of evaluation to know outcome of the programme. The evaluation used to answer the following questions:

   i) Are the programme implementation proceeding in right direction? It may point out omissions, recommended changes and suggest new directions.

   ii) are the outcomes of the programme good enough and on expected line?

   iii) is the implementation programme as planned?

   Evaluation is a waste of time and money unless the results have an influence in improving the future extension decisions. The main concern in the evaluation of extension programme is to know what happened to the results of extension programme? Are the results as per our expectations or there are unexpected results? Besides, we also want to know whether all planed inputs required for the programme implementation are made available in time or not?

8. **Reconsideration and revision of the programme :** The systematic and periodic evaluation of the programme will reveal the weak and strong points of the programme. Based on these points the programme is reconsidered and the necessary adjustments and changes should be made in order to make it more meaningful and sound. On the basis of evaluation results, if needed, the programme should be revised for further consideration to implement. If the programme evaluation results are as per the project objectives, new project objectives may be added and extension programme may be redesigned to implement the programme. If the programme evaluation results are not as per the project objectives, then necessary corrective steps may be introduced based on our past experiences to modify the extension programme for better implementation.

Extension Programme Planning Model Proposed by Sandhu

Sandhu (1965) developed a model for planning extension and rural development programmes. This model has six phases with a number or steps to be followed under each phase.

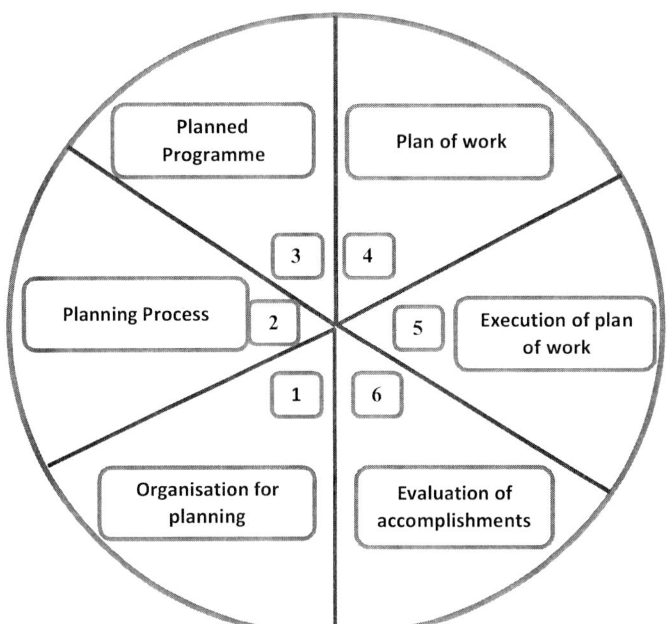

Extension Programme Planning Model

The various phases and steps involved in this model are:

I. Organisation for Planning

The concept of involving potential clientele in the planning of extension programmes has received widespread acceptance. Involvement of people in making decisions about educational objectives not only results in better decisions about educational objectives, but also speeds up the process of educational change. By participating in the analysis of the local situation, the people's representatives are better informed and are better prepared for positive action.

The following conditions should be met in order to ensure that a good organisation has been set up

1. All social systems and special interest groups are identified.
2. Members of the planning committee represent all major interest groups, various economic and social levels of people, major vocations of the locality and other important elements in the area.
3. Each member of the planning committee clearly understands
   a) the purpose of the group;
   b) how the group should function in attaining its purpose; and
   c) his individual role as a member.
4. Members of the planning committee have been elected, nominated or co-opted by appropriate democratic procedures.

II. Planning process

a) Reaching understanding regarding principles, procedures, roles and time schedule

It is necessary that all staff and the people's representatives are familiar with the principles and procedures of programme planning for the purposes of clarity and uniformity of action.

The following conditions should be met in order in fulfil the spirit of this step:

i) A clearly defined statement of purpose and roles of each member is given by the planning committee.

ii) The block, district and state level extension workers and programme planning committee members have understood:
   a) the roles of extension workers in programme planning;
   b) the role of programme planning committee members;
   c) the purpose of programme planning;

d) the scope of extension's educational responsibilities;
e) the procedures to be followed;
f) the principles to be kept in view; and
g) the time schedule to be followed.

b) Analyse situation

Situation analysis involves collection, analysis and interpretation of the existing facts. Good planning depends on the availability of adequate and reliable data and scientific elaboration and interpretation of the same.

The following criteria should be met in order to ensure that this step has been adequately followed.

- Facts needed to evaluate the accomplishment of the previous year's programme are collected.
- Local facts needed to define correct and projected needs and interests and problems of the area are assembled
- The basic facts assembled and collected about background information are analysed and interpreted.
- The major needs and problems of the area, which are within the scope of extension's educational responsibility, are identified.

c) Determine objectives

It is essential in the programme planning process that before deciding on the projects to be undertaken, basic objectives of the programme are determined by the villagers in consultation with the extension staff.

The following conditions or qualities will exist when objectives have been determined adequately and properly

- Objectives have been determined relating to major problems, need and/or interests as determined by the programme planning committee.
- Both immediate and long-term objectives have been determined.

d) Select problems with due regard to priorities

Selection of problems to be tackled will involve identification, classification and selection with due regard to priorities. Identification of problems will be done on the basis of situation analysis. Once the problems have been identified, it is desirable that they be properly classified into the following categories:

- Problems which can be solved by the people themselves with no outside financial aid.

- Problems which can be solved by the people with the aid of the Panchayat Samiti
- Problems which can only be solved with the help of Government funds

The following conditions will exist when the requirements of this step have been adequately met:

- Of the identified problems, the most felt and of widest concern are selected by the extension agents and people's representatives.
- Selected problems are related to the family, community block and situation.
- For tackling the selected problems, the time is scheduled on greatest priority basis.

e) Find solutions to problems

The Village Level Workers at the village level and the concerned Extension Officer at the block level are two most important functionaries who advise the village families and the village institutions regarding solutions to their problems. The other Extension officials at various levels may join with the team in finding solutions to problems. Experiences of the farmers and suggestions of the specialists will help in arriving at a joint decision.

The following conditions will exist when this step has been properly carried out

- All the available research findings in the State are collected and projected.
- Block level and district level specialists make suitable solution to the problems according to the research findings.

III. Planned Programme

As Leagans (1961) pointed out, it is of utmost importance that the staff and the people in each area not only develop an extension programme, but also prepare the programme in a written form that is readily understood and is suitable for obtaining approval and use as a guide for officials and non-officials.

The problems should be stated from the viewpoint of the farm, the home and the community. They should not be stated in terms of solutions. The objectives should also be stated at a lower level in specific and measurable terms. They should include details about the learners to be reached subject matter to be taught and the behavioural changes to be effected. The objectives may also be stated from the point of view of the extension organisations and the extension public.

The following conditions will be met in order to have a good programme statement :

- The written programme should be suitable for use by the staff, planning groups and other individuals or groups concerned with the programme.
- It should clearly state the important problems or needs identified by the staff and the people in the programming process.
- It should specify the subject matter related to each objective that is highly significant to the people, socially or economically or both.
- It should be used as the basis for developing annual plans of work.

IV. Plan of Work

Preparing a plàn of activities directed towards solving selected problems is an important step. A plan of work is the listing of activities by which the objectives already decided upon are to be achieved.

The following conditions should exist in a good plan

- The plan of work is in written form.
- It has been developed co-operatively by the extension workers and people's representatives.
- It identifies the specific educational job to be done.
- The plan indicates for each educational job.
    - How it will be done
    - When it will be done
    - Where it will be done
    - Who will do it
    - What people are to be reached
- The subject matter is appropriate considering the people's level of interests, knowledge, attitude and available time and technology.
- The plan provides for the needed training of extension workers and leaders.
- Specific changes to be achieved or evidence of accomplishment are indicated clearly.

V. Implementation Phase

a) Make advance arrangement for inputs and teaching aids

The conditions to meet the requirements of this step are

- Realistic needs of inputs such as fertiliser, seeds, credit facilities etc. have been worked out jointly by the areas extension staff and the Panchayat Raj institutions.

- Needed inputs have been procured well in time and stocked at proper places.
- Teaching aids to be used by the extension workers have been prepared and/ or procured in sufficient quantity, well in time.

b) Interpret the approved programme to the staff and the people's representatives.

The following criteria will be met to ensure that this step has been adequately undertaken

- The approved programme has been explained adequately.
- The plan of work has also been explained adequately.
- They have been explained to all the block staff, all the people's representatives and other important leaders.

d) Carry out the plan of work

The approved programme should be carried out, step by step, according to the plan of work and in a co-ordinated manner. The success of a programme depends on the methods used to implement it.

It should be ensured that -

- the plans for coordination including calendar of activities within and outside extension agency system
- the techniques, methods and materials vary appropriate to the situation and clientele
- the subject matter used was appropriate considering the people and their objectives
- the plans for shared responsibilities were followed.

VI. Evaluation of Accomplishments

Concurrent and ***ex-post facto*** review of progress towards the objectives is an essential phase of extension programme planning. This keeps the extension agency on the right track and helps in differentiating means from ends. Evaluation of the activities should be undertaken jointly by the extension staff and the people's representative organisations at different levels.

Conditions that will exist when this guideline is met are as under

- Evaluation plans were developed for each of the phases of the programme to be evaluated as indicated in the annual plan of work.

- A report of accomplishments and implications was made to the extension governing group. The governing group in projecting their plans for extension activities gave the findings from the report of accomplishments and implications.

Extension Programme Monitoring and Evaluation

Monitoring

Mobile Veterinary Unit (MVU) is a programme launched by Government of Odisha and implemented by the Department of Animal Husbandry and Veterinary Services of Odisha. The main objectives of the programme are to provide door step veterinary services to the poor and needy people of the state. At Gram Panchayat level, the Livestock Inspector keep record of number of animal treated, number of farmers availed the benefits, number of vaccination, deworming and AI conducted, etc. He also periodically submits record and attend meeting at Block level veterinary office. Similarly, at block level, veterinary doctor makes arrangement of vehicle, medicine, staffs, etc. for the programme. He also periodically sends reports and attend meetings at the district level. treatments. At district level, the Chief District Veterinary Officer, makes budget provision, provides veterinary staff, conducts field visits, etc., for successful implementation of the programme. All these functionaries at Gram Panchayat, Block and District levels, what are they doing for this programme? In fact, besides implementation, they are actively involved with the monitoring of the programme. They are monitoring to compare the actual progress in activities and results against the objectives formulated in the programme.

In extension programme, provision of monitoring mechanism is made to get feedback on the progress of the project. For any veterinary extension project, higher officers other than those who are implementing the project are assigned the responsibilities of monitoring the implementation of the project. Monitoring is undertaken or performed while a project or a programme or a scheme is being implemented. It is done with the aim of improving its design and functioning while in action.

Meaning of Monitoring

The word "monitor" is derived from the Latin word meaning to 'warn'. *Monitoring* is an integral and important part of a project management information system. Extension workers require information to keep track of development, to guide its course of action.

Monitoring is a continuous / periodic review and surveillance by the management team, at every level of the implementation of an activity to ensure that input deliveries, work schedules, targeted outputs and other required actions are proceeding according to plan. Availability of a 'plan' is a pre-condition for monitoring.

We may define monitoring is that it is a process of measuring, recording, collecting, processing and communicating information to assist project management decision-making. To be precise and brief, "monitoring system is an information system for management decision making".

According to Shapiro "Monitoring is the collection and analysis of information as a project progresses. It is aimed at improving the efficiency and effectiveness of a project or organization. It is based on targets set and activities planned during the planning phase of work. It helps to keep the work on track and can let management know when things are going wrong. If done properly, it is an invaluable tool for good management and it provides a useful base for evaluation."

Monitoring of programme activities begins with the start of a project and ends with the completion of the project, but it is a continuous process during the implementation of project. The key requirement for Monitoring is an 'ACTION PLAN' without which monitoring is not possible. The whole gamut of monitoring is explained in the Table below.

Gamut of Monitoring

What ?	Check, review, overview, keep track, observe, control, guide, correct, inspect, supervise, verify, feed-back, follow up of the activities	Progress of programme implementation with reference to action plan
Why?	To ensure successful implementation of the project by identifying shortfalls, deviation, problems and the reasons there to	Take appropriate corrective/ remedial action to keep the project on track
When?	During the implementation of the project continuously / periodically	From the inception till completion of the project (concurrently with project implementation)
Who ?	BY the project management team at different levels	Including beneficiaries (participatory monitoring).

A project's operation, performance, and impacts are the aspects of concern in monitoring with a view to keep track on the technical and economic 'efficiency' of the project.

Monitoring is a management function, and all those who are involved in the project implementations are to be involved in the monitoring process. This may include, even the beneficiaries when local groups / organizations have been formed as part of project strategy (e.g.: Farmers' group, Self Help Group, Water Users Committee, Education Committees, User Groups, etc.). It is important to appreciate that monitoring is not an individual's function but a collective function. When all stakeholders, including beneficiaries are involved in monitoring, then it paves way for participatory monitoring.

Basic Concepts and Elements in Monitoring

Four concepts are basic to monitoring and evaluation.

They are:

1. Operational investment (e.g., investment per family),
2. Operational efficiency (e.g., the number of visits, meetings, demonstrations, and trials, per extension worker),
3. Technical efficiency (e.g., output, and value added), and
4. Extension-induced changes (e.g., income, and income distribution)

Capability, effectiveness, efficiency and impact are monitored and evaluated

i) **Capability** is the command that programme has over physical, financial, and human resources, enabling it to serve its clients (e.g. livestock farmers, SHG members). It is reflected by outreach, intensity, technical competence, and physical and financial resources.

ii) **Effectiveness** is defined as "the degree to which goals are attained". It is the adequacy of endeavour to accomplish a purpose for producing intended or expected result. Every developmental project has to take into consideration the effectiveness in order to produce desired result with the given time period. Monitoring the project effectiveness is quite crucial.

iii) **Efficiency** means functioning in the best possible manner with the least waste of time and effort. Lon Roberts defines efficiency as "to the degree of economy with which the process consumes resources especially time and money". Monitoring of efficiency is essential as it will check wastage of resources and ensure completion of project in right time.

iv) **Impact** can be measured by a simple indicator, like Adoption Rate, Learning Achievement, etc. Such indicators provide ultimate tests for the success of any sectoral programmes.

Basic Elements in Monitoring

i) **Input:** Goods, Funds, Services, Manpower, Technology and other resources provided in a project with the expectation of OUTPUTS.

ii) **Results:** Certain things happen immediately, and certain things ultimately, while certain things in between these two (intermediate). According to sequence, the result of a livestock project can be grouped into three broad categories, such as productivity, production and income.

iii) **Output** (Immediate results)**:** Specific products or services, which an activity is expected to produce from its inputs in order to achieve the set objectives. Example: Increased milk production, vitamin use, Group formation, etc.)

iv) **Impact:** Outcome of Project Effects (broad long term objectives: Standard of living and reducing poverty both at individual and community level) - Ultimate results. Impact is described as the outcomes for a community or region than on individuals. It may include direct and indirect as well as primary, secondary and tertiary level.

Types of Monitoring

Beneficiary Contact Monitoring

Beneficiary contact monitoring is done to measure the delivery of services and inputs as per the project guideline. It is taken up to keep records of project beneficiaries, response of beneficiaries and analyse periodically the penetration of the service in the project area.

Process Monitoring: Project implementation begins with deployment of inputs/ resources to realize some specific outputs. The conversion of inputs into outputs will involve certain methods, activities, and completion of certain events. This happens in a sequence as below.

Process: It is the way in which activities are conducted. Processes are continuous and cuts across activities. For example, rapport building as a process is relevant to poultry group formation activities, training, etc.

Milestones: These are a series of achievements that leads to a completion of stage in an activity (an event). For example: Formation of 100 SHGs in the project area.

Activities: These are what we do to deliver the output. Activities always have a beginning and an end and are associated with numbers linked to a budget. For example: Conduction of 10 training programmes on improved dairy farming in the project villages.

Output: This is what a project delivers before the close of the project

Process monitoring is an approach that ensures that processes are steered to achieve the desired results and that quality is maintained throughout. As long as there is a focus, not only on the inputs and outputs, but the way in which the outputs are being delivered, and quality indicators are devised and tracked, process monitoring would be useful and successful.

Tools and Techniques of Monitoring

Following tools are used for the purpose of monitoring:

i) **Regular progress report :** Monthly or quarterly progress reports related to physical and financial progress against the stated target is an important tool for monitoring the progress of the project. From the financial and physical progress report, it is often possible to make a rapid assessment of whether, and to what extent, the original activities of the scheme have been fulfilled, and whether it is working successfully within the allocated budget.

ii) **Monitoring staff performance (review) Monitoring :** As per the requirement of the project, monthly or weekly review meeting of the project staffs are conducted to monitor the performance of staff in meeting the project objectives.

iii) **Tour reports by field staff :** Tour report of the project staff will indicate their activities in the field as per the project guideline.

iv) **Participant observation :** The field staff may stay in the villages and observe the groups closely so as to obtain sensitive, first-hand insights which will be useful for monitoring the progress of the project.

v) **Reports from visitors :** The tour reports of the visitors to the project area (Project Director, State Level Officials, researchers, etc) provide required information to the project management team for its better implementation.

vi) **Interviews :** Group members and community leaders should be interviewed on their attitude towards the scheme and resultant behavioural changes.

vii) **Participatory Monitoring :** In his process, the beneficiaries are made partners in monitoring and evaluation. Project staff and beneficiaries discuss and assess the performance together, in order to understand how they have performed, what the problems are and what the future holds for them. The project staff mainly plays a guiding role to formulate appropriate questions and eliciting answers. For example, while monitoring the performance of a SHG along with the members of the group, the group members and project staff can be prompted to draw inferences from their meeting book, attendance register, and savings books, etc. regarding their progress.

viii) **Key informants :** In addition to our regular contacts, we must try to interact with other people who may be useful sources of information. e.g. Teachers, Postmaster, Kirana Shop, SHGs etc.

ix) **Complaints / grievances :** Many a times, complaints and grievances petition from people in general and target group in particular may throw some light on the actual performance of the scheme. Every project should make provisions for such source of information as part of monitoring mechanism.

Indicators of Monitoring

Following types of indicator are used in monitoring:

i) **Quantitative indicators :** Provide numeric information about a change in a situation. For example, number of farmers trained in the programme, number of SHG formed, etc.

ii) **Qualitative indicators :** Are largely descriptive statements about processes and outcomes? For example, what is the level of participation of livestock farmers in meetings? How are feed and fodder requirement of goat farmers are assessed?

iii) **Direct indicators :** Provide information, which expressly relates to what is being measured. If, for example, information regarding functioning of farmers' producer group is required then their functioning is measured.

iv) **Indirect indicators :** Essential information, chosen from amongst many types of information to serve as substitutes (or proxy indicators) for answering questions or responding to statements that are difficult to measure. For example, if we are interested in measuring the level of poverty in a community, instead of choosing direct indicators for income, indirect indicators for poverty may be chosen, e.g. persons are poor if they go for MGNREGA work as unskilled labour.

v) **Process indicators :** Steps involved in planning, designing, construction of sheds, supply of animals and marketing of milk are the process involved in a dairy farming for example, are the processes involved in dairy development programme.

vi) **Progress indicators :** It measures or monitor changes against stated targets in the project plan. The number of dairy farmers assisted, number of training programmes conducted, number of sheds conducted, number of vaccination programmes conducted, number of awareness camp organised, etc.

Evaluation

Evaluation is a process for determining systematically and objectively the relevance, efficiency, effectiveness and impact of project activities in the light of their stated objectives. Unlike monitoring, 'evaluation' is more comprehensive. In a literal sense, evaluation is the determination of value to an object or a phenomenon. Evaluation is a study of the outcome of a project (changes in income, housing quality, benefits distribution, cost-effectiveness, etc.) with the aim of improving the design of future projects. Evaluation studies can assess the extent to which the project produced the intended impacts (increase in income, better housing quality, distribution of the benefits between different groups, etc.) and can evaluate the cost-effectiveness of the project as compared with other options. Extension programmes are mostly funded with public money and are planned and implemented by an organization, which in most cases is a Department of a government. In order to justify the appropriation of public funds and continuing support from the people, it is necessary that their management as well as impact be properly and adequately evaluated from time to time.

The word 'evaluation' has its origin in the Latin word "*valere*" meaning to be strong or valiant. Its dictionary meanings are the determination of the value, the strength or worth of something, an appraisal, an estimates of the force of or making a judgement of something.

Evaluation as applied to the field of extension education, may be defined as "a process of systematic appraisal by which we determine the value, worth or meaning of an activity or an enterprise". It is a method for determining how far an activity has progressed and how much further it should be carried to accomplish objectives'. Thus to an extension worker evaluation means determining the results of his extension programmes in order to know the extent to which objectives have been achieved and why and what changes would be needed in case the programme is planned again, or in its implementation.

Definitions of evaluation

More specific definitions of evaluation are given by persons involved in rural development programmes. While most of these definitions refer specifically to the assessment of the results of programmes of extension education, they can also be applied to the training aspect of such programmes. Some definitions of evaluation are:

- It is a process, which enables the administrator to describe the effects of his programme and thereby make progressive adjustments in order to reach his goal more effectively (Jahoda and Barnit, 1955).
- Programme evaluation is the determination of the extent to which the desired objectives have been attained or the amount of movement that has been made in the desired direction (Boyle and Johns, 1970).
- Programme evaluation is the process of judging the worth or value of a programme. The judgement is formed by comparing the programme should be (Steele, 1970).
- Evaluation is the process of delineating, obtaining and providing useful information for judging decision alternative (Stufflebeam, 1971).
- Evaluation is a co-ordinated process carried on by the total system and its individual subsystem. It consists of making judgements about a planned programme based on established criteria and known, observable evidence (Boone, 1985).

Monitoring consists of routine collection of information relating to the on-going programmes, schemes or projects. Both, monitoring and evaluation are indispensable vis-a-vis a prorgramme, a scheme or a project. The main purpose of evaluation is to improve the programme by identifying merits and demerits of the programme but not to discourage the workers and the programme. It is a process concerned with final checking and improving the programmes. Evaluation covers pre-planning, planning and implementation stages of the programmes. In other words, evaluation deals with such aspects that occur before the implementation of the programme, during the operation of the programme and after the completion of the programme. In scientific terms, evaluation is an important procedural basis for discovering what has been accomplished, which intended outcomes have been achieved, what weaknesses or failures have occurred and what importance should be ascribed to each of these.

Based on the above discussion, we can now clearly summarise the general objectives of monitoring and evaluation as follows:

i) to identify the merits and demerits.
ii) to provide feedback to the implementing agency.
iii) to know the physical arrangements being made.
iv) to find out the problems to be remedied.
v) to know the extent of achievement of the set targets.
vi) to find out the appropriateness of utilization of the allocated funds
vii) to know whether the project or programme is going on right lines.

Nature of Monitoring and Evaluation

Monitoring and evaluation mechanisms assume great significance in the following context/situations:

- Provide constant feedback regarding the extent to which the projects are achieving their goals.
- Identify potential problems at an early stage and propose possible solutions.
- Monitor the accessibility of the project to all sections of the target population.
- Monitor the efficiency with which different components of the project are being implemented and suggest improvements, if any, required.
- Help in formative evaluation on the extent to which the project is able to achieve its general objectives.
- Form the basis for formulation of effective guidelines for the planning of future projects

- Improve project design: Past experience helps in better designing of the project
- Show need for mid-course corrections: A reliable flow of information during implementation enables managers to keep track of progress and suitably adjust the operations.

Features of Evaluation

Some of the basic features of evaluation are as follows:

- It is always with reference to stated criteria
- It is always with reference to a point of time
- It starts where progress reporting/monitoring/estimation surveys end
- It establishes relationship between policies/methods and results
- It investigates and find out factors for success/failure and suggest remedies
- More qualitative in approach and emphasis is on variability than standardization
- More purposive and less aggregative
- Its focus is - policy issues, problem formulation, organizational forms, administrative practices, and extension of technical contents of the programmes, people cooperation, attitude and impact

Difference between Appraisal, Monitoring and Evaluation

These three words, appraisal, monitoring and evaluation are used inter-changeable yet distinction can be established among these three concepts.

Appraisal

Appraisal is usually taken to mean a critical examination of a proposal of a programme or project, normally before it is approved for implementation and funding. Sometimes, evaluation and appraisal are used interchanging as if they are synonymous. Appraisal deals with economic viability, technical feasibility and social desirability of a project that is being contemplated. Thus, appraisal is basically a planning and project formulation activity. Appraisal may be guided by evaluation findings of similar projects / components, which have already been implemented.

Monitoring and Evaluation

As far as distinction between monitoring and evaluation is concerned, both monitoring and evaluations are undertaken to find out how a programme or project performs or has performed. The basic difference between monitoring and evaluation is given in Table.

Basic Differences between Monitoring and Evaluation

Continuous: Starts and ends with a programme	One shot operation: At a point of time (usually at completion or mid-way of programme)
Required for immediate use and mid-course correction expansion	Used for future planning/ replication/ expansion
Done by implementing personnel	Usually by outside agency
Quick but covers all units	In-depth; covers a sample
Correcting / managing	Learning process
Symptomatic, early warning system	Diagnostic

Types of evaluation

Once a project or programme is launched, its implementation involves many aspects -physical, human, financial and technical - which are subjected to certain processes directed at achieving the objectives in the form of outcome, product or improvement. And an evaluation may take into account all these as a whole or may focus on selected aspect(s) of a given programme. Evaluation can, however, be done by internal people (those involved in implementation of a policy, a scheme, project or a programme) or by outside persons or agencies, so as to ensure more validity, objectivity and fairness in the process of evaluation.

Evaluation is of different types depending upon different aspects or criteria considered thereof and are discussed in detail below.

1. Types of evaluation based on the different aspects of the Programme/ Project

Based on the aspect(s) of the programme or project covered, evaluation can be categorized into the following types:

i) Context evaluation

It evaluates or studies the context and the feasibility of developing a programme or a project. It is done prior to developing a programme based on the perceived need. It takes into account different aspects of the existing situation and the ground realities in terms of the -. needs, requirements of the people and the physical aspects of the area in the given context.

ii) Input evaluation

It takes into account different types of inputs - physicall material, human, financial, technical - involved since beginning of implementation of a programme or a project. It helps in assessing the nature, quantity, quality, adequacy and timeliness of different inputs into the programme.

iii) Process evaluation

This involves judging the nature and quality of activities or strategies of the project. It evaluates what has been done, who has done what and to what extent, the range and quality of the activities, etc. It seeks answers to questions such as the following.

- Are all the project activities going on as per the schedule plan? If not, why?
- Were any changes made to the intended activities? If' so, why?
- Are materials, information and their presentation in good quality?
- Is the project reaching the intended target people through appropriate activities?
- Are the involved participants and the key functionaries satisfied?

iv) Impact / outcome evaluation

This involves judging the extent to which the project had shown its effects vis-a-vis those expected or sought. In other words, the extent to which the relevant project has realized its goal and objectives. Thus, impact evaluation judges how far and how well the objectives were achieved and outcome evaluation judges how well the goal has been achieved. It seeks answers to questions such as:

- To what extent has the project met its objectives?
- How effective has the project been at producing desired/intended changes.
- Are there any factors outside the project that have contributed to or prevented the desired change?
- What progress has been made towards achieving the goal?
- Has the project resulted in any unintended change or effect?

2. Types of evaluation based on the stages of the Programme/Project

Evaluation may be done at the beginning or at the end or after completion of the project.

Accordingly, the evaluation may be classified as:

i) Formative Evaluation

Formative evaluation is done to assess the strength and weaknesses of the project before and during implementation. Some time we do pre-testing before a small group to know the responses of the members so that they are incorporated in the programme before implementation in a large scale. Its intent is to assess the ongoing project activities and provide information to monitor and improve the quality of the project. It is done at several points during the developmental period of a project and its activities. The purpose of formative evaluation is to provide information and judgments, which will be useful in making improvement in project.

ii) Summative Evaluation

Summative evaluations are conducted after the completion of the programme or project or scheme. It is meant to summarise and inform decisions about whether to continue the project (or parts of it), whether it is valuable to expand it into other settings. It involves seeking answers to questions such as:

- What were the main benefits and disappointments?
- What factors helped and hindered the project?
- What could be the advice to others willing to embark on something similar?
- What aspects can and will be sustained and how?
- Is it worth continuing in its current form? Why/ why not? '
- What recommendations have emerged about where to from here?

Summative evaluation is thus holistic and collects information and makes judgments about all related aspects - strategies, processes, activities and outcomes - thus provide an insight into resultant impact/outcome.

3. Types of evaluation based on the Agency conducting the Evaluation

Based on the agency involved in conducting evaluation, it is conveniently divided into the following two types.

i) ***Internal evaluation:*** It is the evaluation conducted by the implementing agency itself to know the progress of the programme and its outcomes.

ii) ***External evaluation:*** It is the evaluation conducted by an external agency by following the same procedures and guidelines of evaluation in measuring the programme and its outcomes.

Extension evaluation process

There are several models of evaluation available in the literature. However, a very simplified version of most of these models may be quite workable for evaluating extension programmes since, as Bhatnagar (1987) has pointed out, any extension evaluation process has to be based on certain assumptions. For example, if some inputs are provided in the form of a programme, specific outputs can be expected and if these outputs happen, then the purpose of the programme can be achieved; if the purpose is achieved, then the development goal is realised. This means that evaluation has to be so designed that the quality types and adequacy of the input measures, outputs and their impact in achieving the programme objectives have to be evaluated systematically.

Steps involved in an Extension Programme Evaluation Process

i) Formulation of Evaluation Objectives

What objectives this evaluation is going to achieve, must be specified in clear terms form the very beginning of the evaluation process. Thereafter, it would be easier for us to proceed further.

ii) Understanding programme objectives

Each extension programme, when formulated and implemented, will have specific well-defined objectives. Since evaluation is basically a process of determining the extent to which various extension activities were organized and managed and the extent to which they contributed to achieving the goals, programme objectives must be clearly understood before starting the evaluation process. This is a crucial step as all further efforts will be directed towards collecting evidence related to these objectives.

iii) Identification of indicators

The kind of evidence necessary to evaluate achievement in relation to specified programme objectives, it is necessary that specific beneficiaries of the programme be identified, the kind of changes expected in them be clearly stated for evaluation. Some examples include: % reduction of poultry mortality, number of beneficiaries benefited, number of training programmes conducted, etc. Once indicators are identified and specified than measurement of achievement will not be difficult.

iv) Decision on kind of information required

Once the indicators for evaluating the management and performance of a programme have been indicated, specific information to be collected may be worked out. Since there is usually more information than an extension worker can collect, he has to be very discriminating about the kind and amount of information that should be collected. Timing for collection of information may also need to be specified.

v) Sampling

The purpose of sampling is to take a relatively small number of units from the project population in such a way that the evidence collected from them becomes representative evidence of the entire project population. Although there are several sampling methods, perhaps stratified sampling procedures may be most suitable for extension evaluation studies as they allow inclusion of all interested groups and ensure enough heterogeneity in the sample.

vi) Deciding on the design of evaluation

The survey is most commonly used on conducting extension evaluations. An ideal design of evaluation may be an experimental one. This would allow separating the effect of the programme from other factors, by setting control and treatment groups. Several experimental designs, such as one-group pre-test-post-test design, static groups comparison, pre-test, post-test control group design, Solomon four-group design, longitudinal study design, etc. are available in literature and can be used. However, in actual practice, extension progammes are seldom run in a way that allows an experimental design of evaluation. In pilot Projects, it might be possible to use an experimental design of evaluation. By and large, a survey method is use. This method can be used for evaluating ongoing progress or as an ex-post facto evaluation of the programme after it has completed its tenure.

vii) Collection and analysis of evaluation data

Selection of the right kind of data collection method will depend on the objectives of the evaluation, kind of information needed, time and resources available and the type of respondents from whom information is to be collected. There are many methods for collection of information for evaluation purposes, such as the questionnaire, interview, observations, interviews, focus group discussion, case studies, systematic field observations, study of secondary data etc. After collection of data, it has to be tabulated, summarized and analyzed with adequate care. Help of computer may be taken to analyse the date.

viii) Interpretation of the results

The analysed data must be interpreted correctly to derive meaningful conclusions about the evaluation. The findings of evaluation may be discussed with the interpreters as well as with programme planning and implementation officials, so that the results of evaluation are put in a proper perspective. The evaluation results must clearly state the achievements, failures and future adjustments needed. A written report of the evaluation findings should be prepared and made available to all concerned.

Various aspects of evaluation

i) Efficiency Evaluation

This may be defined as the amount of outputs created and their quality in relation to the resources (capital and personnel) invested. It is, then, a measure of how productively the resources/inputs have been used.

Effectiveness Evaluation

This expresses to what extent the planned outputs; expected effects (immediate objectives) and intended impacts (development objectives) are being or have been produced or achieved.

Impact Evaluation

Impact means long-term effect-positive and negative, intended and unintended. These are the longer-term, largely indirect consequences of the programme or project for the intended beneficiaries and any other people. The main impacts are, of course, expected to be positive. Example: Improvement of socio-economic condition of dairy farmers due to dairy development programme. However, there may be negative impacts as well, on beneficiary groups or others. Example: Migration of traditional dairy farmers to other occupation. These should also be analysed. Sometimes, negative impacts on some people may have been suspected or even expected at the planning stage. These might then have been mentioned and even specified in the plan documents, with or without counteracting measures. In other cases, they may have been entirely unforeseen. They may then be more difficult to trace for evaluators. Impacts are normally generated through complex relations and processes and they, therefore, need to be analysed through broad-focusing investigations. Impact evaluation can use quantitative or qualitative methods or both.

Evaluation of Sustainability Aspect Evaluation

This means the maintenance, continuation or augmentation of positive changes induced by the programme or project after it is terminated. Sustainability may relate to all the levels of the project intervention framework. Sustainability of the project effect may mean:

- Maintenance of physical facilities produced (for instance, a Chilling plant);
- Continued use of physical facilities (for instance, a Chilling plant) or intangible qualities (for instance, knowledge);
- Continued ability to plan and manage similar development work with the help or assistance from the previous agency/institution.

- Continued production of the kinds of outputs created (for instance, packaged milk from a dairy society)
- Maintenance of impacts created (for instance, improvement of socio-economic condition of new dairy farmers associated with the project); and
- Multiplication of effects and impacts (formation of new dairy societies in other localities).

Evaluation of Result Oriented Aspects

The five main aspects in project operation and evaluation are input – activities - output - effect (outcomes) -impact sequence and their need for monitoring at different stages of the projects' progress. There is change in approach, in recent times; new approach is called Result Oriented/ Result based evaluation, an improvement over the activities to outputs in impact approach is used.

The focus here is to ensure that resources 'invested' in any development activity generate their intended results objectively as possible. Projects are now only deemed successful, if the measured results achieve the projected quantified indicators. This approach lays emphasis on 'results' and benefits at every stage. The concept is to link development resources to the objective of societal benefits, along with the means of achieving them, impact measures and the risks involved in the process.

Suggested Readings and References

1. Ahmed, M.R. (1991). Planning and Designing Social Forestry Project. In Ahmed, M.R. (ed.) Social Forestry and Community Development, pp. 109-116. FAO, FTPP.
2. Leagans, J.P. (1961). Programme Planning to Meet People's Needs. In: Extension Education in Community Development, Directorate of Extension, Ministry of Food and Agriculture, Government of India, New Delhi.
3. Kelsey L.D. and Hearne C.C. (1966). Cooperative Extension Work. New York: Constock Publishing Associates.
4. Roling, N. (1988). Extension Science: Information Systems in Agricultural Development, Cambridge University Press.
5. Van den Ban, A.W. and Hawkins, H.S. (2002). Agricultural Extension, CBS Publishers and Distributors, New Delhi.
6. Misra, D.C. (1999). Monitoring Extension Programme and Resource, in Improving Agricultural Extension; A Reference Manual: Ed: FAO, Rome.
7. Murphy, J., & Marchant, T.J. (1988). Monitoring and Evaluation in Extension Agencies, World Bank Technical Paper No.79, DC: World Bank, Washington.

8. Participatory Monitoring and Evaluation (1990). A Handbook for Training Field Workers, 1998 Bangkok: Regional Office for Asia and the Pacific (RAPA), FAO.
9. World Bank (2004). Monitoring & Evaluation: Some Tools, Methods and Approaches, Washington, DC: World Bank.
10. Dennis J. Casley & Krishna Kumar (1990). Project Monitoring and Evaluation in Agriculture, TheWorld Bank.
11. Kamath, M.G. (1961). Extension Education in Community Development (Ed), Pub. Directorate of Extension, Ministry of Food and Agriculture GOI, New Delhi.
12. Slade, R.H., & Feder, G. (1985). Training and Visit Extension: A Manual of Instruction (mimeo), Washington, DC: World Bank.
13. Casley, D.J., & Kumar, K. (1987). Project monitoring and evaluation in agriculture, Johns Hopkins University Press (published for the World Bank), Baltimore and London.
14. Cemea, M.M., & Tepping, B.J. (1977). A system for monitoring and evaluating agricultural extension projects. World Bank Staff Working Paper No.272. DC: World Bank, Washington.

11

Data Collection and Report Writing

1. What is data ?
   a) Primary data
   b) Secondary Data
2. Levels of Measurement of Data
   a) Nominal level of Measurement (Nominal or Classificatory scale)
   b) Ordinal level of Measurement (Ordinal or Ranking Scale)
   c) Interval level of Measurement (Interval Scale)
   d) Ratio Level of Measurement (Ratio Scale)
3. Methods of data collection
   1. Questionnaire
      i. Characteristics of a Good Questionnaire
      ii. Types of questionnaires
         a) Structured questionnaire:
         b) Unstructured questionnaire
      iii. Advantages of Questionnaire Method
      iv. Limitations of Questionnaire Method
      v. Designing a Questionnaire
   2. Interviews
      i. Characteristics of an Interview:
      ii. Types of Interview
         a) Structured interviews
         b) Unstructured interviews
         c) Semi-structured interviews
      iii. Merits of Interview:
      iv. Disadvantage of Interview:
   3. Schedules
      1. Kinds of Schedule
         a) Observation Schedule
         b) Interview Schedule
         c) Document Schedule
         d) Rating Schedule
      2. Important Features of Schedule
      3. Points to be kept in mind while designing schedule
      4. Essentials of a Good Schedule
      5. Merits of a Schedule
      6. Limitations of a Schedule
4. Pilot testing or Pre-testing the Questionnaire / Schedule

5. Procedure for Data Collection
6. Sampling
    1. Importance of Sampling
    2. Universe or Population
    3. Sample
    4. Statistic and parameter
    5. Advantages of Sampling
    6. Disadvantages or Limitation of Sampling
    7. Sample Size
    8. Characteristics of a good Sample
    9. Methods of Sampling
        a) Probability Sampling
            i. Simple Random Sampling
            ii. Stratified Random Sampling
            iii. Cluster sampling
        b) Non-probability sampling methods
            i. Convenience sampling
            ii. Purposive sample
            iii. Accidental Sampling
            iv. Quota Sampling
            v. Snowball Sampling
            vi. Double sampling
            vii. Volunteer sampling
7. Social Survey
    1. Instruments of Survey Research
    2. Merits of Survey Method
    3. Limitation of Survey Method
8. Data Processing and Analysis
    1. Data processing
    2. Editing of data
    3. Coding of data
    4. Classification of data
    5. Tabulation
    6. Graphical presentation of data
        a) Diagrams and Graphs
            i. Line Diagrams
            ii. Simple Bar Diagram
            iii. Multiple Bar Diagrams
            iv. Sub divided bar diagrams
            v. Deviation Bars
            vi. Histogram
            vii. Pie Diagram
            viii. Pictograms
            ix. Line Graph
9. Report Writing
10. Constituents of Research Report
11. Suggested Readings and References

Data Collection and Report Writing

Many a times you may be asked questions like what is the average milk production of deshi cows of your area? What is the average lactation period of CB cows of your area? or maybe what is the impact of AI programme in your area? etc., by your higher officers. How to answer all these questions? All these questions may be answered scientifically if you possess elementary knowledge on statistics. We have to frame a research design and to collect data to answer these questions.

What is Data ?

Data is a collection of facts, such as numbers, words, measurements, observations or even just descriptions of things. Example: 5, Ram, Kilogram, Good, Male, etc. Independently they do not produce any meaning.

These are special types of information, generally obtained through observation, surveys, enquiries or are generated as a result of human activities.

> **Data**
>
> Independently do not produce meaning
>
> e.g.: 25, Boy, Sex, etc.
>
> **02 types:** Qualitative and Quantitative
>
> **Qualitative data**
>
> Can be counted and cannot be computed
>
> **Quantitative data**
>
> Can be counted but can be computed

Once you have decided what to study and how to study, you are faced with the task of systematically collecting reliable and valid evidence upon which you can base your findings. Data (singular datum) are facts which are observed and measurable phenomena. The purpose of gathering and summarizing data is to transform them into information. The data collected in the research study may be quantitative or qualitative in nature. Quantitative data can be counted and can be computed. Such as age of a boy, marks scored by a student, distance, etc. Quantitative data are easier for analysis. We also collect qualitative data like sex of a person as Male or Female or Transgender. The qualitative characteristics can be counted, but as such cannot be computed. For example, we may get "Yes' or "No" to a question to farmers about vaccination of his animals. For this "Yes" or "No" , we may assign 0 to "Yes" and 1 to "No" in an artificial or nominal way to categorise these qualitative data, and go for computation. So, quantitative data are expressed in the form of numerals and are amenable to statistical analysis readily. Whereas, qualitative data are descriptive in nature and can be statistically analysed only after processing and after having them classified into some appropriate categories. Data is required to make a decision in any business situation. The researcher is faced with one of the most difficult problems of obtaining suitable, accurate and adequate data. Utmost care must be exercised while collecting data because the quality of the research results depends upon the reliability of the data. There are basically two sources from which we obtain data for our research works. They are known as primary data and secondary data.

Primary Data

The Primary data are original data which are collected for the first time for a specific purpose. For your research work, you are going and directly collecting the information from the dairy owners about the milk production data-these data are known as the primary data. These data are gathered at the first hand and the responsibility remain with the authority that originally gathered them. Data from primary sources may be gathered by observation, personal interview, conference, correspondence, questionnaire and other devices.

> **Primary Data**
>
> Collected by the investigator for first time
>
> **Secondary Data**
>
> Published or unpublished data collected by other than the investigator.

Secondary Data

The Secondary data are those which have already been collected by some other agency and which have already been processed. Secondary data may be available in the form of published or unpublished sources. For instance, information collected from Annual Reports of the Department for your research work may be known as the secondary sources of data. Here, the information you have taken from the report has not been collected by you rather the same has been collected by someone else for their research purpose.

Levels of Measurement of Data

As we know that the data may be quantitative or qualitative-they need to be measured. The measurement is the process of assigning numbers to the variables according to rules. Ways to assign these numbers include counting, ranking and comparing objects or events. Measurements, as used in research implies qualification of information, that is the assigning of some type of number to the data and numbers are then become the means of computing the information. The aim of measurement is to provide accurate and objective description of phenomena that you can communicate to others. There are four different types of data and four different levels of measurements.

Nominal level of Measurement (Nominal or Classificatory scale)

The term nominal means to "insignificant' or "minimal". This level of measurement is the lowest and simple level of measurement. This indicates that with this type of data very minimum level of mathematical calculation can be done. Nominal data are numerical in name only, because they do not share any of the properties of the numbers, we use in ordinary mathematics like addition, subtraction, division, etc. For example, the dairy farmers may be classified as male-female, rural-urban, etc., and number may be assigned to them, say 1 for male and 2 for female. The number 1 assigned to male is a category and cannot say that 1< 2 or we cannot write also 2-1=1. The numbers assigned in this level of measurement indicate serial order only. The data are classified only and the measurement is known as nominal level of measurement or classificatory measurement. With this type of data, we may do statistical operations like frequency, percentage, mode, chi-square test, etc.

> **Measurement:**
>
> Assigning number to the variables according to certain rules
>
> **Types of Measurement:**
>
> Nominal, Ordinal, Interval and Ratio
>
> **Nominal:** Do not share any properties of number
>
> No addition, subtraction, division, multiplication
>
> **Ordinal:** Ranked, ordered compared according to standard. E.g.: Grades in a class

Ordinal Level of Measurement (Ordinal or Ranking Scale)

Ordinal data are discontinuous data that are ranked, ordered or compared according to a predetermined standard. They are ordered in to a greater or less than scale. For example, grades obtained by a student in the class as "A", "B", "C" and "D" are of ordinal in nature. Here, data indicate less than or greater than relationship. In ordinal level of measurement, numbers are assigned to objects or events not only to categorise them, but also to indicate greater than or less than relationship. The ordinal scale places events in order but there is no attempt to make the intervals of the scale equal in terms of some rule. The scale has no absolute value. For example, Ram's position in the class is 1, Hari's position is 2 and Pradeep's position is 3, then it cannot be said that Ram's position is 2 times as good as that of Hari. This statement makes no sense at all. However, we may say that the Ram's position is better than that of Hari. Similarly, we cannot say the difference between Ram and Hari's position is equal to Hari and Pradeep's position.

Interval level of Measurement (Interval Scale)

In case of Interval level of measurement, the intervals are adjusted in terms of some rules that have been established on the basis as a basis for making the units equal. The zero point is set arbitrarily. The primary limitation of the interval scale is the lack of a true zero. That means it does not have the capacity to measure the complete absence of a trait or characteristics. For example, the scores on an English test of four students are-

Rani-75, Reeta- 50, Bani- 25, Meeta- 0

Here, Meeta has received a 0 on the test, that does not mean that Meeta has no (zero) English language ability, as the zero point was set arbitrarily. Addition and subtraction are permissible operations but because of arbitrary zero, multiplication and division are not permissible.

Another example, the Fahrenheit scale is an example of an interval scale. One can say the that an increase in temperature from 30^0 to 50^0 involves the same increase in temperature as increase in temperature from 60^0 to 80^0, but one cannot say that the temperature of 60^0 is twice as warm as the temperature of 30^0 because both numbers are dependent in the fact that the zero in the scale is set arbitrarily at the temperature of the freezing point of water. The ratio of the two temperatures, 30^0 and 60^0, means nothing because zero is an arbitrary point.

Interval: Intervals are adjusted in terms of some rule.

Zero point is arbitrary

Addition and subtraction permissible

Multiplication and division are not permissible E.g.: Fahrenheit scale

Ratio Scale:

Highest level of measurement

Having absolute zero value

All mathematical calculations and statistical techniques can be applied

Ratio Level of Measurement (Ratio Scale)

Ratio level is the highest level of measurement. They are distinguished from internal scales by virtue of having an absolute zero value. Ratio scale provides information regarding: Rank Ordering, interval between object, absolute zero value. Ratio scale represents the actual amounts of variables. All statistical techniques are usable with ration scales and all manipulations that one can carry out with real numbers can also be carried out with ratio scale values. Multiplication and Division can be carried out with this scale but not with other scales mentioned earlier.

Methods of Data Collection

We collect data from the respondents to answer research questions. The collection of data requires a great deal of deliberation and expertise. If we don't collect data carefully then the research result would be erroneous. Some of the important and widely used tools by the researchers for data collection are:

1. Questionnaires
2. Interviews
3. Schedules
4. Observation Techniques
5. Rating Scales
6. PRA/FGD
7. Case Study

In this chapter, we will discuss about only questionnaire, interviews and schedules.

Questionnaire

> **Questionnaire:**
> Contains number of questions used for data collection

A questionnaire is a systematic compilation of questions that are submitted to a sampling of population from which information is desired. In general, the word questionnaire refers to a device for securing answers to questions by using a form having number of questions which the respondent fills in him. The questionnaire is probably most used and most abused of the data gathering devices It is easy to prepare and to administer. The questionnaire is a form prepared and distributed to secure responses to certain questions. It is a systematic compilation of questions. It is an important instrument being used to gather information from widely scattered sources. Normally used where one cannot see personally all of the people from whom he desires responses or where there is no particular reason to see them personally.

Characteristics of a Good Questionnaire

a) Purpose

i) Collect data precisely to answer the research questions (test the hypothesis)

ii) questionnaire must motivate the respondents to communicate the required information.

b) Language

i) Language should be concise and directed towards producing uniformity in understanding among the respondents.

ii) The vocabulary should be simple and within the easy grasp of the least intelligent of the group under study.

iii) The syntax should be clear and straightforward.

iv) Proverbs and quotations should be avoided. Subjective words, such as 'bad', 'good', 'fair' should not be used.

c) Frame of reference

i) Complex questions that require the respondent to go through several steps of reasoning before answering is undesirable and have often resulted in misleading information.

ii) Questions on controversial issues should be broken down into components so that the researcher can determine the respondent's feeling about various aspects of the problem, including those which he/she refuses to comment upon.

iii) The required answers of the question should be within the informational domain of the respondents.

Characteristic of a good questionnaire

a) Purpose
b) Language
c) Frame of reference
d) Arrangement of questions
e) Length of questionnaire
f) Arrangement of questions
g) Length of the questionnaire
h) Form of response

d) Arrangement of the questions

The arrangement or ordering of questions should receive special attention. It should appear logical to the respondents. The questions placed first in the questionnaire should be the easiest to answer. 'Interest-generating' questions should be asked at the beginning. A proper sequence of questions proceeds from the general to specific, from simple to complex one, from those that will create favourable attitude to those that may be somewhat delicate or sensitive

e) Length of the questionnaire

A questionnaire should not be longer than necessary. The total number of questions must not be too large to tire or bore the respondents. If too many questions are asked and the respondent becomes tired, the questions at the end of the series may not be well answered. If it is necessary to include a large number of questions, it is advisable to have separate questionnaires.

f) Form of response

The form in which the responses are recorded must be integrated with the form of the questions. There should be no hesitation in asking for responses in different forms in the same questionnaire, since it is frequently found that one form is better than another for questions about different aspects of the same subject. Questions requiring answers like "Yes" or "No" are subject to least bias. These responses are easy to tabulate. However, they do not always yield sufficient information on the subject under study. In such cases, the use of multiple choice responses is desirable. Questions that present multiple choices to the respondent are effective when the choices are few and easy to follow.

Types of questionnaires

Questionnaires can be classified in various ways. Here, we confine ourselves to structured and unstructured questionnaires.

> **Types of questionnaire**
>
> a) Structured
>
> b) Unstructured
>
> **Structured Questionnaire**
>
> a) Close ended: Limited choice
>
> b) Open ended:
>
> Unlimited choices to answer
>
> **Unstructured Questionnaire**
>
> Interview guides

Structured questionnaire

Structured questionnaires are those which pose definite, concrete and pre-ordained questions, i.e., they are prepared in advance and not constructed on the spot during the questioning-period. This questionnaire uses highly standardized techniques and a set of pre-determined questions. It includes both closed end and open ended questions. Closed questions are used when categorised data are required or when the researcher wants to make various classifications for his study. For an example a question in the questionnaire is: "How many milch animals do you have?" To this question, a farmer may respond either one only/ two/three/four/five or more than five. He has to answer to the options given against the question. The respondent goes through all those given responses and chooses one which is true for his situation. Closed-form of questionnaires are used when categorised data are required. They include a set of questions to which a respondent can reply in a limited number of ways–'yes', 'no', 'no-opinion', or an answer from a short list of possible responses. He/she is asked to put a tick (") mark in a space provided on the answer sheet or is requested to underline a response.

Example: Close-ended items

1. Have you ever attended a training programme on Improved Dairy Farming?
   ( ) Yes
   ( ) No
2. How important you think to have a topic on "Marketing age of Sheep and Goat" in your training Programme?
   ( ) Extremely important
   ( ) Very important
   ( ) Some what important
   ( ) Not at all important

The open end questions provide a proper space for the respondent to answer. The open end responses are free and spontaneous expression on the part of the informant who is not limited in his replies to a particular question posed on him". Suppose a question was asked to a farmer- What is your thinking about dairy entrepreneurship development programme of Government? The answers to this type of question are varied and qualitative in nature. Farmers may give different types opinion about the programme. Open ended questions are very much essential for exploratory research where you want to probe about an event. The open-ended questions have also its demerits. Since it does not provide any direction and restriction for the respondents to answer, a wide range of answers is usually given, some meaningful and some meaningless, and obviously those meaningless, non-directed and irrelevant answers create some problems of classification and analysis.

Example: Open-Ended items

1. In your opinion what are the causes of low productivity in animals?
2. Why do opt dairy farming as an income generating activity?

Unstructured questionnaire

Unstructured questionnaires are frequently referred to as "interview guides". They aim at precision and contain definite subject matters area that are covered while conducting an interview. Flexibility is the chief advantage of the unstructured questionnaire. It is designed to obtain viewpoints, opinions, attitudes and to show relationships between various types of information which might escape notice under more mechanical types of interrogation. No predetermined responses are provided; instead, free responses are solicited. This is characterised by a greater flexible approach in questioning the respondents. It is of non-directive type which involves relatively much less standardization of techniques and operation. Here the respondents have the freedom to express any event that seems significant to them, to give their own definition of an event or a situation and to narrate any particular incident of his life. In unstructured questionnaire the researcher is also having a greater freedom to ask any supplementary question of the respondents.

Advantages of Questionnaire Method

1. It's very economical.
2. It's a time saving process.
3. It covers the research in wide area.
4. It's very suitable for special type of responses.
5. It is most reliable in special cases.
6. Greater validity

Limitations of Questionnaire Method

1. Through this we get only limited responses.
2. Lack of personal contact.
3. Questionnaire cannot be used with illiterate people
4. Greater possibility of wrong answers.
5. Chances of receiving incomplete response are more.
6. Sometimes answers may be illegible.
7. It may be useless in many problems.
8. Impossibility to probe deeper problem

Designing a Questionnaire

Main aspects of questionnaire

- General Form
- Question Sequence
- Question Wording

A questionnaire is a proforma containing a sequence of questions to elicit information from the interviewees. The questionnaire is used for personal interview. At the same time the questionnaire is also mailed to individuals who are requested to write the answers against each question and to return the completed proforma by post. The questionnaire is the heart of the primary data collection technique. Hence; its drafting requires utmost skill. The questions must be clear, simple and to the point. They must be well organised from the point of view of the respondent and be formulated in such a manner as to provide the data in so far as possible in the desired form. This is especially true of a mail questionnaire which essentially has to speak for itself. If it is not clear; not only the replies may be vague and of little value but many potential respondents may not bother returning the questionnaire at all.

A questionnaire may be said to possess three main aspects:

General Form

Question Sequence

Question Wording

General Form

The form of a questionnaire will depend partly on the type of data being sought and partly on the data collection method to be used. The choice lies between two extremes. On the one hand, there is the highly structured questionnaire in which all questions and answers are specified. At the other end is the unstructured questionnaire in which the interviewer is provided with a general brief on the sort of information to be obtained but the exact question is largely his own responsibility.

Question Sequence

The introduction to the questionnaire should be as short and simple as possible. The introductory letter accompanying the mailed questionnaire should also be made very brief. The introduction lays the foundation for establishing the rapport with the respondent in addition to making the interview possible. Once the rapport is established the questions will generally seek substantive information of value to the study. As a general rule, questions that put too great a strain on the memory or the intellect should be reserved till later. Likewise, questions relating to personal wealth and personal character should be avoided in the beginning.

Question Wording

It has been stated that the question wording and formulation are more of an art than a science. The wording of the questions should be impartial so as not to give a biased picture of the true state of affairs. Colourful adjectives and undue descriptive phrases should be avoided. In general, the questions should be worded such that:

a) they are easily understood

b) they are simple

c) they are concrete and conform to respondents' way of thinking.

Multiple choice questions constitute the basis of a structured questionnaire, particularly in a mailed questionnaire method. But in addition to these questions various open ended questions are generally inserted to provide a more complete picture of the respondent's feelings and attitudes.

Interviews

The Interview is a two-way method which permits an exchange of ideas and information between interviewee and interviewer. It is a systematic method by which a person enters more or less imaginatively into the inner life of a comparative stranger to get the required information.

> **Interview**
>
> It is a two-way method which permits exchange of ideas

Characteristics of an Interview

1. The interviewer can probe into casual factors, determine attitudes, discover the origin of problem.
2. It can make cross questioning possible.
3. It helps the investigator to gain an impression of the person concerned.

4. It can deal with delicate, confidential and even intimate topics.
5. It has flexibility.
6. Sincerity, frankness, truthfulness and insight of the interviewee can be better judged through cross questioning.
7. It is applicable in survey method, but it is also applicable in historical, experimental, case studies and clinical studies.

Types of Interview

Structured interviews: They are based on a strict procedure and a highly structured interview guide, in which case it is no different from a questionnaire. The instrument allows no freedom to make adjustments to any of its elements, such as content, wording or order of the questions. Such interview is based on a schedule, and strict adherence to the questions and the instructions is paramount. The interviewer is expected to act in a neutral manner, keeping the same tone of voice, offering the same impression to the respondents, using the same style, appearance, prompts, probes etc., and showing no initiative, spontaneity or personal interest in the research topic. The purpose of this is to reduce interviewer bias to a minimum and achieve the highest degree of uniformity in procedure.

Types Interview

- **Structured Interviews**-Strict adherence to the questions
- **Unstructured interviews**- No restriction to adhere to the questions
- **Semi-structured interviews**-Between structured and unstructured interviews

Unstructured interviews: They have no strict procedures to follow the instructions given in the questionnaire. There are no restrictions in the wording of the questions, the order of questions or the interview schedule. The interviewer acts freely in this context, on the basis of certain research points, formulating questions as and when required and employing neutral probing. The structure of these interviews is flexible and the restrictions minimal, being presented in most cases in the form of guides rather than rules.

Semi-structured interviews: They lay somewhere between structured and unstructured interviews. They contain elements of both, and while some are closer to structured interviews, others are closer to unstructured interviews. The degree to which interviews are structured depends on the research topic and purpose, resources, methodological standards and preferences and the type of information sought, which can be either quantitative or qualitative techniques. The researchers i.e. the interviewers hold a central place in the research process.

Merits of Interview

1. Direct research.
2. Deep research
3. Knowledge of past and future.
4. Knowledge of special features.
5. Mutual encouragement is possible.
6. Supra-observation is possible.
7. Knowledge of historical and emotional causes.
8. Examination of known data.

Disadvantage of Interview

1. May provides misleading information.
2. Defects due to interviewee (low level of intelligence or may be emotionally unbalanced)
3. Result may be affected due to prejudices of interviewer.
4. Result may be affected due to the difference in the mental outlook of internee and interviewer.
5. One sided and incomplete research.
6. Art rather than science.

Schedules

> **Schedules**
>
> Set of questionnaires used for interview purpose

When a researcher is using a set of questionnaires for interview purpose it is known as schedule. It is a list of questions which is used to collect the data from the field. This is generally filled in by the researcher or the enumerators. If the scope of the study is wide, then the researcher appoints people who are called enumerators for the purpose of collecting the data. The enumerators go to the informants, ask them the questions from the schedule in the order they are listed and record the responses in the space meant for the answers in the schedule itself. For example, the livestock census all over the country is conducted through this method. The difference between questionnaire and schedule is that the former is filled in by the informants, the latter is filled in by the researcher or enumerator.

The purpose of schedule is to provide a standardised tool for observation or interview in order to attain objectivity.

Kinds of Schedule

The schedules used in the social research may be classified into following four groups according to their use.

1. **Observation Schedule:** These schedules are used for observation purposes. They contain specific topics upon which the observer record data.
2. **Interview Schedule:** These are the schedule used for interview purposes. These schedules contain standard questions and blank spaces that the interviewer has to fill up after getting information from the respondents.
3. **Document Schedule:** These schedules are used to recording the data from different written documents like annual reports, case history, dairies, official records, etc.
4. **Rating Schedule:** They are mostly used sociological and psychological research works. They are used when there is need of measuring the attitude or opinion of the respondents.

Features of Schedules

- Presented by interviewer
- Questions asked to interviewee
- Responses noted down
- Questions are pre planned

Important Features of Schedule

1. The schedule is presented by the interviewer. The questions are asked and the answers are noted down by him.
2. The list of questions is a mere formal document; it need not be attractive.
3. The schedule can be used in a very narrow sphere of social research.
4. It aids to delimit the scope of the study and to concentrate on the circumscribed elements essential to the analysis.
5. It aims at delimiting the subject.
6. In the schedule the list of questions is preplanned and noted down formally and the interviewer is always armed with the formal document detailing the questions. Thus interviewer not to depend upon the memory.

Points to be kept in mind while designing schedule

1. Interviewer should not frame long, complex, defective questions.
2. Unrelated and unnecessary questions should not be asked.
3. Schedule should not contain personal and upsetting questions.
4. Its questions should be simple, clear and relevant to topic.
5. Questions be suitable to respondent's intelligence level.
6. Impersonal, indirect and unambiguous questions should be included in schedule.

Essentials of a Good Schedule

There are two essential conditions of a good schedule.

a) Accurate Communication

b) Accurate Response

Accurate Communication

The questions asked to the respondents are answered in the line it is expected. The respondents should clearly understand the questions and answer accordingly. There should not be any ambiguity in answering the questions.

Accurate Response

Accurate response is said to have been achieved when replies contain the information sought for. This information should be unbiased and true. The respondents may also cooperate in filling the schedule.

Merits of a Schedule

1. It is a useful method in case the informants are illiterates.
2. Removal of doubts is possible because face to face interaction is there.
3. The researcher can overcome the problem of non-response as the enumerators go personally to obtain the information.
4. It is very useful in extensive studies and can obtain more reliable data.
5. It is possible to know about the defects of the interviewee.
6. Higher percentage of response

Limitations of a Schedule

1. It is a very expensive and time-consuming method as enumerators are paid persons and also have to be trained.
2. Since the enumerator is present, the respondents may not respond to some personal questions.
3. Reliability depends upon the sincerity and commitment in data collection.

The success of data collection through the questionnaire method or schedule method depends on how the questionnaire has been designed.

Pilot testing or Pre-testing the Questionnaire / Schedule

Before finalising the questionnaire and schedule, it is desirable to carry out a preliminary testing on a sample basis. The investigator should examine each question to ensure that the question is not confusing, leading to biased responses etc. The real test of a questionnaire is how it performs under actual conditions of data collection. This test can be carried out among small groups of subjects in order to provide an estimate of the time needed for responding to the questions. Necessary modifications and corrections may be made on tested questionnaire to make it a final tool for data collection.

Procedure for Data Collection

Before we entre in to the process of data collection, it is necessary to make a meticulous plan, so that the data collection is completed smoothly. We have already developed questionnaire/ interview schedule and now we know (i) what data are to be collected, (ii) from whom the data to be collected (sample size), (iii) who will collect the data- researcher by himself or by his/her team. If it is going to be collected by other than the researcher, they should be properly advised and trained on how to collect the data from the respondents, (iv) from where data to be collected- it is the place from which you want to collect the data, and (v) when the data to be collected – during summer or winter, before or after harvest, etc.

Sampling

Sampling is the process of obtaining information regarding the entire research population or aggregate or totality by examining only a part of it. It is a picture in miniature to represent the larger whole, to enable the researcher to make a judgment or inference about the whole with the presumption that the sample data will provide valid and reliable conclusions. Sampling is not only typical to the field of science, rather in our day-to-day life, we take to such method. For example, a cook presses a few pods of boiled rice in the cooking pot to be able to know that it is ready to be served. Similarly, while examining the quality of food grain one need not examine each and every grain contained in the bag. Rather an examination of a handful of grains gives the impression regarding the entire bag. So, when a small group is taken as the representative of the whole, the study is called sampling study.

Sampling

Representative small part of a population

Importance of Sampling

- Complete coverage of population not possible
- Save time, resources and manpower
- When high degree of accuracy is not required

Importance of Sampling

A large population cannot be studied in its entirety for reasons of size, time, cost or inaccessibility. Limited time, lack of large amount of funds, and population scattered in a very wide geographical area often make sampling necessary. These are the following purposes of sampling:

1. Population in many cases may be so large and scattered that a complete coverage may not be possible. Suppose, the Director of AH and VS wants to find the reactions of dairy farmers towards the responses of Veterinary Doctors towards the farmers in providing veterinary services at door steps . For this, thousands of dairy farmers are to be contacted in different districts. Some of these farmers may be residing in inaccessible areas and hence it would be impossible to collect information within a short span of time.
2. It offers a high degree of accuracy because it deals with a small number of persons.
3. In a short period of time valid and comparable results can be obtained. A lengthy period of data collection generally renders some data obsolete by the time the information is completely in hands.
4. Sampling is less demanding in terms of requirements of investigators since it requires a small portion of the target population.
5. It is economical since it contains fewer people. Large populations would involve employing a large number of interviewers which will increase the total cost of the research.

Universe or Population

The two terms universe and population are used interchangeably in our research work and we have to understand it correctly. A population may be defined as the totality of a particular characteristic for any specified group of individuals or objects. Thus, all the dairy farmers of the State, all the calves born under calf rearing scheme, all the dairy entrepreneurs of the state etc. are examples of population.

A population may be finite or infinite. A population is said to be finite if it consists of a fixed number of elements so that it can be easily counted. For instance, the population of dairy farmers or the population of a village or city etc. But an infinite population is one whose size is unlimited and, therefore, its members cannot be counted. The population of fishes in a river, the number of crows in a country are examples of infinite population.

Universe or Population

Totality of a particular characteristics of any specified group of individuals or objects.

Sample

Selected number from population

Statistics

Characteristics of Sample

Parameter

Characteristics of population

Sample

A sample may be defined as a selected number from a population to represent it. Generally, this selection is done according to some rule or plan. By studying the sample, some inferences may be made about the population.

Statistic and parameter: A statistic is a characteristic of a sample, but a parameter is a characteristic of a population. The word parameter is used to indicate various statistical measures like mean, median, mode, standard deviation, correlation etc. in the population or universe. Such statistical measures describe the characteristics of a population. For example, the population mean is a parameter. Whereas, when we work out certain measures such as mean, median, mode or the like ones from samples, then they are known as statistics as they are based on the characteristics of a given sample. The sample mean is a statistic.

Advantages of Sampling

Sampling has a number of advantages and some of them are listed below.

1. It is not possible to study large number of people scattered in wide geographical area. Sampling will reduce their number.
2. It saves time and money.
3. It saves destruction of units.
4. It increases accuracy of data (having control on the small number of subjects).
5. It achieves greater response rate.
6. It achieves greater cooperation from respondents.
7. It is easy to supervise few interviewers in the sample but difficult to supervise a very large number of interviewers in the study of total population.
8. The researcher can keep a low profile.

Disadvantages or Limitation of Sampling

1. Scope of biasness. (Less accuracy)
2. Problem of representative Sample-Difficulty in selecting a truly representative sample.
3. Need of eligible researchers.
4. Instability of sample subjects or changeability of units i.e. in heterogeneous population.
5. There are certain situations where sampling is possible.

Sample Size

For a sample to have the study, the questions are often asked: how many persons should be included in the sample, i.e., how large or small must the sample be to be representative? Some people say, the most common size is one-tenth of the total population. Some other say that a minimum of 100 subjects is required to allow statistical inferences. However, these estimates are not always correct. The sample size has to be based on the following considerations:

1. **The size of the population**, i.e., whether the total population to be studied is very large, large or small.
2. **Nature of population**, i.e., whether the population is homogenous. In the former, a small sample may suffice but in the latter, a larger sample is required.
3. **Purpose of study**, i.e., whether the study is descriptive, exploratory or explanatory.
4. **Whether the study is qualitative or quantitative**. In qualitative studies, sampling does not resort to numerical boundaries to determine the size of sample. Similarly, when purposive or accidental samplings are employed, the researcher himself can decide the „sufficient number of respondents. In such cases, generalizations are concerned with quality rather than with quantity.

> **Characteristics of a good Sample**
> - Representative
> - Free from bias
> - Objective
> - Accurate
> - Comprehensive
> - Practicability for research

5. **Accessibility of the elements**. Many a time it is difficult to contact respondents at time and place convenient to the researchers.
6. **Cost of obtaining elements**. With more resources, an adequate number of investigators can be appointed and a large sample may be considered.
7. **Variability required.** Sometimes the respondents required have to be persons of different groups, e.g., of different age, different income, different educational background, different occupations and so on.
8. **Desired accuracy or confidence level**. For high degree of accuracy, large samples need to be drawn. One has to think of the level at which one will be confident that his sample is representative.
9. **Sampling error or desired risk level.** The minimum the sample error, maximum will be the samples representativeness. For example, the study of parents (with children of school-going age) who want to send their children to English medium private schools or to government schools. If

the average annual family income of parents in the area in which the study is to be conducted is Rs. 40,000, then, the researcher should make sure that his samples average income is as close to Rs. 40,000 as possible. Smaller the percentage error, greater the chance of proving (through the selected sample) that income is one factor that affects parents' choice.

10. **Stratification :** It has to be kept in mind that how many times the sample has to be sub-divided during the data analysis. This is to ensure an adequate size for each sub-division. In stratified sampling, the researcher should draw a sample having some characteristics as population. In the study of parents willing to send their children to private or government schools, of the total population (of parents), if 75 percent have annual income of over Rs. 40,000 and 25 percent less than Rs. 40,000, the researcher should be sure that his sample also has the same distribution of income.

Characteristics of a good Sample

1. A good sample is the true representative of the population corresponding to its properties.
2. The population is known as aggregate of certain properties and sample is called sub-aggregate of the universe.
3. A good sample is free from bias; the sample does not permit prejudices, the learning and pre-conception, imaginations of the investigator to influence its choice.
4. A good sample is an objective one; it refers objectivity in selecting procedure or absence of subjective elements from the situation.
5. A good sample maintains accuracy. It yields an accurate estimates or statistics and does not involve errors.
6. A good sample is comprehensive in nature. This feature of a closely linked with true-representativeness. Comprehensiveness is a quality of a sample which is controlled by specific purpose of the investigation. A sample may be comprehensive in traits but may not be a good representative of the population.
7. A good sample has the practicability for research.

Methods of Sampling

The method used for drawing a sample is significant to arrive at dependable results or conclusions.

Sampling methods can be broadly classified into two categories:

i) Probability Sampling.

ii) Non-probability Sampling.

Probability Sampling

> **Probability Sampling**
> Every unit of the population has an equal chance of being selected

Probability sampling is one in which every unit of the population has an equal probability of being selected for the sample. It offers a high degree of representativeness. However, this method is expensive, time-consuming and relatively complicated since it requires a large sample size and the units selected are usually widely scattered. the probability sampling requires following conditions to be satisfied:

1. Complete list of subjects to be studied is available
2. Size of the universe must be known
3. Desired sample size must be specified, and
4. Each element must have an equal chance of being selected.

Major types of probability sampling are: simple random sampling, stratified random sampling and cluster sampling.

Simple Random Sampling

A process that gives each element in the population an equal chance of being included in the sample is termed as simple random sampling. The elements are selected, using a list of random numbers appended with most textbooks of research and statistics. Before using the table of random numbers, it is first necessary to number all the elements in the population to be studied. The table is marked at some point and the cases whose numbers come up as one from this point down the column of numbers are taken into the sample until the desired number of elements is obtained. The selection of any given element places no limits on other element being selected, thus making equally possible the selection of any one of the many possible combinations of elements.

Stratified Random Sampling

Stratified random sampling are two types (i) Proportionate stratified random sampling and Disproportionate stratified random sampling.

i) Proportionate Stratified Random Sampling

In stratified random sampling, the population is first divided into strata. The strata may be based on a single criterion or on a combination of two or more criteria. After, stratification a simple random sample is taken from each stratum, and the sub samples are then joined to form the total sample. In case the researcher is interested in the study of some characteristics of a phenomenon he uses a proportionate stratified random sampling plan. Of course, this sampling design presupposes that the investigator has some knowledge concerning the population characteristics such as age, sex, marital status etc. In the sampling plan the sample will have specified characteristics in exact proportion to those same characteristics which are distributed in the population. To understand this sampling plan we will consider the following example. Let us consider the Dairy farmers of the State taken loan under the Dairy Entrepreneurship Programme. The researcher wishes to have proportionate stratified random sample of them taking year of their availing loan for this programme Let us suppose that the dairy farmers of the State are distributed as is shown in Table.

Table : Distribution of the Dairy farmers availed loan in different years

Year	Population	Proportion of each class
Dairy Farmers on 1st year loan	50	0.25
Dairy Farmers on 2nd year loan	40	0.20
Dairy Farmers on 3rd year loan	30	0.15
Dairy Farmers on 4th year loan	40	0.20
Dairy Farmers on 5th year loan	40	0.20
Total	200	1.00

Suppose that the researcher decides to have a sample size of 60 dairy farmers for his study. First, he determines the proportion of dairy farmers in each class (as shown in the second column). Then he calculates the composition of the sample taking each proportion of the stratifying characteristics in the population and multiplying it by the desired size of the sample. Thus, he multiplies 60, the desired sample size by .25, the proportion of Dairy farmers of 1st year loan in the population is

(60) (.25) = 15

As such, he has to include 15 dairy farmers availing loan in the first year in his sample.

This procedure is repeated for each year as described below:

(60)(.25) = 15

(60) (.20) = 12

(60)(.15) = 9

(60) (.20) = 12

(60) (.20) = 12

Sample Size (N) = 60

Table : Distribution of Dairy farmers by Proportion

Year	Sample Break-up	Proportion of each class
Dairy Farmers on 1st year loan	15	0.25
Dairy Farmers on 2nd year loan	12	0.20
Dairy Farmers on 3rd year loan	9	0.15
Dairy Farmers on 4th year loan	12	0.20
Dairy Farmers on 5th year loan	12	0.20
Total	60	1.00

ii) Disproportionate Stratified Random Sampling

This sampling plan is almost similar to proportionate stratified random sampling except that the sub samples are not necessarily distributed according to their proportionate weight in the population from which they were drawn. It is possible that some sub samples are over represented while other sub groups are underrepresented.

Let us suppose that the researcher stratifies the population into two sub strata using income as the criteria. He would get the following break-up of the population:

Table : Distribution of Dairy Farmers by Income

Income	Number of Dairy Farmers	Percentage
Low income	160	30
High Income	40	20
Total	200	100

If the researcher -wants to draw a disproportionate stratified random sample of 60 from this population, stratified by income of the dairy farmers, then he has to draw 30 from each substratum, this means low income group farmers (30) will be under represented and high income group farmers (30) will be over represented in the sample. In other words, disproportionate sampling gives equal weights to each substrata. There is a clear improvement over simple random sampling when the sampling is based on a stratification of population on certain attributes. With this kind of stratification, we get a marked increase in the size of samples that yields statistics very close to the population parameters if selected on the basis of Proportionate Stratified Random Sampling.

Cluster sampling

In case the area of study is wide spread, a large expense is involved if simple and stratified random sampling are used. For example, in the preparation of sampling frame from the population and in covering the widespread areas by interviewers, a large amount of expenditure is required. The more widely spread the area of study, the greater are the travel expenses, the greater is the time spent in travelling, and hence expensive - and the **tasks** of administering, monitoring and supervision of the research project and in particular supervising the field staff become more complicated. For the reasons mentioned above and few other reasons, large-scale research studies make use of the methods of cluster sampling.

In cluster sampling, first the whole research area is divided into sub area, more commonly known as "clusters". The simple random or stratified method is used to select clusters. Finally, researcher arrives at the ultimate sample size to be studied by selecting sample from within the clusters, which is carried out on a simple or stratified random sampling basis.

Suppose for example, we want to do a survey of beggars in urban areas of a state. We may proceed as follows: prepare a list of districts and group them into clusters, and select a simple or stratified random sample from each clusters. For each of the districts included in the sample, list the cities/towns and take a simple or stratified random sample of them. If some or all of the towns/cities thus selected for the sample have more numbers of beggars that can be studied, we may take a sample of these towns/ cities in each district. The beggars in these towns/cities will be the sample of the beggars. Characteristically, the procedure moves through a series of stages-hence the common term, "multistage" sampling-from more inclusive to less inclusive sampling units until we finally arrive at the population elements that constitute the desired sample.

Non-probability sampling methods

> **Non-probability Sampling**
>
> Items of the samples are selected deliberately without using the technique of random sampling

Non-probability sampling is that sampling procedure in which there is no way of assessing the probability of the elements of population being included in the sample. In this type of sampling, items for the sample are selected deliberately by the researcher instead of using the techniques of random sampling. Non-probability sampling is based on the judgement of the researcher. The guiding factors in non-probability sampling include the availability of the units, the personal experience of the researcher and his/her convenience in carrying out a survey. Since these samples are not prepared through random sampling techniques, they are known as non-probability samples.

Non-probability sampling procedures do not employ the rules of probability theory, do not claim representativeness, and are usually used for qualitative exploratory analysis.

The different types of non-probability samplings used for research works are as follows:

a) Convenience sampling

This is also known as "accidental" or "haphazard' sampling. In this sampling, the researcher studies all those persons who are most conveniently available or who accidentally come in contact during a certain period of time in the research. The most obvious advantage of convenience sample is that it is quick and economical. But it may be a very biased sample. The possible sources of bias could be: (i) the respondents may have a vested interest to serve in cooperating with the interviewer, and (ii) the respondents may be those who are vocal and/or want to brag. Convenience samples are best utilized for exploratory research when additional research will subsequently be conducted with a probability sample.

b) Purposive sampling

A purposive sample is also known as a judgement sample. This type of sample is chosen because there are good reasons to believe that it is a representative of the total population. This also reflects certain controls identified as representative areas like a city, state or district; representative characteristics of individuals like age, sex, marital status, etc.; or types of groups like school administrators, elementary school teachers, secondary school teachers, college teachers, etc.

c) Accidental Sampling

Accidental sampling refers to a method of selecting respondents who happen to meet the researcher and are willing to be interviewed. Thus, a researcher may take the first hundred people he meets who are willing to be interviewed. For example, let us consider the situations where a programme director, wishes to make some generalisation about the programme in progress, selects beneficiaries who have come to the agency for a service or a community organiser, trying to know how "the people" feel about health status in that community, interviews available community dwellers like shop-keepers, daily wage earners, barbers and others who are presumed to reflect public opinion. In both the situations those who are available for study are included in the samples. This is exactly what we call accidental sampling. It is very obvious that the sample so collected are biased and there is no known way (other than by doing a parallel study with a probability sample) of evaluating the biases introduced in such samples. However, in the situation illustrated above, most probably, accidental sampling is the only way out because of the reason that the population parameters of the beneficiaries or the community people are not available with the researcher.

d) Quota Sampling

Quota sampling insures inclusion of diverse elements of the population in the sample and make sure that these diverse elements take account of the proportions in which they occur in the population. For example, we take a sample from a population with equal number of boys and girls, and that there is a difference between the two groups in the characteristic we wish to study and we fail to interview any girl, the results of the study would almost certainly be extremely misleading generalisations about the population. In practice, elements in small numbers are frequently underrepresented in accidental samples. In anticipation of such possible exclusion of small groups, quota sampling ensures inclusion of enough cases from each stratum in the sample. It should be noted here that the major goal of quota sampling is the selection of a sample that is a replica of the population to which one wants to generalise. Hence it should be clear that the critical requirement in quota sampling is not that the various population strata be sampled in their correct proportions, but rather than there be enough cases from each stratum to make possible an estimate of the population stratum value.

e) Snowball Sampling

Snowball sampling is externally helpful in studying some special sampling situation like getting a sample of drug abusers, or alcoholics or pickpockets. In snowball sampling we start with a few respondents of the type we wish to include in our study and who in turn are expected to guide us to get more respondents and so on. Like the rotating snowball, sample increases in its size as we continue to get more units of study. The technique is especially useful in the investigation of sensitive topics mentioned above because this sampling technique depends on sampled cases having knowledge of other similar cases. Another argument in favour of using this sampling technique is that, the victims might be hesitant to identify themselves if approached by a stranger but might be friendly to someone who they know and share their experiences or deviant status.

f) Double sampling

Double sampling is defined as drawing a small sample of respondents from a bigger sample of them. For example, the researcher wants to study the knowledge of newly started poultry farmers towards the importance of vaccination programme through mailed questionnaire. For this purpose, he mails questionnaire to five hundred poultry farmers residing in different localities. He finds that only 50 percent, that is 250 questionnaires are returned. From these 250 persons he draws a random sample of 100 and mails another set of questionnaire to get their in-depth knowledge about poultry vaccination. This method is known as double sampling. This method has the disadvantage of taking much time and labour of the researcher.

g) Volunteer sampling

This is the technique in which the respondent himself volunteers to give information he holds.

Social Survey

> **Survey Method**
>
> Collection of information through interviews, questionnaire, etc. for research purpose

The word survey has been derived from the word 'Sur' or 'Sor' and 'Veeir' or 'Veoir' which means 'over' and 'see' respectively. Therefore, the literal meaning of a survey is to see something. The term is used for technique of investigation by direct observation of phenomena or collection of information through interviews, questionnaire, etc. Social survey may be defined as Process by which quantitative facts are collected about the social aspects of a community's composition and activities (Mark Abrams). A social survey is usually an enquiry into the composition, activities and living conditions of a group of people. The main characteristics are –

a) It is directly concerned with social life as it exists here and now, what is observed, described, collected as a body of facts about current situations and problems

b) It focuses on a locality or a geographical area

c) It leads to measures of reform as the data assembled both for improvement and means to obtain them

d) It must be conducted in an objective spirit, that is, subjective ideas, opinions and bias should be avoided.

Survey research is basically a method of gathering information from a population on a given subject. Unlike qualitative research, survey research invariably covers a large population; but it does not imply that it collects information from each and every individual. There are various methods of drawing a representative sample from a given population, which can reveal trends for the entire population.

Quantitative research methods are often classified into two types, namely, census and sample based survey research. When information is gathered from each and every member of the population, or in other words, when all units of the population are covered for information, it is called census. But it is an expensive, lengthy and time-consuming process. Therefore, we focus on a portion (or unit) of the population; it is from the study of apart that we arrive at an understanding of the whole. When a part (or section, or unit) of a population is studied, it is called 'sample survey research. The term 'sample' is used for the part of a population that is subjected to study. Identifying such a portion or sample population is not easy. In order to make a survey scientific and representative, one must follow a scientific procedure.

Instruments of Survey Research

The main work in a survey research is collection of data and it should be collected from original and reliable sources. For this, major methods are:

- Observation
- Interview
- Questionnaire or
- Any combination of these.

Instrument of Survey Research

- Observation
- Questionnaire
- Interview
- Telephone survey
- Electronic survey

Telephonic Surveys

Now a days mobile and land line telephones are used increasingly to get data and opinions for social surveys form the willing respondents. These are ultimately economic in terms of time and money.

Advantages

- It is interactive, and not frozen like a printed questionnaire.
- Clarifications can be sought and given in case a question is not clear.
- Many people prefer to speak out than give something in writing.
- Interviews can be conducted at a mutually convenient time.
- Response rate is high.

Problems

There cannot be detailed discussions, as in a face-to-face meeting. These have to be concise. There is no check if later the respondent denies having said so. For the latter problem telephonic conversation may also be tape-recorded. It is not possible to collect data from them those who are not having telephone.

Electronic Surveys

The modern electronic gadgets like internet, SMS, WhatsApp, etc. are also used very frequently for the purpose of data collection.

Merits of Survey Method

Survey method has the following merits in comparison to other methods:

i) Survey research is relatively inexpensive (especially self-administered surveys).

ii) A survey permits the researcher to come in direct contact with the people to whom he wants to study

ii) Survey research is useful in describing the characteristics of a large population, demographic structure of a population, and its emerging trends and patterns.

iii) Survey research can be administered from remote locations using mail, e-mail or telephone. Consequently, very large samples are feasible, making the results statistically significant even when analysing multiple variables.

iv) In survey research one can ask many questions about a given topic, which gives considerable flexibility to the analysis.

v) We can choose different ways of administering a survey. From face-to-face interviews to telephones and e-mails one can use any mode · of collecting data depending on one's requirements and limitations.

vi) Unlike the qualitative methods, survey research is carried out through standardized questions, which makes measurement more precise by enforcing uniform definitions upon the participants. Standardisation ensures that similar kinds of data are collected from groups and then interpreted comparatively (between-group study), implying more objectivity and higher reliability.

Limitation of Survey Method

i) It is expensive in nature.

ii) Survey research is inflexible in the sense that it requires a precise study design. Everything must be worked out in advance, the tools to be used and the method of administering the tools.

iii) In order to make a survey viable and meaningful the researcher has to make sure that a large proportion of selected respondents agree to respond. This, however, may not always be an easy task to achieve. In such situations carrying out a survey becomes difficult.

iv) Survey method is a prolonged and time consuming process.

v) Surveys also demand a great deal of attention and honesty on the part of respondents, particularly when a questionnaire is being used and the survey is self-administered. Respondents may not always be willing to give such attention to filling the questionnaire. Sometimes, it may be hard for participants to recall certain information or to take a clear position on controversial issues.

vi) Survey method is not suitable for problems that require the study in the historical retrospect.

Data Processing and Analysis

Data Processing

The mass of raw data collected by us is difficult to understand its meaning unless it is processed and analysed. We have to condense or summarise them in the form of tables and graphs. The main purpose of data processing and analysis is to identify whether research assumptions were correct or not, and to highlight possible new views on the problem under study. The processing of data involves:

Editing

Coding

Classification

and Tabulation

Editing of Data

The editing of data is a process of examining the raw data to detect errors and omissions and to correct them, if possible, so as to ensure completeness, consistency, accuracy and homogeneity. This will facilitate coding and tabulation of data. In fact, the editing involves a careful scrutiny of the completed questionnaires.

Editing of Data:

Examining the raw data to detect errors and omissions and to correct them

The editing can be done at two stages: field editing and central editing.

Field editing: The field editing consists of review of the reporting forms by the investigator for completing or translating what the latter has written in abbreviated form at the time of interviewing the respondent. This form of editing is necessary in view of the writing of individuals, which vary from individual to individual and sometimes difficult for the tabulator to understand. This sort of editing should be done as soon as possible after the interview, as it may be necessary sometimes to recall the memory. While doing so; care should be taken so that the investigator does not correct the errors of omission by simply guessing what the respondent would have answered if the question was put to him.

Central Editing: Central editing should be carried out when all the forms of schedules have been completed and returned to the headquarters. This type of editing requires that all the forms are thoroughly edited by a single person (editor) in a small field study or a small group of persons in case of a large field study. The editor may correct the obvious errors, such as an entry in a wrong place, entry recorded in daily terms whereas it should have been recorded in weeks/months, etc, Sometimes, other information recorded in the schedule. If necessary, the respondent may be contacted for clarification. All the incorrect replies, which are quite obvious, must be deleted from the schedules.

The editor should be familiar with the instructions and the codes given to the interviewers while editing. The new (corrected) entry made by the editor should be in some distinctive form and they be initialed by the editor. The date of editing may also be recorded on the schedule for any future references.

Coding of Data

Coding is the process of assigning some symbols (either) alphabetical or numerals or (both)to the answers so that the responses can be recorded into a limited number of classes or categories. The classes should be appropriate to the research problem being studied. For example, if we assign 1 for women farmer and 2 for male farmer, it is a form of coding. Coding must be exhaustive and must be mutually exclusive so that the answer can be placed in one and only one cell in a given category. Further, every class must be defined in terms of only one concept.

> **Coding of Data:**
>
> Assigning some symbols (either) alphabetical or numerals or (both) to the answers so that the responses can be recorded into a limited number of classes or categories.

The coding is necessary for the efficient analysis of data. The coding decisions should usually be taken at the designing stage of the questionnaire itself so that the likely responses to questions are pre-coded. This simplifies computer tabulation of the data for further analysis. It may be noted that any errors in coding should be eliminated altogether or at least be reduced to the minimum possible level. One standard method is to code in the margin of the interview schedule/questionnaire with a pencil. The other method is to transcribe the data in a coding sheet.

Classification of Data

After the data has been systematically collected and edited, the first step is to reduce it into homogeneous groups for any meaningful analysis. This necessitates classification of data, which in simple terms is the process of arranging data in groups or classes on the basis of some similarities and dissimilarities. Classification helps in making comparisons and drawing meaningful conclusions. Classification can either be according to attributes or according to numerical characteristics.

Objectives of Classification

The principal objectives of classifying data are:

- to condense the mass of data in such a way that salient features can be readily noticed
- to facilitate comparisons between attributes of variables
- to prepare data which can be presented in tabular form
- to highlight the significant features of the data at a glance.

Types of Classification

Some common types of classification are:

1. Geographical i.e., according to area or region.
2. Chronological, i.e., according to occurrence of an event in time.
3. Qualitative, i.e., according to attributes.
4. Quantitative, i.e., according to magnitudes.

Geographical Classification. In this type of classification, data is classified according to area or region. For example, when we consider production of egg state wise, this would be called geographical classification. The listing of individual entries is generally done in an alphabetical order or according to size to emphasise the importance of a particular district or region

Chronological Classification. When the data is classified according to the time of its occurrence, it is known as chronological classification. For example, milk production of State for last six years are given below:

Year	Production (000' tonnes)	Year	Production (000' tonnes)
2001-02	929	2004-05	1283
2002-03	941	2005-06	1342
2003-04	997	2006-07	1431

Qualitative Classification. When the data is classified according to some attributes (distinct categories) which are not capable of measurement is known as qualitative classification. In a simple (or dichotomous) classification, an attribute is divided into two classes, one possessing the attribute and the other not possessing it. For example, we may classify population on the basis of employment, i.e., the employed and the unemployed. Similarly, we can have manifold classification when an attribute is divided so as to form several classes.

For example, the attribute education can have different classes such as primary, middle, higher secondary, university, etc.

Quantitative Classification. When the data is classified according to some characteristics that can be measured, it is called quantitative classification. For example, the employees of a company may be classified according to their monthly salaries. Since quantitative data is characterised by different numerical values, the data represents the values of a variable. Quantitative data may be further classified into one or two types: discrete or continuous. The term discrete data refers to quantitative data that is limited to certain numerical values of a variable. For example, the number of employees in an organisation or the number of machines in a factory are examples of discrete data.

Continuous data can take all values of the variable. For example, the data relating to weight, distance, and volume are examples of continuous data. The quantitative classification becomes the basis for frequency distribution.

When the data is arranged into groups or categories according to conveniently established divisions of the range of the observations, such an arrangement in tabular form is called a frequency distribution. In a frequency distribution, raw data is represented by distinct groups which are known as **classes.** The number of observations that fall into each of the classes is known as **frequency.** Thus, a frequency distribution has two parts, on its left there are classes and on its right there are frequencies.

When data is described by a continuous variable it is called continuous data and when it is described by a discrete variable, it is called **discrete data.** The following are the two examples of discrete and continuous frequency distributions.

No of Dairy Farmers	Litre of milk production of their animals	Age of the dairy Farmers	Years of dairy farming
100	7	30-35	10
110	9	35-40	8
120	10	40-45	6
130	5	45-50	9

Discrete frequency distribution **Continuous frequency distribution**

Construction of a Discrete Frequency Distribution

The process of preparing a frequency distribution is very simple. In the case of discrete data, place all possible values of the variable in ascending order in one column, and then prepare another column of 'Tally' mark to count the number of times a particular value of the variable is repeated. To facilitate counting, block of five 'Tally' marks are prepared and some space is left in between the blocks. The frequency column refers to. the number of `Tally' marks, a particular class will contain. To illustrate the construction of a discrete frequency distribution, consider a sample study in which 50 dairy farmer's families were surveyed to find the number of children per family. The data obtained are:

3	2	2	1	3	4	2	1	3	4
1	2	3	3	2	1	1	2	3	0
4	3	5	5	4	3	6	5	4	3
5	4	3	1	2	0	1	2	3	5
5	0	2	3	2	1	1	0	6	5

To condense this data into a discrete frequency distribution, we shall take the help of 'Tally' marks as shown below:

No of Children	No of Dairy Farmers	Frequency
0	IIII	04
1	~~IIII~~ IIII	09
2	~~IIII~~ ~~IIII~~	10
3	~~IIII~~ ~~IIII~~ II	12
4	~~IIII~~ I	06
5	~~IIII~~ II	07
6	II	02

Construction of a Continuous Frequency Distribution

In constructing the frequency distribution for continuous data, it is necessary to clarify some of the important terms that are frequently used.

Class Limits. Class limits denote the lowest and highest value that can be included in the class. The two boundaries (i.e., lowest and highest) of a class are known as the lower limit and the upper limit of the class. For example, in the class 60-69, 60 is the lower limit and 69 is the upper limit or we can say that there can be no value if! that class which is less than 60 and more than 69.

Class Intervals. The class interval represents the width (span or size) of a class. The width may be determined by subtracting the lower limit of one class from the lower limit of the following class (alternatively successive upper limits may be used). For example, if the two classes are 10-20 and 20-30, the width of the class interval would be the difference between the two successive lower limits, i.e., 20-10 = 10 or the difference between the upper limit and lower limit of the same class, i.e., 20-10 = 10.

Class Frequency. The number of observations falling within a particular class is called its class frequency or simply frequency. Total frequency (sum of all the frequencies) indicate the total number of observations considered in a given frequency distribution.

Class Mid-point. Mid-point of a class is defined as the sum of two successive lower limits divided by two. Therefore, it is the value lying halfway between the lower and upper class limits. In the example taken above the mid-point would be (10+20)/2 = 15 corresponding to the class 10-20 and 25 corresponding to the class 20-30.

Type of Class Interval. There are different ways in which limits of class intervals can be shown such as:

Exclusive and Inclusive method, and Open-end

Exclusive Method. The class intervals are so arranged that the upper limit of one class is the lower limit of the next class. The following example illustrates this point.

Income of the farm	No of farm	Income of the farm	No of farm
20-24.999	25	35-39.999	33
25-29.999	20	40-44.999	31
30-34.999	18	45-19.999	16

In this example, there are 25 farms whose sales are between Rs. 20,000 and Rs. 24,999. A firm whose sales are exactly Rs. 25,000 would be included in the next class. Therefore, in the inclusive method, it is presumed that upper limit is included.

It may be observed that both the methods give the same class frequencies, although the class intervals look different. Whenever inclusive method is used for equal class intervals, the width of class intervals can be obtained by taking the difference between the two lower limits (or upper limits).

Open-End. In an open-end distribution, the lower limit of the very first class and upper limit of the last class is not given. In distribution where there is a big gap between minimum and maximum values, the open-end distribution can be used such as in income distributions. The income disparities, of residents of a region may vary between Rs. 800 to Rs. 50,000 per month. In such a case, we can form classes like: Less than Rs. 1,000

1,000-2,000

2,000-5,000

5,000-10,000

10,000-25,000

25,000 and above

Remark. To ensure continuity and to get correct class intervals, we shall adopt exclusive method. However, if inclusive method is suggested then it is necessary to make an adjustment to determine the class interval. This can be done by taking the average value of the difference between the lower limit of the succeeding class and the upper limit of the class. In terms of formula:

$$\text{Correction factor} = \frac{\text{Lower limit of second class- Upper Limit of the first class}}{2}$$

This value so obtained is deducted from all lower limits and added to all upper limits. For instance, the example discussed for inclusive method can easily be converted into exclusive case. Take the difference between 25 and 24,999 and divide it by 2. Thus correction factor becomes (25-24,999)/2 = 0.0005. Deduct this value from lower limits and add it to upper limits. The new frequency distribution will take the following form:

Income of the farm	No of farms	Income of the farm	No of farms
19.9995 -24.9995	25	34.9995-39.9995	33
24.9995-29.9995	20	39.9995-44.9995	31
29.9995-34.9995	18	44.9995-19.9995	16

Guidelines for Choosing the Classes

The following guidelines are useful in choosing the class intervals.

1. The number of classes should not be too small or too large. Preferably, the number of classes should be between 5 and 15. However, there is no hard and fast rule about it. If the number of observations is smaller, the number of classes formed should be towards the lower side of this limit and when the number of observations increase, the number of classes formed should be towards the upper side of the limit.
2. If possible, the widths of the intervals should be numerically simple like 5, 10, 25 etc. Values like 3, 7, 19 etc. should be avoided.
3. It is desirable to have classes of equal width. However, in case of distributions having wide gap between the minimum and maximum values, classes with unequal class interval can be formed like income distribution.
4. The starting point of a class should begin with 0, 5, 10 or multiples thereof. For example, if the minimum value is 3 and we are taking a class interval of 10, the first class should be 0-10 and not 3-13.
5. The class interval should be determined after taking into consideration the minimum and maximum values and the number of classes to be formed. For example, if the income of 20 employees in a company varies between Rs. 1100 and Rs. 5900 and we want to form 5 classes, the class interval should be 1000

$$\frac{(5900 - 1100)}{1000} = 4.8 \text{ or } 51000$$

Cumulative and Relative Frequencies

It is often useful to express class frequencies in different ways. Rather than listing the actual frequency opposite each class, it may be appropriate to list either cumulative, frequencies or relative frequencies or both.

Cumulative Frequencies. As its name indicates, it cumulates the, frequencies, starting at either the lowest or highest value. The cumulative frequency of a given class interval thus represents the total of all the previous class frequencies including the class against which it is written. To illustrate the concept of cumulative frequencies, consider the following example.

Income of the farm	No of farm	Income of the farm	No of farm
19000-24000	25	35000-40000	33
24000-30000	20	40000-45000	31
30000-35000	18	45000-50000	23

If we keep on adding the successive frequency of each class starting from the frequency of the very first class, we shall get cumulative frequencies as shown below:

Income of the farm	No of farm	Cumulative frequency
19000-24000	25	25
24000-30000	20	45
30000-35000	18	63
35000-40000	33	96
40000-45000	31	127
45000-50000	23	150

Relative Frequencies. Very often, the frequencies in a frequency distribution are converted to relative frequencies to show the percentage for each class. If the frequency of each class is divided by the total number of observations (total frequency), then this proportion is referred to as relative frequency. To get the percentage for each class, multiply the relative frequency by 100; For the above example, the values computed for relative frequency and percentage are shown below:

Income of the farm	No of farm	Relative frequency	Percentage
19000-24000	25	0.2	16.7
24000-30000	20	0.1	13.3
30000-35000	18	0.1	12.0
35000-40000	33	0.2	22.0
40000-45000	31	0.2	20.7
45000-50000	23	0.2	15.3
	150	1.0	100.0

There are two important advantages in looking at relative frequencies (percentages) instead of absolute frequencies in a frequency distribution.

1. Relative frequencies facilitate the comparisons of two or more than two sets of data.
2. Relative frequencies constitute the basis of understanding the concept of probability.

Tabulation

Tabulation

Summarization and condensation of data

The tabulation is used for summarization and condensation of data. It aids in analysis of relationships, trends and other summarization of the given data. The tabulation may be simple or complex. Simple tabulation results in one-way tables, which can be used to answer questions related to one characteristic of the data. The complex tabulation usually results in two way tables, which give information about two interrelated characteristics of the date; three way tables which give information about three interrelated characteristics of data, and still higher order tables, which supply information about several interrelated characteristics of data. In boarder sense the tabulation is an orderly arrangement of data in columns and rows.

Tabulation is essential because of the following reasons.

1. It conserves space and reduces explanatory and descriptive statement to a minimum.
2. It facilitates process of comparison
3. It facilitates the summation of items and the detection of errors and omissions.
4. It provides a basis for various statistical computations.

Following are the important characteristics of a table:

i) Every table should have a clear and concise title to make it understandable without reference to the text. This title should always be just above the body of the table.
ii) Every table should be given a distinct number to facilitate easy reference.
iii) Every table should have captions (column headings) and stubs (row headings) and they should be clear and brief.
iv) The units of measurements used must always be indicated.
v) Source or sources from where the data in the table have been obtained must be indicated at the bottom of the table.
vi) Explanatory footnotes, if any, concerning the table should be given beneath the table along with reference symbol.

vii) The columns in the tables may be numbered to facilitate reference.

viii) Abbreviations should be used to the minimum possible extent.

ix) The tables should be logical, clear, accurate and as simple as possible.

x) The arrangement of the data categories in a table may be a chronological, geographical, alphabetical or according to magnitude to facilitate comparison.

x) Finally, the table must suit the needs and requirements of the research study.

Tabulation can be done by hand or computer. The choice depends on the size and type of study, funds availability, facilities and trained personnel.

Graphical Presentation of Data

The table may present clear and concise picture of the mass of data. But, the figures in the table may not be readily intelligible. The visual aids, like diagrams and graphs are helpful in understanding the facts of numerical data easily. Comparison of data is also made easier by such diagrams and graphs.

Diagrams and Graphs

The different diagrams used for displaying facts. Some of them are discussed which can be used for presentation of data

a) Line Diagram
b) Simple Bar Diagram
c) Multiple Bar Diagram
d) Sub-divided Bars
e) Deviation Bars
f) Histogram
g) Pie diagram
h) Pictogram
i) Line graph

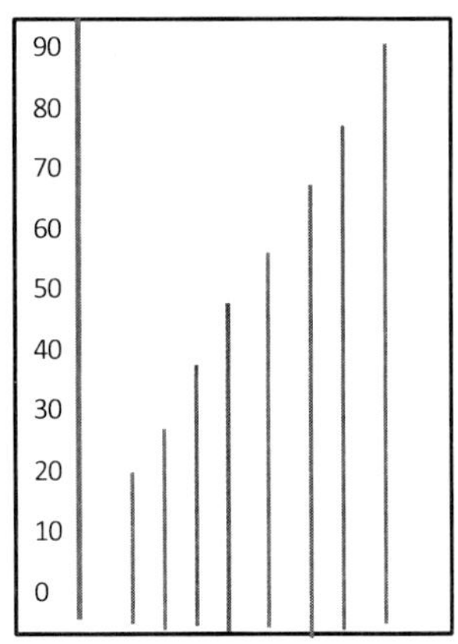

Line Diagram

a) Line Diagrams

In these diagrams only lines are drawn for the purpose of comparison.

Illustration

The following data relate to expenditure of eight kids of dairy farmers on purchase of books. Represent it by line diagram. **Line Diagram**

Expenditure: 20, 30,50,70,90,60, 40,80

Solution: Arrange the expenditure in the ascending order as given below

20, 30, 40, 50, 60, 70, 80, 90.

b) Simple Bar Diagram

Simple bar diagrams are very popular. we may see numerous such diagrams in newspapers, journals, exhibitions, and even on television to depict different characteristics of data. For example, population, per capita income, sales and profits of a company can be shown easily through bar diagrams. It may be noted that a bar is a thick line whose width is shown to attract the viewer. A simple bar diagram may be either vertical or horizontal with equal width. The simple bar diagrams are used only in those cases where one comparison has to be made. The bars are separated from each other by equal intervals. The bars may be coloured to make it attractive and distinctive.

In order to draw a simple bar diagram, we take the characteristic (or attribute) under consideration on the X-axis and the corresponding value on the Y-axis. It is desirable to mention the value depicted by the bar on the top of the bar.

Illustration

Represent the following data of FMD outbreaks in different years in the district of Cuttack

Year	**2013**	**2014**	**2015**	**2016**	**2017**	**2018**	**2018**	**2020**
No. of outbreaks	44	55	30	50	62	35	25	40

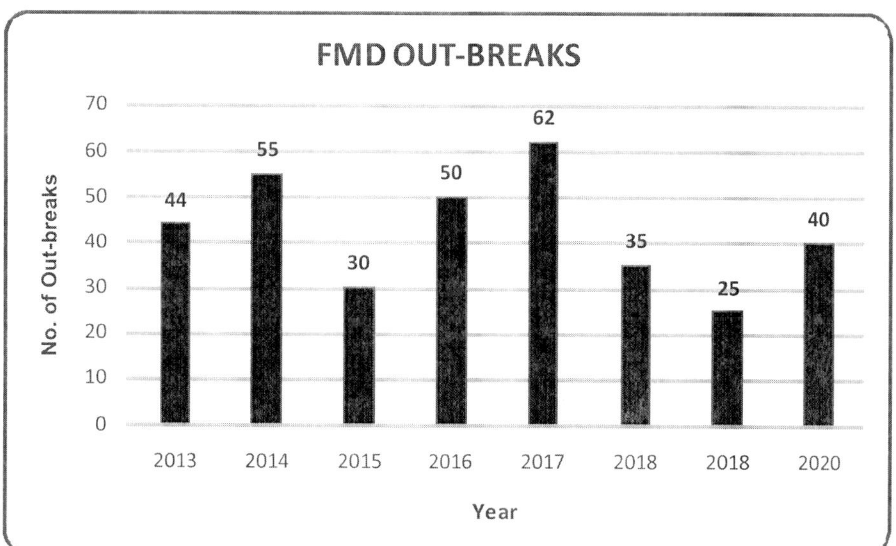

c) Multiple Bar Diagrams

When more than one comparison is required to be made then multiple bar diagrams are used. The method of drawing is the same as in case of simple bars.

Illustration

Represent the following data of FMD, HS and Anthrax outbreaks in different years in the district of Cuttack

Year	FMD	HS	Anthrax
2015	30	18	11
2016	50	22	16
2017	62	34	22
2018	35	22	10
2019	50	29	12
2020	40	28	14

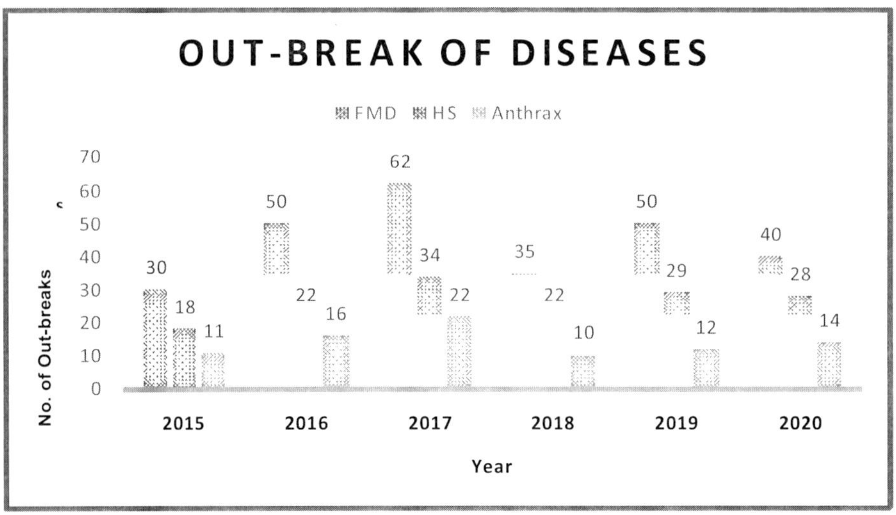

d) Sub divided bar diagrams

Sub-divided bars serve the same purpose as multiple bars. The only difference between two is that is in case of multiple bars each part is shown independently and is represented by a separate bar, but in case of sub-divided bar each group is taken as the part of the whole and different bars of the same group are placed one upon the other. In order to draw these barsm first all bars representing the total are drawn. Then each bar is divided in to sub parts as required.

Illustration

Represent the following data of FMD, HS and Anthrax outbreaks in different years in the district of Cuttack in a sub-dived bar.

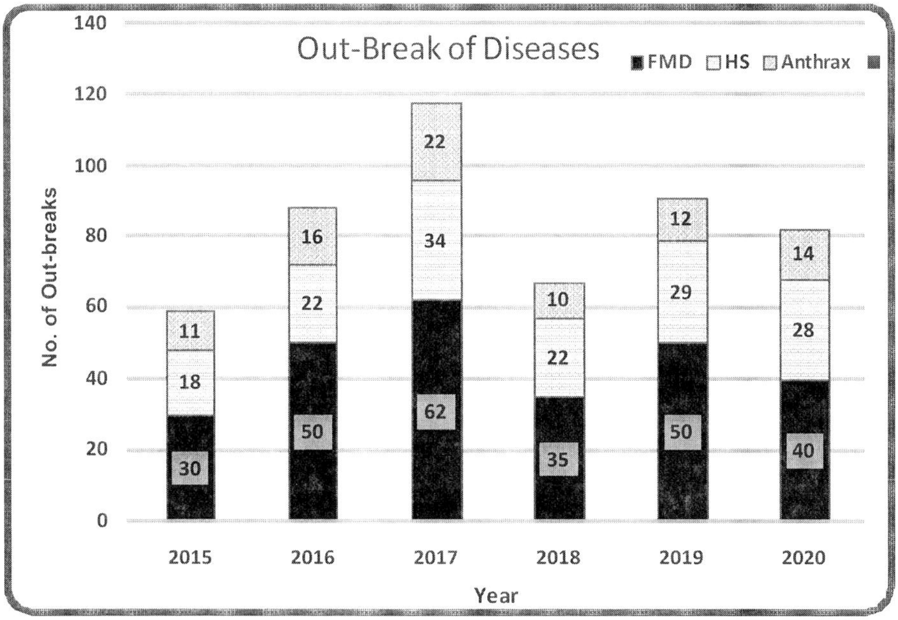

e) Deviation Bars

Bars representing positive and negative deviations are drawn above and below the base line. The differences may be towards positive or towards negative side. The base line is therefore, drawn in the centre and may be vertical or horizontal. If the base line is horizontal, plus values are shown upwards and minus values are shown downwards. If base line is vertical, the plus values are shown in the left side and minus values are shown in the right side.

Illustration

Change in the number of dairy animals in 10 Gram Panchayats from 2000 to 2020

GP-1	900
GP-2	750
GP-3	1000
GP-4	500
GP-5	600
GP-6	-250
GP-7	-350
GP-8	-450
GP-9	-400
GP-10	-200

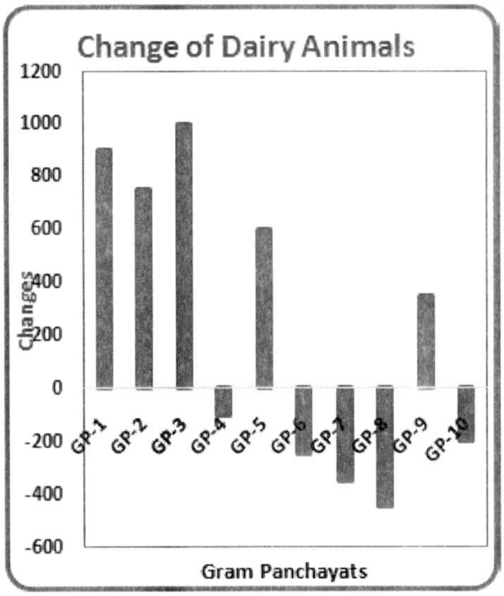

Horizontal Deviation Bars

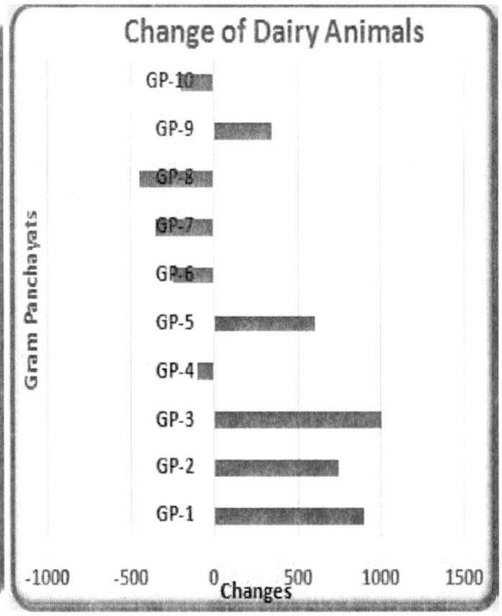

Vertical Deviation Bars

f) Histogram

Histogram is drawn to represent relative frequency size of different groups. Numerical data are often presented in histogram, which are very similar to the bar diagrams which are used for categorical data. An important difference is that in a histogram the bars are connected (as long as there is no gap between the data) whereas un a bar chart the bars are not connected, as the different categories are distinct entities.

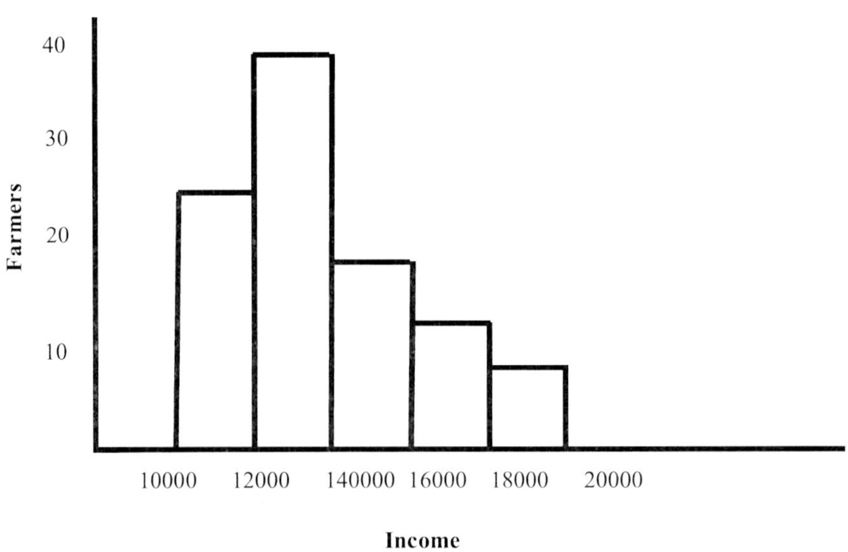

Illustration

Income of 100 dairy farmers from dairy business

Income	No of dairy farmers
10000-12000	24
12000-14000	38
14000-16000	18
16000-18000	12
18000-20000	8

g) Pie Diagram

A Pie Chart is a type of graph that displays data in a circular graph. The pieces of the graph are proportional to the fraction of the whole in each category. In other words, each slice of the pie is relative to the size of that category in the group as a whole. The entire "pie" represents 100 percent of a whole, while the pie "slices" represent portions of the whole. It is used to emphasise relative proportion or shares of each category. The relative frequency in each category or sector is proportional to the arc length of that sector or the area of that sector or the central angle of that sector.

Illustration

The distribution of 4000 livestock population in a village in 2020 as follows:

Cattle : 1250

Sheep : 350

Goat : 1100

Pig : 250

Buffalo : 125

Draw a pie diagram.

Solution: The angle of a circle is 360^0. We have to find out the proportionate arc value for each category of livestock to represent in the circle. Besides, we have to find out the percentage of the area for each category of livestock species for better presentation of data.

- $\text{Angle value of the sub-group} = \dfrac{\text{Value of the sub-group}}{\text{Total Value}} \times 360$

- $\text{Percentage of the sub-group} = \dfrac{\text{Angle value of the sub-group}}{360} \times 100$

Livestock	Number	Angle of the circle	Percentage area of circle
Cattle	1500	135^0	37.5
Sheep	550	49^0	13.75
Goat	1200	108^0	30
Pig	450	40^0	11.25
Buffalo	300	27^0	7.5
	4000	360^0	100

Year	2001-02	2002-03	2003- 04	2004-05	2005-06	2006-07	2007-08	2008-09	2009-10
Milk Production 000' tones	929	941	997	1283	1342	1431	1625	1598	1651

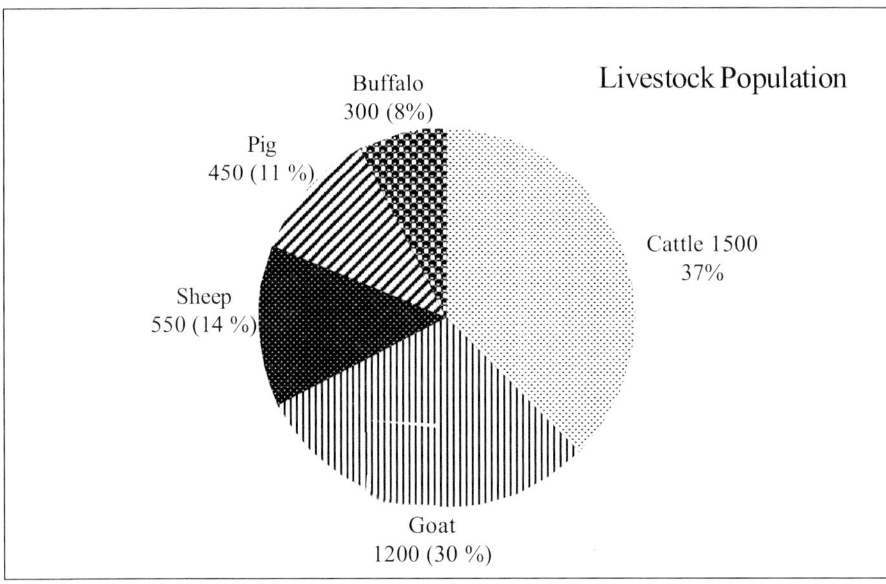

h) Pictograms

Diagrams representing different data may be expressed in the form of pictures. Pictures may be less precise but never less attractive and interesting. Highly suitable for semi-literate and illiterate farmers. A pictogram showing more number of goats than cattle could be easily recognised by the farmers of which species is more.

i) Line Graph

Sometimes the data may be taken repeatedly over time. Such chronological data are known as time series data. For example, total milk production of the State over a period of time, the out-break rate over a period of time, etc. are time series data.

Illustration: Line graph with the data of milk production of Odisha State since 2001

Year	2001-02	2002-03	2003-04	2004-05	2005-06	2006-07	2007-08	2008-09	2009-10
Milk Production 000' tones	929	941	997	1283	1342	1431	1625	1598	1651
Year	2010-11	2011-12	2012-13	2013-14	2014-15	2015-16	2016-17	2017-18	2018-19
Milk Production000' tones	1671	1721	1724	1861	1903	1903	2003	2088	2311

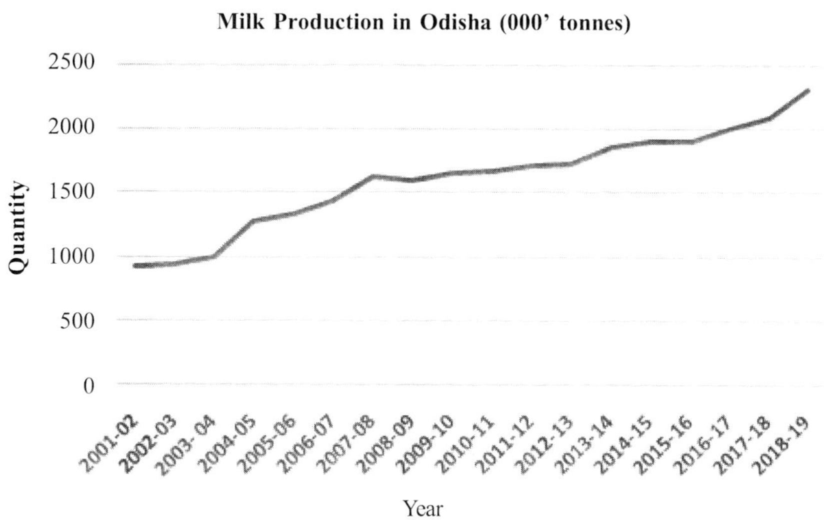

Report Writing

After collecting data and analysis the data, the researcher has to accomplish the task of drawing inferences followed by report writing. The researcher is in obligation to submit the research report after completion of research work. The report helps us to know what has been done, why it has been done, how it has been done, what results were obtained, what conclusion and recommendations have been arrived at, etc. Research reports vary greatly in length and depending on the subject. Research investigation are presented like a technical report, a popular report, an article, a monograph or even sometimes in the form of an oral presentation. In the technical report, the main emphasis is on: (i) the methods employed; (ii) assumptions made in the course of study and; (iii) the detailed presentation of the findings, including their limitations and supporting data. Social and development research reports need to:

- have a logical, clear structure
- be to the point
- use simple language, and have a pleasant layout

Constituents of Research Report

This is an indicative guideline of what should constitute a project report. There are variations widely found in different research reports.

1. Title and cover page
2. Forward
3. Preface
4. Acknowledgement
5. Table of contents
6. List of table
7. List of figures
8. List of abbreviations
9. Executive summary
10. Introduction
11. Objectives of the study
12. Research/Project area
13. Materials and Methods (Methodology)
14. Results and Discussion
15. Conclusion and recommendation
16. References/Bibliography
17. Appendices/Annexures

Title and Cover Page

The title and cover page contains the name of the author with their designation, the institution to whom they are affiliated, month and year of publication.

Forward

Forward may or may not be there in the report. It is some time written by an expert appreciating the work.

Preface

A preface, in contrast, is written by the author of the research work. It covers the story how this research report has been prepared.

Acknowledgement

In acknowledgement portion, the author(s) acknowledge the contribution made by the people, organisation and others who contributed or helped in the conduct of research and preparation of the report on various ways.

Table of Contents

A table of contents is essential. It provides the reader a quick overview of the chapters with major sections and sub sections of your report, and page references, so that the reader can go through the report in a different order, or skip certain sections.

List of Tables

If you have many tables or figures, it is essential to list these also in a table of contents with formatted with page numbers. The initial letters of the key words in the title are capitalized and no terminal punctuation is used.

List of Tables

S.No	Name of the Table	Pages
1.1	Milk Production in the State	xxxx
2.1	Sampling Pattern	xxxx
3.1	Income of households	xxxx
3.2		
3.3....		

List of Figures

The list of figures appears in the same format as the list of tables, titled List of Figures.

List of Abbreviations

AI	:	Artificial Insemination
BVO	:	Block Veterinary Officer
LI	:	Livestock Inspector
SDVO	:	Sub-Divisional Veterinary Officer
______	:	______________________
______	:	______________________

Executive Summary

The Executive summary enables the readers to have an essence of the research/ project carried out. It should contain

- a very brief description of the problem (**Why** this study was needed)—

- the main objectives (**What** has been studied)
- the place of study (**Where**)
- the type of study and methods used (**How**)
- the major findings and conclusions
- the major (or all) recommendations.

Introduction

Introduction should certainly contain some relevant (environmental/administrative/economic/social) background data and information about the topic on which you are carrying out research for example if you are doing research on livestock production, then a brief about the status of livestock production in the country, state-wise break up, etc., need to be described. The purpose of introduction is to introduce the topic to the readers in a comprehensive way stating the importance of problems you have studied.

Review of Literature

A literature review is a body of text that aims to review the critical points of current knowledge and or methodological approaches on a particular topic. Literature reviews are secondary sources, and, as such, do not report any new or original experimental work. Its ultimate goal is to bring the reader up to date with current literature on a topic, and forms the basis for another goal, such as future research that may be needed in the area.

Objectives of the Study

A clear statement of objectives is very important for any research works. We should not have many objectives for a research work. Objectives should be framed in a such way that it would be useful to reach the problem. For example-to study the existing pattern of credits to the livestock sector.

Research/Project Area

In this chapter, information regarding the geographical area of the State/District/Block where the research has been conducted is furnished. A map of the study area indicating locations from where data have been collected may be given.

Materials and Methods (Methodology)

The methodology adopted in conducting the study must be fully explained. The scientific reader would like to know about the basic design of the study, the methods of data collection, information regarding the sample used in the study, the statistical analysis adopted and the factors limiting the study .The methodology section should include a description of :

- the study type
- major study themes or variables (a detailed list of variables on which data was collected may be annexed)
- the study/ target population(s), sampling method(s) and the size of the sample(s)
- data collection techniques used for the different study populations
- duration of data collection
- how the data was collected and by whom?
- procedures used for data analysis, including statistical tests (if applicable)
- any constraints and its management
- limitations of the study

Results and Discussion

The systematic presentation of your findings in relation to the research objectives is the crucial part of the report. The list of data by objectives will help you to decide how to organise the presentation of data. The decision concerning where to put what can best be made after all data have been fully processed and analysed. Tables and figures are commonly used here to support and supplement the textual materials. Discussion helps to interpret the results of the study in proper perspective and leading in to meaningful conclusions and possible recommendations. The discussion may also include findings from other related studies that support or contradict the present findings.

Conclusions and Recommendations

The conclusions and recommendations should follow logically from the discussion of the findings. Conclusion is a reasoned judgement or insights that provides a deep insight about the study. On the basis of findings and discussion, the researcher puts forward some suggestions for consideration and action by the appropriate authority. It is advisable to present conclusion and recommendations in specific sections related to issues of importance/under investigation/ objectives of the study for better clarity to different stake holders. The conclusions should be given in bullets so that it can easily catch the attention of the reader.

References/Bibliography

This is the list of publications which the researcher has referred while conducting the study and writing the report. The references in the report should be numbered author wise alphabetically.

Appendices/ Annexures

The annexures / appendices should contain essential supporting materials of the study which cannot be given in detail in the report. Information that would be useful to special categories of readers but is not of interest to the average reader can be included in this section. .

Suggested Readings and References

1. Kothari C.R. and Garg G. (2015). Research Methodology: Methods and Techniques. New Age International(p) Limited, New Delhi.
2. Ray G.L. and Mondal S. (2004). Research Methods in Social Sciences and Extension Education, Kalyani Publishers, New Delhi-110 002.
3. Rangaswamy R. (2014). A Textbook of Agricultural Statistics, New Age International (p) Limited, New Delhi.
4. Goode W.J. and Hatt P.K. (1981). Methods in Social Research. McGraw- Hill Book Company, Singapore.
5. Kerlinger F.N. (1973). Foundations of Behavioural Research. Holt, Rinebart and Winston Inc., New York.
6. Young P.V. (1996). Scientific Social Surveys and Research. Prentice –Hall of India Pvt. Ltd., New Delhi.
7. Bajpai S.R. (1993). Methods of Social Survey and Research, Kitab Ghar, 87/ 259, Kanpur-3.
8. Cohen, L., Manion, L. and Morrison, K. (2000). Research Methods in Education 5th Edition. London: Routledge Falmer
9. Hansraj (1990). Theory and Practice in Social Research. Asia Publishing House, Culcutta.
10. Reddy, S.V., and Praveena, C. (1985). An Invitation to Research Methodology in Behavioural Sciences, EEI, Hyderabad.
11. Siegel S. (1956). Nonparametric Statistics for the Behavioural Sciences. McGraw-Hill Book Company Inc., New York.
12. Moser C.A., Kalton G. (1989), Survey Methods in Social Investigation. Hants, UK: Gower Publishing Company.
13. Ranjit K. (2011). Research Methodology, a step-by-step for beginners, Sage Publication, Mathura Road, New Delhi-110044.

SECTION-II: RURAL DEVELOPMENT

12

Rural Development : Concept and Meaning

Rural Development : Concept and Meaning

Mahatma Gandhi said, *"India lives in its villages. If the village perishes, India will perish too"*. This saying about the social, economic and political development of rural areas justifies that India is predominantly an agrarian country with more than 70 percent of its population living in more than five lakh villages. Agriculture is the predominant livelihood occupation and the rural population largely consists of small and marginal farmers, agricultural labourers, artisans and scheduled castes and scheduled tribes. A large part of this rural population is still living below the poverty line and is the focus of rural development programmes. Rural Development is not a new concept for India rather it is a very basic principle of our culture. The famous epics like Ramayana and Mahabharata teach us the dignity of humanity and benevolence and justice to people. In ancient days, our villages were self-sufficient and requiring very little assistance from outsiders. However, during British rule, the rural economy was destroyed and the rural mass was made dependent on goods and services provided by outsiders. There was no rural development policy as such to make the people self-reliant. Some of the rural development activities were taken up by the British Government in India during the Great Bengal Famine. These attempts were of very limited scale without having legal sanctions behind the move.

Meaning of Rural Development

Rural

Rural is an area, where the people are engaged in primary industry in the sense that they produce things directly for the first time in cooperation with nature. It is sparsely settled places away from the influence of large cities and towns. Such areas are distinct from more intensively settled urban and suburban areas. Occupation of rural area is predominantly agriculture in India. (For more difference between rural and urban areas, student may refer to the Rural Sociology chapter of this book).

Development

Development refers to the changes in the quality of life due to different interventions. It implies change in physical quality of life which encompasses economic as well as social aspects. Development does not only mean economic growth but also mean the equitable distribution of the gains made from economic growth. The meaning of development and growth is not same. The growth in the rural development context may be increase in livestock population, increase in production, number of new houses constructed, etc. These are all quantitative improvement. Growth mainly focuses on quantitative improvement which are visible, measurable while development is associated with both qualitative and quantitative improvement. Therefore, development is inclusive of growth. In other words, development implies growth with justice. It means an improvement in the quality of life through better health, education, housing and overall material and social welfare. The basic elements of development are the following:

i) Removal of inequality and poverty;

ii) Increase in material welfare of the people;

iii) Increase in social well-being (education, health, housing, etc.);

iv) An equitable distribution of the gains of development among different groups of people in a region or country;

v) An enhancement in technology and the capacity to produce a wider range of goods and services in the economy leading to a better quality of life;

vi) Building institutional structures which permit participation in decision-making at all levels, equalization of opportunities for development and removal of disparities.

Characteristics of Underdevelopment

Most developing countries are characterized by the following conditions:

i) Mass poverty;

ii) Low levels of income and concentration of incomes in a few hands;

iii) High levels of unemployment and under-employment;

iv) Poor nutrition, health, housing, literacy and welfare status;

v) Preponderance of primary sector and low levels of industrialization; and

vi) Lower status of women.

Rural Development

According to Ensminger (1974) rural development is a process of transformation from traditionally oriented rural culture towards an acceptance and reliance on science and technology.

Lela (1975) defined rural development as an improvement in the living standard of the masses of low-income population residing in rural areas and making the process of self-sustaining.

According to Agarwal (1989), rural development is a strategy designed to improve the economic and social life of a specific group of people, the rural poor.

According to World Bank (1997), "Sustainable Rural Development can make a powerful contribution to four critical goals of poverty reduction, wider shared growth, household, national and global food security and sustainable natural resource management"

According to United Nations, "Rural Development is a process of change, by which the efforts of the people themselves are united, those of government authorities to improve their economic, social and cultural conditions of communities in to the life of the nation and to enable them to contribute fully to national programme ".

The term 'rural development' is used very frequently by planner, policy maker, academician, researcher, social worker, common man, etc. across the globe in different ways, and vastly in divergent contexts. It is very difficult to find out a universally acceptable definition. The concept of rural development encompasses a wide spectrum of fields of development.

Rural Development is a concept, a phenomenon, a strategy and a discipline.

As a Concept, it connotes overall development of rural areas with a view to improve the quality of life of rural people (Singh, 1999, p.18). In this sense, it is a comprehensive and multidimensional concept and encompasses the development of agriculture and allied activities – village and cottage industries and crafts, socio economic infrastructure, community services and facilities, and above all, human resources in rural areas.

As a Phenomenon, it is the result of interaction between various physical, environmental, technological, economic, socio-cultural and institutional factors in the rural areas of a nation (Mathur, 2008, p.2).

As a Strategy, it is the approach or operational design to bring about the desired positive changes in the socio-economic and cultural life of the rural people (Mathur, 2008, p.2).

As a discipline, it is multi-disciplinary in nature, representing an intersection of agricultural, social, behavioural, engineering and management sciences (Chamabers, 1983, p.147).

Thus rural development is planned, designed and deliberate interventions to influence the socio-economic situations to achieve improved living standard of low-income population residing in rural areas and making the process of their development sustainable and self sustained. It is a process that enhances the capacity of the rural people to improve their lives and environment, accomplished by wider distribution of benefits resulting from such improvement. Rural development includes both agricultural and non-agricultural aspects of life. It includes economic growth as well as development of various sections and sectors of rural society.

Economists distinguish among the terms development, economic growth and economic development. Sing (2008) explains the term development, "Generally speaking, the term development implies a change that is desirable. Since what is desirable at a particular time, place and in a particular culture may not be desirable at other places, or at other times at the same place and in the same cultural milieu, it is impossible to think of a universally acceptable definition of development. At best, development in the context of society could be conceptualized as a set of desirable societal objectives which society seeks to achieve. Thus defined, development is cherished by all individuals, communities and nations, irrespective of their culture, religion and spatial location". Economic growth means sustained increase in per capita real income. But, economic development is a much wider term. It includes economic growth and at the same time encompasses other issues like pattern of production, distribution of national income, consumption behaviour of the people and concern for environment. The concept of sustainable development advocates economic progress in an environmentally responsible manner. To quote, "Sustainable development is development that meets the needs of the present without compromising the ability of future generation to meet their own needs (WCED 1987, p.43)." Sustainable development attempts to strike a balance between the demands of the economic development and the need for protection of the environment. It seeks to combine the elements of economic efficiency, intergenerational equity, social concerns and environmental protection. Although, the term sustainable development has many interpretations, it is generally referring to non-declining human well-being over time (Government of India, Economic Survey, 1998-99, p. 156).

Rural development is a strategy to enable a specific group of people, poor rural women and men, to gain for themselves and their children more of what they want and need. It involves helping the poorest among those who seek a livelihood in the rural areas to demand and control more of the benefits of rural development. The group includes small farmers, tenants and landless. Hence, rural development is defined as a process of sustainable improvement in the quality of life of rural people, especially the poor (Singh, 2008, p. 21).

Rural development is utilization, protection and enhancement of the natural, physical and human resources needed to make long-term improvements in rural living conditions. It involves provision of jobs and income opportunities while maintaining and protecting the environment of rural areas.

Rural development is a national necessity and has considerable importance in India because of the following reasons:

- To develop living standard of rural population
- To develop facilities like rural road, drinking water, rural market, education, transport, electricity, irrigation, telecommunication, etc., in the rural areas.
- To develop agriculture, animal husbandry and other agricultural related activities
- To develop rural industries through the development of handicrafts, small scaled industries, village industries, rural crafts, cottage industries, etc.
- To develop rural youths, women and farmer's associations.
- To develop and empower human resource of rural area in terms of their psychology, skill, knowledge, attitude and other abilities.
- To develop rural area as whole in terms of culture, society, economy, technology and health.
- To develop rural institutions like panchayat, school, cooperatives, post, banking and credit.
- To restore uncultivated land, provide irrigation facilities and motivate farmers to adopt improved seed, fertilizers, package of practices of crop cultivation and soil conservation methods.

Problems in Rural Development in India

1. Human induced problems

i) Traditional way of thinking.

ii) Low level of education

iii) Low scientific orientation.

iv) Poor level awareness.

2. Agricultural problems

i) Lack of awareness, knowledge, skill and attitude related to improved technologies

ii) Small size land holding

iii) Unavailability of inputs.

iv) Poor marketing facility.

v) Non-remunerative of agricultural products

3. Infrastructural problems

Poor infrastructure facilities like water, electricity, transport, educational institutions, communication, health, storage facility etc.

4. Economic problems

i) Unfavourable economic condition to adopt high cost technology.

ii) High cost of inputs.

iii) Underprivileged rural industries

5. Social and Cultural problems

i) Rigid cultural norms and traditions

ii) Conflict within and between groups, castes, religions, regions, languages.

6. Administrative problems

i) Target oriented approach

ii) Top to bottom planning approach to rural development

iii) Political interference.

iv) Low budget allocation to rural development

v) Unwillingness of employee to work in rural area.

vi) Improper utilization of budget.

Suggested Readings and References

1. Singh, Katar (2008). Rural Development: Principles, Policies and Management, New Delhi, Sage Publications.

2. Mukundan, N. (2009). Rural Development and Poverty Eradication in India, New Century Publications, Ansari Ganbj, Daryaganj, New Delhi-110 002.

3. Ensminger, D. (1957). A Guide to Community Development, Ministry of Community Development and Cooperation, Govt. of India, New Delhi.

4. Dahama, O.P., Bhatanagar, O.P. (1985). Education and Communication for Development, Oxford & IBH Publishing Company, New Delhi.

5. Environment for Cooperatives, Reading Materials prepared for Higher Diploma in Cooperative Management by NCCT of NCUI, New Delhi.

6. B.D. Singh (1992). Planning for Rural Development and Poverty Alleviation, Mittal Publications, New Delhi.

7. Nagpal C.S. & Mittal A.C. (1993). Rural Development, Anmol Publications Pvt. Ltd., New Delhi.

8. Government of India (1973). Community Development Programme in India 1952-72, Monograph Published during 25th Anniversary of Indian Independence, Ministry of Agriculture, Department of Community Development.

9. Government of India (1957). A Guide to Community Development, Ministry of Community Development, Government of India.

10. Arora, R.C. (1979). Integrated Rural Development, New Delhi: S.Chand and Company Limited.

13

Rural Development During Pre and Post Independence Period

1. Pre-Independence Rural Development Programmes
2. Development Initiatives by Philanthropists
    a) Rural Reconstruction Programme (1890)
    b) Scheme of Rural Reconstruction (1903)
    c) Servants of Indian Society (1905)
    d) Economic Conference of Mysore (1914-18)
    e) The Gurgaon Experiment (1920)
    f) Marthandam Attempt (1921)
    g) Sriniketan Rural Reconstruction Programme (1921)
    h) Sevagram Project (1923)
    i) Rural Reconstruction Programme in India (1932)
    j) Rural Development Programme (1935)
    k) Grow More Food Campaign (1943)
    l) Indian Village Service (1945)
    m) Firka (Village) Development Scheme (1946)
3. Post-Independence Rural Development Programme (Before Planned Strategies of Rural Development)
    a) Etawah Pilot Project (1948)
    b) Sarvodaya Scheme (1948)
    c) Nilokheri Project (1948)
    d) Paul Hoffman-15 pilot projects (1951)
    e) Chester Bowels (1951)
4. Suggested Readings and References

Pre-Independence Rural Development Programmes

Rural development traces back its history to the seventeenth century when voluntary efforts to serve the mankind were initiated by a religious society of people known as 'Friends' or 'Quakers' in England, then the other parts of World including India. It aimed at providing services to mankind transcending bonds of religion, territory and culture. During the British period, the British government was never serious about the rural development. But, they acted under compelling situation like famines and economic distress. During 1800 to 1825, it was reported that there were five famines; during 1825 to 1850, two famines; during 1850 to 1875, six famines; and during 1875 to 1900, there were eighteen famines in different parts of the country. Famines forced the British government in to action. The Famine Commission of 1880, 1898, 1901, the Irrigation Committee of 1903, the Commission on Co-operation of 1915 and the Royal Commission on Indian Agriculture were the efforts of the Government to improve the economic condition of the common man, but seldom were the reports of the commissions implemented in right spirit. However, during these periods, the most active role in the field of rural development was played by the Christian missionaries who aimed at the all-round development of their Christian converts. In the year 1987, British Government heeding to the representation made by Manchester Cotton Supply Association established the Department of Revenue, Agriculture and Commerce. But, this department did not do much related to agriculture development except the collection of agricultural statistics.

Based on Famine Commission's (1880) recommendations, Agriculture Department was established in most of the States, and as per the Famine Commission (1901) report, the Imperial Agricultural Research Institute, livestock farms and experimental stations were stated established at Pusa which marked the beginning of an organized agricultural research in India. The Indian Agricultural Service was constituted at the centre. The Government of India Act 1919 empowered the transfer of all the Development Departments connected with rural development to the major provinces and there after agricultural development become a state subject. The Royal Commission on Agriculture (1928) suggested the government to establish a body for agricultural research at the national level for promotion, guidance and co-ordination of agricultural research. The commission observed that agricultural research can be of no help to the cultivators until its results are given to them in a form in which they become a part of their agricultural practice.

Development Initiatives by Philanthropists

Prior to independence of the country, many reformers and philanthropists started various innovative rural development programmes either alone or with association with other organisations for the benefit of the poor people. Some of them are:

1. Rural Reconstruction Programme (1890) in Borada

The rural reconstruction programme was started in Borada province by Maharaja Sayaji Rao. The programme emphasized on establishment of village Panchayats; education of children; adult education; improving agriculture production through expansion of irrigation facilities; production, distribution and use of better quality seeds, etc.

The important approaches of the Programme

a) Integrating and collaborative works of various departments

b) Proactive administrative approaches to different social issues

c) Working together of different local bodies, associations, voluntary agencies, etc at village level for speedy development.

2. Scheme of Rural Reconstruction (1903)

Daniel Hamilton launched a scheme of creating model village in an area of 'Sunderban' near West Bengal on co-operative principles. In 1934, a Rural Reconstruction Institute was also established. He established Cooperative Credit Society, Central Cooperative Bank, Cooperative Marketing Society and Rural Reconstruction Institutes in their adopted villages for overall development of the rural people. The rural reconstruction institute provided various training facilities to the villagers on cottage industries. Through these institutions an effort was made to organize people into groups. When people come together, there is bound to happen something. This something happening is contributing for development. Through Cooperative Banks, society was served with financial support, which was very essential for bringing changes. Even today financial support is a key element of ensuring development. The latest examples of financial support for the weaker sections of society include Pradhan Mantri Jan Dhan Yojana, Life insurance schemes just paying Rs.1.00 per month etc.

3. Servants of Indian Society (1905)

The person who brought to and taught political life to Gandhiji was Gopal Krishna Gokhale. He was also having concern for introducing developmental initiatives in rural areas. The servents of Indian Society was funded by Gopala Krishna Gokhale as a political society at Poona. It laid strong emphasis on socio-economic and educational activities. Later Gokhale started training centres in Madras State(Chennai), United Province and Central Province (Madhya

Pradesh) and published booklets on the basic education and labour problems, etc. The training centres in villages imparted training on agriculture and cottage industries. There is organic relationship between the agriculture and cottage industries in villages. Cottage industries support agriculture by proving implements and other inputs. In turn agriculture provides raw materials to cottage industries. Hence, all development thinkers emphasized on development of small scale and cottage industries. Compared to other nations, India is having maximum number of people dependent on agriculture. Hence, the issues become more pertinent in this regard. Village should be the centre of development, otherwise there will be imbalanced growth in the nation. It happened to majority of extent. Now the institutions are opening their eyes and making all possible efforts to provide urban facilities in rural areas. Even though the sangha was established in Pune, Maharashtra, it was operational in the states of Madhya Pradesh, Uttar Pradesh and Orissa. The beauty of the organization is, it is still active in these areas and working for the cause of development. Apart from these developmental initiatives Sangha published books on basic education, labour problems, indebtedness etc.

4. Economic Conference of Mysore (1914-18)

This was launched by Dr. M.S. Visweswarya as the Divan of Mysore state. It was planned to have an overall development of the locality. Agriculture was given priority in the scheme. Various committees were formed with officials to survey the needs and formulate plans for implementation. The committee used to survey the needs and prioritise the problems for addressing. The main aim of the programme was to achieve the all-round progress of rural areas by giving emphasis on agriculture development. The scheme was wound up later due to immense load of the programme.

5. The Gurgaon Experiment (1920)

The Village Development Programme was started by F.L. Brayne, a Britisher, in Gurgaon district of Punjab and Haryana. The programme included establishment of school of rural economy to train the village guides for rural uplift work; setting up of domestic school of economics to train the village women; taking up rural sanitation works; agricultural development programmes, etc. He especially visualized the role of village school teacher as beyond teaching in the school and as a person who can solve the simple problems of the villagers. After the transfer of Brayane, there was a lack of interest and the scheme did not make much headway. Again this programme gathered momentum after 1933 when Brayane was appointed as the Commissioner of Rural Reconstruction in Punjab.

6. Marthandam Attempt (1921)

This programme was started by Dr. Spencer Hatch in 1921 at Marthandam (place nearer to Kanyakumari in Tamil Nadu) with the help of YMCA (Young Man Christian Association). The main objectives of this project were five-fold, namely, mental, spiritual, physical, economic and social development. The importance was given in the programme from the very beginning not to depend on Government assistance rather on self-help and self-reliance. Rural Reconstruction Centre at Marthandam had demonstration units having activities on honey production, cottage industries, livestock, poultry, seed production, etc. for giving training to local people. The programme through YMCA facilitated the marketing of rural products through cooperative organisations. Different clubs like egg selling club, honey club, seed club, weaver's club were organised under this programme. The programme successfully changed the attitude of the rural people on their dependence on Government for their welfare. It created desire among the people to change their situation through mutual cooperation and self-help.

7. Shriniketan Rural Reconstruction Programme (1921)

The Poet Rabindranath Tagore set up an Ashram at Shantinikatan (West Bengal), a peaceful place away from Calcutta. He started his rural development activities with L.K. Elmhirst from his institute of reconstruction established in the year 1921 with objectives of to improve village situations and developing interest among youth in rural development works. The institute of rural reconstruction conducted several demonstrations on farmers' holding on improved agricultural practices, established a dairy and poultry to supply milk, eggs, better animals and birds to the farmers for breeding. The programme emphasized on helping villagers to develop agriculture, livestock, formation of cooperatives and improving village sanitation. The activities of the institute were development of agriculture, cooperatives, industries and education through village organisations. His emphasis was on education as it will change the outlook of the people and focused on the slogan of 'Education for all'. Following were the objectives of the programme:

- To create a real interest in people for rural welfare work;
- To study rural problems and to translate conclusions into action;
- To help villagers develop their resourcks; and
- To improve village sanitation.

These objectives were desired to be achieved by: a) Creating a spirit of "self help and mutual help" b) Developing village leadership, c) Organizing village scouts called Brati Balika, d) Establishing training centres for handicrafts, and e) Establishing a demonstration centre at Shantiniketan.

His programme was limited to only 8 villages of his Zamindari and yielded very little result.

8. Sevagram Project (1923)

This project was started by the Father of Nation, Mahatma Gandhi in 1923 but it had really started in 1920 as All India Spinners' Association. The project was based on the principles of 'Truth and Non-Violence' and aimed at social and economic development. The objectives of the project were to provide service to the underprivileged section of the society for self dependency. The main activities of the project were organisation of training centre for cottage industries, prohibition, removal of untouchability, stressing women education and basic education and preaching and practicing of communal unity. Gandhiji believed in a philosophy of life which would achieve the welfare of all people (Sarvodaya). For the emancipation of villagers, he formulated an 18-point programme, which included the promotion of village industries, basic and adult education, rural sanitation, uplift of backward tribes, uplift of women, education in public health and hygiene, propagation of national language, love for the mother tongue, economic equality, organisation of Kisans, labourers and students, and so on. He sought to make the villagers self-sufficient and to develop in them that moral stamina which was essential to stand up against oppression and injustice. Truly speaking, the Gandhian constructive programme was a movement of the people, by the people and for the people. His small works became big organisations and institutions, and the simple ideas of that time became philosophies. His emphasis. on Khadi became the Charkha movement and then, the All-India Khadi and Village Industries Board. His thought, against untouchability and the caste system, resulted in the organisation of Harijan Sewak Sangh. Similar mention may be made of Hindustani Prachar Sangh, Sarvodaya, Bhudan Movement, etc. He created leaders like Vinoba, Nehru, Jayaprakash Narayan, Mira Ben, etc., who came from common stock, but got inspiration from Gandhiji. The Satyagrah Ashram at Sabarmati, and later Sevagram in Wardha, became not only places of trgining but of pilgrimage (Dahama and Bhatnagar, 2007).

9. Rural Reconstruction Programme in India (1932)

The project was started by V.T. Krishnamachari in Boroda state in 1932. The programme aimed at developing a will to live better and to develop capacity for self help and self reliance. The programme included the activities like digging of water wells, distribution of agriculture inputs and establishment cooperatives, panchayats, etc. The rural reconstruction centre established in 1932 worked in a group of villages round Kosamba (in Navsari District). The basic concern of the programme was that how to provide work to the people during lean agriculture period. Millions of people who remained unemployed during that period were provided various vocational skills for earning income from other than agricultural activities.

The centre aimed at:

1. Effecting an improvement in all aspects of rural life i. e. changing the outlook of the agriculturists, the problem being "the development of the desire for a higher standard of living,"
2. To undertake intensive work to release this aim,
3. To develop best type of village leadership; and to undertake the following programme:

a) Economic Programme consisted of

i) Development of subsidiary occupation like kitchen gardening, weaving, poultry farming, sericulture, bee-keeping etc.

ii) Farm improvements in cotton and other crops

iii) Co-operative society to inculcate thrift and

iv) The village panchayats to provide for sanitation, village roads and drinking water supply.

b) Education and Moral Programmes

Included Adult Education, development of community sense and of a feeling of solidarity in the village; propaganda against evils like early marriages and unreasonable customs connected with social observances; the proper use of village libraries; the scout movement and other educative work through lantern lectures; in short, making village life full and interesting. The village school should be the centre of all such activities. The programme of rural reconstruction was to be part of a wider programme for bringing about a rapid increase in standard of living. Increased agriculture production lay at root of all development. Therefore, the programme was progressively expanded to cover measures such as provision of irrigation facilities; conservation of soil; production of nucleus seed; their multiplication and distribution; education in agriculture and supplementary occupations.

10. Rural Development Programme (1935)

This is a Government Programme initiated in 1935-36 with the announcement of a grant of Rs. 1 crore by the Government of India for distribution to the provinces for the economic development and improvement of rural areas. The programme aimed at encouragement of village industries, improvement of village communication, rural sanitation and recreation, medical aids, agricultural improvements, etc. Rural reconstruction centres were organised for intensive work in the specially selected areas and various non-official organisation and educational bodies also did lot of work in this direction.

11. Grow More Food Campaign (1943)

This was started in 1942 after the crisis of food grains in Bengal. This campaign was done in an organised way to increase agricultural production. More emphasis was given on use of improved agricultural techniques in farming. Trained field men were employed. Fertilizers and improved seeds were distributed to raise food production. The Grow More Food Campaign Enquiry Committee under the chairmanship of V.T. Krishnamachari observed that the campaign failed to achieve the expected results due to various shortcomings in the basic strategy like, very narrow and restricted scope of operation, lack of integrated approach and the short-term objectives of increasing productivity, etc. It was also observed that the movement only touched a fringe of the population, and did not arouse widespread enthusiasm, or became in any sense a national programme. Due to lack of coordination between different departments, the programme did not function effectively. A committee was appointed by Government of India to enquire about the working of this programme and suggest ways and means to improve it. The G.M. F. Enquiry Committee Report (1952) recommendations were:

1. Reorganisation of administrative machinery of the Government to respond to the new concept of India as a welfare state.
2. Mobilisation of the best non-official leadership available in the country to guide the 60 million farm families in the villages in their effort to improve their own condition.
3. Establishment of an Extension organization for rural work, which would reach every farmer and assist in the coordinated development of all aspects of rural life
4. Staffing pattern should consist of a B.D.O., four technical officers and twelve VLWs for a Tahsil or Taluk, with an average of 120 villages.
5. The development activities at the District level will be under the Collector assisted by Specialists. The non-official side will consist of a District Board to which MPs and MLAs should be added as members
6. At the State level there should be a cabinet and a non-official board for facilitating joint action. The Development Commissioner should be in-charge of the entire rural development programme, and

7. The economic aspect of village life cannot be detached from broader social aspect. Agricultural development is, in every respect linked up with a whole set of social problems. All aspects of life are inter-related and no lasting results can be achieved if individual aspects of it are dealt with in isolation.

12. Indian Village Service (1945)

This was a mission project and was operated in U.P. districts in 1948 under the direction of Dr. W.H. Wiser. The main objectives of the scheme were to motivate people regarding cooperation for development work, give chance to rural people for their help in rural uplift works and enable villagers to solve their own problems. For creation of awareness of the different government programmes, various means like personal contact, demonstration, group discussion, informal meetings, use of visual aids etc. were used.

13. Firka (Village) Development Scheme (1946)

Firka Development scheme was a Government sponsored Scheme first started in 34 firkas in the then Madras State by T. Prakasam in 1946. The scheme was later extended to other firkas. Based on Gandhiji's idea of 'Village Swaraj', the programme emphasized on providing housing, education, water supply, developments of roads, improvements of sanitation, etc. The programme was directed in each firka by firka development committee consisting of officials and non-officials. At macro level, the programme emphasized on improvements in agriculture, development of village industries, formation of Panchayat, setting up cooperatives, encouraging social and cultural activities, etc. The administrative structure consisted of Director of Rural Welfare at the State level, the Collector at District level, the Rural Welfare Officer at Firka level and 5 to 10 Gramasevaks under him. Besides these, staffs for Agriculture and Public Works were also provided for every Firka. Later in 1953-54, the Firka Development Scheme was merged with Community Development Programme and National Extension Service Programme.

Merits and Demerits

The above discussed programmes were implemented in different regions of our country under different politico-socio-economic conditions. They varied in area of operation, population coverage, financial position and other resources. They were designed according to the prevailing problems of the area and benevolent individual's perception to the problems. The programmes initiated during pre-independence era had had one or the other shortcomings which are summed up as follows:

1. Attempts were isolated, uneven and discontinuous.
2. Most of the efforts were based on individual initiative.
3. Government backing and financing were not forthcoming.
4. Lack of involvement of people in programme implementation.
5. Plans and programmes were ill-defined and unbalanced.
6. Staff were mostly inexperienced and untrained.
7. No evaluation was carried out; hence the results were not known.
8. Association and coordination other development departments were very limited

Post-Independence Rural Development Programme (Before Planned Strategies of Rural Development)

1. Etawah Pilot Project (1948)

This Project of rural development and welfare was started in Etawah (U.P.) in September 1948 with active assistance of Lt. Col. Albert Mayer and Mr. Horace Holmes of USA. The main objectives of the project were to increase agricultural production and social development. These objectives were sought to be achieved through reclamation of waste land, ravine reclamation and building of upland, construction of sanitary wells, agriculture demonstrations, construction of roads, supply of seeds and manures, horticulture development, etc. Initially, the project was started with 64 villages and later it was extended up to 122 villages. In this project, the village level workers were trained and appointed, co-operation of other department and agencies was enlisted and demonstrations were conducted. The Government of India was very much impressed by the achievements of the project and considered it as a shining example of rural development work. Finally, this project was merged with National Extension Service (NES).

2. Sarvodaya Scheme (1948)

Sri Vinoba Bhave started this programme in 1948, and it was based on Gandhian principles. This programme was worked for village upliftment and it aimed at Bhudan, Gramdan, etc. The land and money collected were distributed amongst the landless labourers in the villages.

3. Nilokheri Project (1948)

This project was started by S.K.Dey to rehabilitate the displaced persons coming from Pakistan (due to partition of the country) by establishing a new township at Nilokheri in Karnal district in Haryana. Dey engaged the refugees in construction work assuring them the right to live, the right to work, and right to earn remuneration for the work they performed. These three rights formed the basis of a scheme known as *Mazdoor Manzil.* The plan included developing medical facilities, sanitation, middle and high school education, vocational farming, horticulture, poultry, fishery, etc. The Nilokheri township developed through this project served the villages around and in turn received the surplus of food and other commodities for the urban population. There was establishment of good relationship between town and nearby villages. The development phase was more or less completed by the end of 1951.

4. Paul Hoffman- 15 pilot projects (1951)

Ford Foundation of USA under the guidance of its president, Paul Hoffman started 15 pilot projects in various states of the country around middle of 1951. Under this project, a centre for training of extension personnel was also opened. The idea was to produce a multipurpose worker who would know how to offer first aid in the various facets of the programme of agriculture. Five training centres attached to five agriculture colleges were started with financial help from ford foundation.

5. Chester Bowels (1951)

Chester Bowles met with Nehru in 1951 and offered 54 million dollar U.S. aid to begin expanding the Etawah work. He agreed to spend the money over three years on approximately 50 projects, each with 300 villages. The planning document specified that each village in the program should be provided with drinking water facility, with agricultural extension and veterinary services, with drainage facilities where needed. He has planned that each group of 25 villages was to be clustered in a market unit, and each five market units would be grouped in a "block," whose central settlement would have accommodations for a thousand families, electricity and telephone services, an agricultural school, a plant nursery, a small hospital, and small-scale industries. Under this programme, fifteen pilot projects were approved in 1951. Each covered 100 villages, and each was under the control of an extension director with a staff agricultural officer, three agricultural technicians, and about a dozen village level workers.

The above mentioned projects had one or more shortcomings which resulted in failure or limited success in achieving the goals of community development. The shortcomings are summed up as follows:

i. Most of the efforts were based on individual efforts and inspired by humanitarian considerations.

ii. Government backing and financial assistance were lacking.

iii. Attempts were isolated, uneven and discontinuous.

iv. Staffs employed were inadequate, inexperienced and untrained.

v. Plans and programmes were very poorly designed, defined and implemented.

vi. Association and cooperation with other departments was very limited.

vii. Involvement of the people in planning and execution i.e. finding out the problems and their solution was very limited.

Suggested Readings and References

1. Singh, Katar (1999). Rural Development: Principles, Policies and Management, Second Edition, New Delhi, Sage Publications.
2. Dey, S.K. (1964), Community Development: A Bird's Eye View, Asia Publishing House, New Delhi.
3. Rural Development. Some Facets, (ed.) NIRD, Hyderabad – 1979.
4. Verma, S.C. (1980). Direct Attack on Rural Poverty, Ministry of Rural Development, Delhi.
5. Desai, Vasant (2009). Rural Development in India, Himalaya Publishing House, Mumbai.
6. Mahajan, R.K. (1991). Integrated Rural Development Programme, Concept Publishing Company, New Delhi.
7. Mehta, Shiv R. (1984). Rural Development Policies and Programmes, Sage Publications.
8. Arora, R.C. (1979). Integrated Rural Development, New Delhi: S.Chand and Company Limited.
9. Lawania, Vinod Kumar (1992). Rural Development in India. New Delhi: Ashish Publishing.
10. Ray, G.L. (2001). Extension, Communication and Management, 4th Edition, Naya Prokash, Calcutta.

14

Planned Strategies for Rural Development in India

1. Community Development
2. Development and Community Development
3. Community Development Programme (CDP)
4. National Extension Service (NES)
5. Evaluation of Community Development Programme
6. Weaknesses in the Community Development Programme
7. Suggested Readings and References

Planned Strategies for Rural Development in India

The Food and Agriculture Ministry appointed a Committee to examine the Grow More Food activities of the Government which were in implementation and to suggest measures for ensuring rapid expansion of agricultural production. The Grow More Food Campaign Inquiry Committee pointed out that there was imperative "Need of an organisation for intensive rural work which would reach every farmer and assist in the coordinated development of rural life as a whole similar in conception to the "extension" or "advisory"' services in the U.S.A., the U.K. and elsewhere." One of the recommendations of the Committee was that an extension agency should be set up for rural work, which would reach every farmer and assist in the coordinated development of rural life. The Planning Commission set up the Government of India in 1950 to formulate the First Five Year Plan summarized the reasons for failure of the earlier efforts by the governmental and voluntary organisations as follows-

i. Most of the schemes are short duration
ii. The activities were not properly planned and coordinated
iii. Initiatives come from the Government side and not from the people
iv. Some basic problems like land tenure, rural credit, etc., remained untouched in the programmes.

On the basis of experiences and reports of earlier rural development programmes, the Planning Commission, gave the highest priority to the development of agriculture and irrigation in the First Five-Year Plan. The Commission fixed substantially high targets of internal production and decided that the drive for food production should form part of plans for overall agricultural development, and that agricultural improvement in its turn should form an integral part of the much wider efforts for raising the level of rural life condition. The Commission prescribed "Community Development" as the method for initiating the process of transformation of the social and economic life of villages and "Rural Extension" as its agency. On the basis of experiences, reports of earlier rural development programmes, enquiry committee report and successful experiences of Etawah Pilot Project, the Planning Commission of India suggested a systematic, planned and country wide community development programme in its First Five Year Plan report to address the issues of rural community. One of the initial moving forces for launching the Community Development Programme in India was First Prime Minister, Pt. Jawaharlal Nehru. He felt that the undeveloped human resource of the country could be involved in building new India through community development programme. It was out of this background that India's Community Development Programme (CDP) was born in 2nd October, 1952 with the aim to promote better living of the whole community in rural areas.

Community Development

The term "Community Development" has been frequently used to indicate any efforts towards the advancement of community interests. It is described as a:

- **process** of change from the traditional way of living of rural communities to progressive ways of living.
- **method** of helping local communities to become more aware of their needs, to assess their resources more realistically, to organize themselves and their resources in such a way as to satisfy some of their needs through action projects.
- **programme** for accomplishing certain activities concerning the welfare of the rural people.
- **movement** for progress with certain ideological contents.

Community

A community is a group of people, who live in a continuous geographical area and have interests in each other for the purpose of making a living. It is a part of a larger social system which meet the basic social needs, through the function of which people have developed a sense of belongingness and ability to work together as an entity.

Some of the important characteristics of the community are

1. Communities are close-knit entities
2. Their customs are interrelated
3. These communities are complexes of sub-group relationship and
4. There is a discernible leadership within the community.

Development and Community Development

The term development connotes growth or maturation. It implies gradual and sequential phases of change.

Cambridge Conference in 1948 defined community development as a movement designed to promote better living of the whole community with the active participation of the community members. On the similar line, United Nations define community development as a process designed to create conditions of economic and social progress of the whole community with its active participation and fullest reliance upon the community initiation.

It is a movement designed to promote better living for the whole community with the active participation, and initiative of the community by organising them to work for their wellbeing. Community development is used as a technique by many governments to reach the village people and to make more effective use of local initiative and energy for increased production and better living of the local people.

By understanding the above terms, we can say that community development programmes means a programme for gradual change in a group of people living in a geographical area and have interest in each other for the purpose of making a meaningful living. It is a process by which the efforts of the people themselves are combined with those of governmental authorities to improve the economic, social and cultural conditions of communities, to integrate these communities into the life of the nation, and enable them to contribute fully to national progress.

Community Development Programme (CDP)

One of the initial moving forces for launching the Community Development Programme in India was First Prime Minister, Pt. Jawaharlal Nehru. He felt that the undeveloped human resource of the country could be involved in building new India through community development programme. The central objectives of India's first planned programme of community development were to secure the total development of the material and human resources of rural areas and to develop local leadership and self-governing institutions.

The CDP was launched on 2nd October 1952 on the birth anniversary of Father of Nation, Mahatma Gandhi in 55 community development projects in the country with active cooperation of Ford Foundation, USA.

It was intended to be the first step in a programme of intensive development which was expected to cover the entire country over a period of time. Initially, the CDP was launched in 55 project areas located in different parts of the country. Each project of Community Development Programme consisted of about, 300 villages covering over 400-500 square miles and having a population of around 2 lakhs. The project area was divided into three development blocks, each comprising 100 villages and population around 60 to 70 thousands. In areas where a full project was considered not feasible, one or two developmental blocks were started to begin with. The blocks were further divided into groups of 5 to 10 villages, and a multi-purpose village level worker was given charge of the villages. Intensive development work was taken up in all fields. The rural people showed great interest in the programme and participated for their economic development. Knowing the beneficial effect of the programme on community development, the Members of the State Legislative Assembly and Parliament demanded the expansion of the programme to their areas. Due to political pressure, the country was forced to implement a new programme which was less ambitious and extensive called as National Extension Service (NES) in 1953 to cover the whole country in eight years and the more extensive CDP in twelve years. The NES scheme was designed to provide the essential basic staff and a small amount of funds with which the pople could start the development work essentially on the basis of self-help whereas intensive development work was taken up in all fields under Community Development Programme. The NES blocks were subsequently converted into CDP blocks.

National Extension Service (NES)

Within a few months of the launching of community development programmes, the people of the project areas responded enthusiastically and indeed much beyond the expectations of the Government and the sponsors of the programme. This success put a pressure on the Government to extend the programme to the other parts of the country. But the country's resources were not sufficient to sustain a comprehensive plan of the same magnitude as contemplated in the community development projects. The Government therefore decided to launch alongside the community development programme another programme which was somewhat less intensive in nature, called the National Extension Service programme. The programme was formulated in April 1953 and was inaugurated one year after the CDP that is, on 2nd October, 1953. The CDP and NES had the same idea and two were integrated under one agency at the Centre as well as in the states. Bothe the programmes were complementary and interwoven and ran concurrently. The idea behind the National Extension Service Programme was to cover the entire country within a period of about 10 years. The National Extension Service was a permanent organization and covered the whole country. It provided the basic organization, official, non-official and a minimum financial provision for development. National Extension Service blocks in which successful results had been achieved with the maximum popular co-operation were selected for intensive development for a period of three years.

The National Extension Service and the community development programmes had uniform unit of operation which was called a development block. It represented on an average 100 villages, with a population of 60,000 to 70,000 persons spread over an area of 150 to170 square miles. But the N.E.S. blocks were not developed with the same intensity as areas under the community development blocks. Out of the areas developed as National Extension Service Blocks, selection was made periodically for intensive development work under the community development programme and the block which were selected were called C.D. blocks. Only those blocks were selected for the second plan period for three years which showed good results.

Activities

a) Agriculture and related matters

1. Reclamation of available virgin and waste land
2. Provision of commercial fertilizers and improved seeds
3. Promotion of fruit and vegetable cultivation
4. Promotion of improved agricultural technique and land utilisation
5. Supply of technical information, improved agricultural implements, improved marketing and credit facilities,
6. Provision of soil surveys and prevention of soil erosion
7. Encouragement of the use of natural and compost manures and improvement of livestock,
8. Establishment of key villages for breeding pedigree stock and the provision of veterinary aid, as well as artificial insemination centres.

For attaining this objective, agricultural extension service will be provided at the rate of one agricultural extension worker for every 5 villages.

b) Irrigation

1. Provision of water for agriculture through minor irrigation works, e.g., tanks, canals, surface wells, tubewells, etc., the intention being that at least half of the agricultural land, if possible, be served with irrigation facilities.

c) Communications

1. Development of road system on the country side to link every village within the Project area up to a maximum distance of half a mile from the village.

d) Education

1. Provision for social education, expansion and improvement of primary and secondary education and its gradual conversion to basic type,
2. Provision of educational facilities for working children and promotion of youth welfare.
3. Vocational and technical training for both rural and urban areas
4. Improved techniques to existing artisans and technicians, both in urban and rural areas.
5. Strengthening existing training centres

e) Health

1. Improvement of environmental hygiene, including provision and protection of water supply

2. Proper disposal of human and animal wastes;
3. Control of epidemic diseases such as Malaria, Cholera, Small-pox, Tuberculosis, etc.
4. Provision of medical aid along with appropriate preventive measures, and education of the population in hygienic living and in improved nutrition.

f) Supplementary Employment

1. Development of cottage and small-scale industries,
2. construction of brick kilns and saw mills and encouragement of employment through participation in the tertiary sector of the economy.

g) Housing

1. Demonstration and training in improved techniques and designs for rural housing. In congested villages, action in the direction of development of new sites
2. Opening of village parks and playgrounds and assistance in the supply of building materials.

h) Training

1. Training of village level workers, project supervisors and other personnel for the Community Development Programme
2. Training of artisans
3. Training of extension personnel

i) Social Welfare

1. Provision of audio-visual aids for instruction and recreation
2. Organisation of community entertainment
3. Organisation of sports activities
4. Organisation of melas (village fairs)
5. Organisation of Cooperative and self-help movement
   (Source : Planning Commission, Govt. of India)

The CDP was to be undertaken by the Government of India(GOI) and the various state governments in cooperation with one another.

Central Level

The GOI formed a Central Committee at the National level with the Prime Minister as the Chairperson, the members of the Planning Commission, and the Minister of Food and Agriculture as member to lay down the broad policies and provide the general supervision for the agreed projects. An administrator was appointed to plan, direct and coordinate the programme through India under the general supervision of the Central Committee and in consultation with appropriate authorities in the various states.

State Level

Each state government established a State Development Committee or similar body consisting of the Chief Minister as the Chairperson, Ministers representing the nation Commissioner who act as Secretary to the Committee. He was responsible for directing the programme in the state and coordinates the activities of the heads of the various departments of the state.

District Level

District Development Officer was responsible for the CDP in the district. He was of the status of an Additional Collector and was responsible for the execution of the community project as well as the general development in the district.

Block Level

At the block level, a Block Development Committee (BDC) was established with Sub Divisional Officer acting as its Chairperson and Block Development Officer (BDO) acting as its Executive Secretary. The BDO was responsible for the implementation of the programme within the block. He was assisted by eight or nine Extension Officers(EOs) in the field of agriculture, animal husbandry, rural engineering, public health, cooperation, social education, women's and children's programme and rural industries.

Village level

At the village level, ten Village Level Workers (VLWs) or Gram Sevaks were responsible for the implementation of the programmes within a cluster of the villages, The VLWs worked under the supervision of the BDO.

Evaluation of Community Development Programme

The CDP has been reviewed from time to time by the Programme Evaluation Organisation of the Planning Commission, the National Institute of Rural Development (now National Institute of Rural Development and Panchayati Raj) and by various research institutes and individual research scholars. The number of studies highlighted the tangible results in terms of distribution of seeds, use of chemical fertilizers, plant protection materials, improved farm tools and equipment, construction of roads, wells, irrigational canals, establishment of rural health centres, etc. However, many of the studies also reported that the CDP failed to achieve the expected increase in agriculture production. The failure was due to the financial, material and administrative resources of the CDP were spread too thinly across the country to produce any tangible impact on agriculture production and rural poverty.

Causes of failure

The causes of the failure of the community development programme are as follows:

1. Lack of people participation in the programme
2. Lack of coordination between different institutions
3. Inadequate allocation of resources
4. Uneven distribution of the benefits of the programme
5. Absence of clearly defined priorities in the programme.
6. Failure to evoke popular response.
7. Unqualified and untrained personnel for implementation of the programme
8. Lack of functional responsibility.
9. Ritualism in implementation of the programme: A spirit of ritualism permeated the block programmes and inauguration, opening or foundation stone laying became the be all and end all at all block activities. The project officers were purposely emphasizing the welfare aspect of the programmes so that they could show to the visiting dignitaries some tangible result of thus efforts. But the creation of these welfare activities only kindled the dissatisfaction with the economic condition of the people.

Weaknesses in the Community Development Programme

A Critical analysis of the Programme with regard to the objective shows that the programme has some weaknesses there are discussed as

1. People did not participate in the programme and perceived it as a government programme.
2. here has been too much emphasis on end result and less emphasis in following the correct methods and process to bring about change in the attitudes of the people.
3. Due to lack of understanding of the objectives of the CD programme there has often been lack of adherence to the real objectives of the C.D Programme there has not been much concentration on essential items.

4. Extension education methods which are so essential for a democratic approach remained mostly as a claim.
5. Lack of uniform understanding about the concept principles methods role function etc, at all levels from village to national level.
6. Lack of proper and adequate supervision and guidance both administrative and technical at various levels.
7. Establishment of superiority by providing democratic leadership is very much lacking to replace autocratic authority.
8. The C.D workers feel unhappy at all levels their moral is not very high unhappy workers or change agents can not a make a good organization.

Suggested Readings and References

1. Mathialagan, P. (2007). Textbook of Animal Husbandry and Livestock Extension, International Book Distributing Co. 7, Meerabai Marg, Lucknow, India.
2. Singh, Katar (1999). Rural Development: Principles, Policies and Management, Second Edition, New Delhi, Sage Publications.
3. Dey, S.K. (1964). Community Development: A Bird's Eye View, Asia Publishing House, New Delhi.
4. Dahama, O.P., Bhatanagar, O.P. (1985). Education and Communication for Development, Oxford & IBH Publishing Company, New Delhi.
5. Rural Development - Some Facets, (ed.) NIRD, Hyderabad – 1979.
6. Five Year Plans (1st -10th), Planning Commission, Government of India, New Delhi.
7. Verma, S.C. (1980). Direct Attack on Rural Poverty, Ministry of Rural Development, Delhi,.
8. NIRD, Fifty Years of Rural Development in India (1998). NIRD, Hyderabad.
9. Desai, Vasant (2009). Rural Development in India, Himalaya Publishing House, Mumbai.
10. Mahajan, R.K. (1991). Integrated Rural Development Programme, Concept Publishing Company, New Delhi
11. Mehta, Shiv R. (1984). Rural Development Policies and Programmes, Sage Publications.
12. Arora, R.C. (1979). Integrated Rural Development, New Delhi: S.Chand and Company Limited.
13. Lawania, Vinod Kumar (1992). Rural Development in India. New Delhi: Ashish Publishing.

14. Ray, G.L. (2001). Extension, Communication and Management, 4th Edition, Naya Prokash, Calcutta.

15. B.S.Mathur (1977). Cooperation in India, Sahitya Bhavan, Agra.

16. Ensminger, Douglas (1957). A guide to Community Development, Ministry of Community Development, Government of India, Coronation Printing Works, Fatehpuri, Delhi-6.

17. Ministry of Agriculture, Government of India (2009). Report of the High Powered Committee on Cooperative.

18. Ray, G.L. (2006). Extension Communication and Management, New Delhi, Kalyani Publishers.

19. Sharma, K.R.G. (2008). Veterinary Extension Education, BSPBS Publications, Hyderabad, Hyderabad.

20. Supe S.V. (1987). An Introduction to Extension Education, Oxford and IBH Publishing Co. Pvt. Ltd. New Delhi.

15

Panchayati Raj System

1. Evolution of Panchayati Raj System in India
2. Panchayati Raj under the 73rd Constitutional Amendment
3. Subjects within the jurisdiction of PRIs
4. Gram Sabha
5. Gram Panchayat
   a) Functions of Gram Panchayat
   b) Sources of funds
6. Panchayat Samiti
   a) Functions of Panchayat Samiti
   b) Committees under Panchayat Samiti
7. Zilla Parishad
   a) Powers and Functions of the Zilla Parishad
8. The Provisions of the Panchayats (Extension to The Scheduled Areas) Act, 1996
9. Suggested Readings and References

Evolution of Panchayati Raj System in India

In January 1957, the Government of India appointed a committee under the chairmanship of Balwantray Mehta to examine the working of the Community Development Programme (1952) and the National Extension Service (1953), and to suggest measures for their better implementation. The committee expressed concern about the lack of participation of people in these programmes and made a string plea for devolution of power. The committee submitted its report in November 1957 and recommended the establishment of the scheme of 'democratic decentralization' through a three-tier system of local government from village to district Level-Gram Panchayat at village level, Panchayat Samiti at block level and Zilla Parisad at district level -which ultimately came to be known as Panchayati Raj in India. The recommendations of the committee were accepted by the National Development Council (NDC) in January 1958. The NDC did not insist on a single rigid pattern of panchayat raj system throughout the country but left it to the states to evolve their own patterns suitable to local conditions. But the basic principles and broad fundamentals of democratic decentralization remained identical throughout the country. Thus, the Panchayati Raj system came into existence in 1959 with two basic objectives. These were (1) democratic decentralization and (2) local participation in planned programmes. The new system of Panchayat Raj Institutions was first adopted in Rajasthan and Andhra Pradesh in 1959, followed by Assam, Tamil Nadu and Karnataka in 1960, Maharashtra in 1962, and Gujarat and West Bengal in 1963 and 1964 respectively. By the mid-sixties, the hype to strengthen the Panchayati Raj Institutions (PRIs) gave way to a growing tendency of centralization and the PRIs descended to ground zero. To revive the working of PRIs, the Janata Government in 1977 appointed a committee headed by Ashok Mehta to study the functioning of PRIs and to suggest measures for improvement. The committee suggested a minor change in the Balwantray Mehta Scheme. Mehta (1978), in the Report of the Committee of Panchayati Raj Institutions (PRIs) identified three phases of Panchayati Raj in India –

1. The phase of ascendancy (1959-64);
2. The phase of stagnation (1965-69); and
3. The phase of decline (1969-77).

The Committee found that stagnation and decline in the Panchayati Raj system during the period were mainly due to:

i. Keeping most of the rural development programmes and activities outside the purview of the PRIs
ii. Making resource base of PRIs weak by reducing the allocation of funds

iii. Lack of adjustment of the bureaucratic administration with the Panchayati Raj system

iv. Frequent postponement of elections and supersession of PRIs' authority

v. Lack of conceptual clarity about Panchayati Raj and its objectives

vi. Lack of political will, as evident in the absence of appropriate laws or if present, in them enforcement;

The Committee observed that the PRIs were dominated by economically or socially privileged sections of society, yielding no benefits to the weaker sections. The performance of PRIs had been vitiated by political factionalism, rendering developmental activities either twisted or diluted. Corruption, inefficiency, scant regard for procedures, political interference in day-to-day administration, parochial loyalties, motivated actions, power concentration, etc, had seriously limited the autonomy and functioning of panchayati raj system in the Indian villages.

The Committee recommended that three tier system of PRIs was to be replaced by a two tier i.e. Zilla Parishad at the district level and Mandal Panchayat (consisting of a number of villages) below it. However, owing to the disintegration of the Janata Government in 1980, the recommendations of the Asoka Mehta Committee could not be implemented. In 1985, another committee under the chairmanship of G.V.K. Rao suggested for appropriate improvement in the representative character and strengthening of the capability of the people's representatives and administrative personnel of PRIs. The major recommendations of the G.V.K.Rao committee were : (i) Zilla Parishads (at district level) should be strengthened, (ii) There should be sub-committees at the district level with proportional representation, (iv) Some planning functions may be transferred to the district level, and(v) Elections of local bodies should be held regularly.

In 1986, the L.M. Singhvi Committee of the Department of Rural Development, Government of India, recommended constitutional status for Panchayati Raj. Some of its major recommendations are of Singhavi committee were : (i)Local self-government should be constitutionally recognized, (ii)· Elections at the panchayat level should be held regularly and without delay, (iii) Panchayati Raj judicial tribunal should be set up in every state to deal with matters related to the working of Panchayati Raj, (iv) There should be adequate financial resources to ensure effective functioning of panchayats , (v)Participation of individuals attached to political parties should be discouraged, and (vi) The Nyaya Panchayat should be given the functions of mediation and settling of issues. In the meantime, the Sarkaria Commission (1988), which was primarily concerned with the *centre-state relationship,* also recommended the strengthening of local bodies financially and functionally. The commission also believed that elections for panchayats must be held regularly. By the end of 1988, a sub-committee of the Consultative Committee of Parliament **Rural Credit and Banking** under the chairmanship of *P.K. Thungon* made recommendations for strengthening the Panchayati Raj system once again. One of its important recommendations was that Panchayati Raj bodies should be constitutionally recognized. Similarly, the Congress Committee headed by *V.N. Gadgil in 1989* recommended a three-tier system of Panchayati Raj with a fixed term of 5 years for the elected members and reservation for Scheduled Castes/Tribes and women.

The recommendations of these various committees and commissions generated a strong realization that there was a need to create a strong panchayat raj system in the country for devolution of power to community. In July-August 1989, the then Congress government introduced the 64th Constitutional Amendment Bill with a view to streamline the Panchayati Raj. However, the bill was defeated in the Rajya Sabha. V.P. Singh government also tried to push a bill in 1990 on Panchayati Raj, it lapsed with the dissolution of the Lok Sabha.

Panchayati Raj Under the 73rd Constitutional Amendment Act, 1992

Sri Rajiv Gandhi as Prime Minister of India revitalized the Panchayat Raj, paving way for realizing Mahatma Gandhi's Gram Swaraj by giving power back to the people. In September 1991, the 72nd Amendment of the Constitution was introduced by the Congress Government. This was referred to a Joint Select Committee of the Parliament in December 1991 for detailed examination. Finally, after including necessary changes, the Amendment was passed with near unanimity in the Lok Sabha on December 22, 1992 and in the Rajya Sabha on December 23, 1992. Finally, on April 20, 1993 the President of India gave it his assent. This Amendment of the Constitution is known as the **Constitution (Seventy-Third Amendment) Act, 1992.** This Act was brought in to force by a notification with effect from April 24, 1993.

The Amendment Act of 1992 also contains provision for devolution of powers and responsibilities to the panchayats to both for preparation of plans for economic development and social justice and for implementation of twenty-nine subjects listed in the Eleventh Schedule of the constitution. By virtue of this Act, no one will be able to take away the powers, responsibilities and finances given to the Panchayats. They are expected to play a much bigger role in the development of their respective areas and people. It is also expected that everyone will be able to take part in this process including the poorest of the poor.

The main features of the 73rd Constitutional Amendment Act are:

i) Constitution of panchayats at village, intermediate (block) and district level; however, panchayats at the intermediate level may not be constituted in a State having a population not exceeding twenty lakhs;

ii) Regular elections to Panchayats at every five years;

iii) Reservation of seats for Scheduled Castes / Scheduled Tribes in proportion to their population. One third of the reserved of SC/ST is reserved for women candidate and overall reservation of seat should not be less than 33% for women;

iv) Setting up of an independent State Finance Commission for strengthening finances of local bodies at all levels to take up developmental activities.

v) Constitution of an independent State Election Commission to hold PRIs elections on a regular basis;

vi) Legal status to Gram Sabhas; and

viii) Addition of Eleventh Schedule to the Constitution listing 29 Subjects within the jurisdiction of PRIs.

Further, the 73rd Constitutional Amendment Act contains provisions for devolution of powers and responsibilities upon panchayats at the appropriate level with reference to (a) the preparation of plans for economic development and social justice; and (b) the implementation of such schemes for economic development and social justice, as may be entrusted to them. The Provision of the Panchayat (Extension to Scheduled Areas) Act 1996 (PESA) extends panchayats to tribal areas in nine States. It enables the tribal society to shape their own development and preserve & conserve their traditional rights over natural resources.

Subjects within the Jurisdiction of PRIS

(Eleventh Schedule, Article 243G)

1. Agriculture, including agricultural extension.
2. Land improvement, implementation of land reforms, land consolidation and soil conservation.
3. Minor irrigation, water management and watershed development.
4. Animal husbandry, dairying and poultry.
5. Fisheries.
6. Social forestry and farm forestry.
7. Minor forest produce.

8. Small scale industries, including food processing industries.
9. Khadi, village and cottage industries.
10. Rural housing.
11. Drinking water.
12. Fuel and fodder.
13. Roads, culverts, bridges, ferries, waterways and other means of communication.
14. Rural electrification, including distribution of electricity.
15. Non-conventional energy sources.
16. Poverty alleviation programme.
17. Education, including primary and secondary schools.
18. Technical training and vocational education.
19. Adult and non-formal education.
20. Libraries.
21. Cultural activities.
22. Markets and fairs.
23. Health and sanitation, including hospitals, primary health centres and dispensaries.
24. Family welfare.
25. Women and child development.
26. Social welfare, including welfare of the handicapped and mentally retarded.
27. Welfare of the weaker sections, and in particular, of the Scheduled Castes and the Scheduled Tribes.
28. Public distribution system.
29. Maintenance of community assets.

The 73rd Amendment Act vests power in the State Government to endow Panchayats with such powers and authority as may be necessary to enable them to function as institutions of self-government such as:

1. Preparation of plans and their execution for economic development and social justice in relation to 29 subjects listed in the XI schedule of the Constitution.
2. Authority to Panchayats to levy, collect and appropriate taxes, duties, tolls and fees.
3. Transfer of taxes, duties, tolls and fees collected by the States to Panchayats.

The panchayats receive funds from:

1. Local body grants, as recommended by the Central Finance Commission
2. Funds for implementation of centrally sponsored schemes
3. Funds released by the State Government in the recommendation of the State Finance Commission.

Gram Sabha

Gram Sabha is a body consisting of persons registered in the electoral rolls of a village or a group of villages which elect a Panchayat. A vibrant and enlightened Gram Sabha is central to the success of the Panchayati Raj system.

State Governments have been urged :

To vest in the Gram Sabha, powers on the lines envisaged in the Provisions of the Panchayats (Extension to the Scheduled Areas) Act, 1996.

To make a mandatory provision in the Panchayati Raj Act for holding Gram Sabha meetings throughout the country on the occasion of the Republic Day, Labour Day, Independence Day and Gandhi Jayanti.

To make a mandatory provision in the Panchayati Raj Act specifying separately, the quorum for Gram Sabha meetings, for ordinary meetings, meetings convened for special purposes and re-convened meetings due to cancellation of earlier meeting for want of quorum.

To make members of the Gram Sabhas aware of their powers and responsibilities with a view to ensuring mass participation, particularly of the hitherto marginalised, groups, such as women and SCs/STs.

To lay down procedures for the Gram Sabha to effectively carry out social audit of beneficiary oriented development programmes of the Ministry of Rural Development, particularly the legal powers of the Gram Sabha to order recovery or punishment for financial mismanagement.

To evolve a plan of action for generating wide publicity for Gram Sabha meetings.

To evolve guidelines/procedures for holding Gram Sabha meetings and a model list of business for such meetings.

To generate awareness as to the rights of the Gram Sabha with respect to control over natural resources, land records and conflict resolution.

The 73rd Amendment Act envisages empowered Panchayats as institutions of self-government at the village level capable of:

Planning and executing village level public works and their maintenance.

Ensuring welfare of the people at the village level including health, education, communal harmony, social justice particularly with regard to gender and caste based discrimination, dispute resolution, welfare of children, especially the girl child.

The 73rd Amendment Act also envisages empowered Gram Sabhas as the Parliament of the People at the grassroots level to whom the Gram Panchayats are solely accountable.

Gram Panchayat

Gram Panchayat is the lowest tier of Panchayat Raj System and the basic institute constituted at the village level for local administration. Every village Panchayat is divided into wards or smaller areas and the number persons to be elected from each area has been determined as per the Election Commission of the State. Each ward elects a representative who is known as the ward member. All the members of the Gram Sabha also elect a sarpanch who is the Panchayat president. The Ward Panchs / members and the Sarpanch form the Gram Panchayat. Among the elected members a vice-chairman is indirectly elected for Gram Panchayat. The Gram Panchayat is elected for five years. There is reservation of seats for women and SC/ST candidates in the Gram panchayat.

The Gram Panchayat has a secretary who is appointed by the state government and responsible for calling the meeting of the Gram Sabha and Gram Panchayat and keeping a record of the proceedings.

The Gram Sabha is the key factor in making the Gram Panchayat play its role and be responsible. It is the place where all plans for the work of the Gram Panchayat are placed before the people. The Gram Sabha prevents the Panchayat from doing wrong things like misusing money or favouring certain people. It plays an important role in keeping an eye on the elected representatives and in making them responsible to the persons who elected them. Gram Panchayat should conduct at least three meetings in a year and quorum for meeting is one third of the total members of panchayat.

Functions of Gram Panchayat

i) Construction and maintenance of roads, drainage, school buildings, water bodies, market places and other common property resources.

ii) Land development and soil conservation

iii) Making provision of drinking water to the village

iv) Registration of death and birth

v) Adoption of preventive measures for control of epidemics in human and animal

vi) Maintenance of pasture land, burial, cremation grounds, etc.

vii) Helping weaker sections of the village like SC/ST, widow, destitute, old person, etc.

viii) Levying and collecting local taxes.

ix) Executing government schemes related to generating employment in the village.

Sources of funds

1. Collection of taxes on houses, market places, ponds etc.
2. Government schemes funds received through various departments
3. Donations for community works.
4. Loans
5. Grants-in-aid from State Government

Panchayt Samiti

Panchayt Samiti is the middle tier of panchayat raj system at block level which is above the gram panchayat and below the Zilla Parishad. The president/ Sabhapati/ Pradhan and Vice-President/ Up-Pradhan of Panchayat Samiti are indirectly elected by the elected samiti members. The chairpersons i.e. sarpanch of all panchayats, members of Rajya Sabha, Lok Shabha, MLA and MLC are Ex-officio members of the Panchayat Samiti. The Block Development Officer (BDO) works as a Chief Executive Officer of the panchayat Samiti. He is entrusted with the responsibility for implementing the resolutions of the Samiti and its Standing Committees. He prepares the budget of the Samiti and places it before the Samiti for approval. Preparing the annual report of the Samiti and sending it to the Zilla Parishad and State Government also comes within the purview of his responsibility. He is accountable to the President of the Samiti for his actions.

Functions of Panchayat Samiti

1. Implementation of all developmental programmes and activities concerning the welfare and development of the rural people in the field of agriculture, animal husbandry, education, drinking water, cottage industries, etc.
2. Construction, repair and maintenance of panchayat samiti roads, elementary schools, markets, etc.
3. Preventive and remedial measures against epidemics and control of dreadful diseases causing loss to human life and animal.
4. Relief and rehabilitation activities during and after natural disaster.
5. Exercise all powers conferred on as per the Act, and performs all other responsibilities entrusted to them by the Government.

Committees under Panchayat Samiti

1. Planning and Production Committee
2. Appointment Committee
3. Co-operation and Industries Committee
4. Education Committee
5. Women Welfare Committee
6. Social Welfare Committee
7. Communication Committee
8. Taxation and Finance Committee, etc.

Each Committee consists of few samiti members including samiti president. The samiti president is the chairman of all the committees. These committees provide guidance and direction for panning, implementation and evaluation of various programmes and activities related to the mandates of the committee.

Zilla Parishad

The District Council or Zilla Parishad or District Panchayat is the topmost tier of the panchayat raj system at the district level. Zilla Parishad is an elected body. Members of Zilla Parishad are elected directly by the electorate of the district for five years.

Besides Zilla Parishad members, panchayat Samiti presidents, all the members of state legislature and members of parliament representing a part or whole of the district are also member of the Zilla Parishad. All members elect chairman and vice chairman of the Zilla Parishad. Seats are reserved in Zilla Parishad for schedule cast, schedule tribe, women and backward class. Chief Executive Officer appointed by the State Government heads the administration in the district.

Powers and Functions of the Zilla Parishad

1. Zilla Parishad functions as advisory body over the Panchayat Samiti with powers to a) approve their budgets b) co-ordinate their plans and c) distribute funds given by the Government among the blocks.
2. It prepares plans for developmental activities in the district
3. Monitor, review and evaluate the implementation of various developmental programmes in the district.
4. The Parishad performs such of the powers and functions of the District Board as are transferred to it by the Government.
5. It advises the Government in all matters relating to rural development in the district.

To improve the quality of living of rural people, Government of India launched various programmes after independence. The important post-independence programmes launched by Government of India in different Five Years Plans are presented below.

The Provisions of the Panchayats (Extension to the Scheduled Areas) Act, 1996

The Provisions of the Panchayats (Extension to the Scheduled Areas) Act, 1996 (PESA Act) came into force on December 24, 1996. This Act extends panchayats to the tribal areas of the states such as Andhra Pradesh, Bihar, Jharkhand, Gujarat, Himachal Pradesh, Maharashtra, Madhya Pradesh, Chhattisgarh, Orissa and Rajasthan. It intends to enable tribal societies to assume control over their destiny and to preserve and conserve their traditional rights over natural resources. The State Governments were required to enact their legislations in accordance with the provisions of the Act within one year, i.e. by December 23, 1997. Most of the states enacted the required state legislation to give effect to the provisions contained in Act 14, 1996.

The salient features of the Act are

1. Every village shall have an elected Gram Sabha and it shall be competent to safeguard and preserve the traditions and customs of the people.
2. Gram Sabha shall approve the plans, programmes and projects for social and economic development before their implementation.
3. It would be responsible for the identification or selection of persons as beneficiaries under the poverty alleviation and other programmes.
4. Every Gram Panchayat shall obtain from the related Gram Sabha a certificate of utilization of funds for the plans, programmes and projects.
5. The reservation of seats in the Scheduled Areas in every panchayat shall be in the proportion of the populations of the communities in the panchayat.
6. Planning and management of minor water bodies in the Scheduled Areas shall be entrusted to panchayats at the appropriate level.
7. Recommendations of the Gram Sabha or the panchayats shall be mandatory for granting i) licenses for mining minerals, and ii) concessions for the exploitation of minor minerals by auction in the Scheduled Areas.
8. The state legislature shall endow panchayats and the Gram Sabha specifically with:

i) the power to enforce prohibition or regulate or restrict the sale and consumption of any intoxicant;
ii) the ownership of minor forest produce;
iii) the power to prevent land alienation in the Scheduled Areas;
iv) the power to manage village markets;
v) the power to control money lending to Scheduled Tribes and social sectors;
vi) the power to control local plans and resources for such plans, including tribal sub-plans; and
vii) the state legislations that may endow panchayats with powers and authority, as may be necessary to enable them to function as institutions of self-government, and contain safeguards to ensure that panchayats at the higher level do not assume the powers and authorit.

Suggested Readings and References

1. Government of India (1994). Renewing Local Self-government in Rural India, Ministry of Rural Development, Government of India, New Delhi.
2. National Institute of Rural Development (1995). Panchayati Raj and Rural Development, National Institute of Rural Development, Hyderabad.
3. National Institute of Rural Development (1995). Panchayati Raj Institutions in Select States: An Analytical Study, National Institute of Rural Development, Hyderabad.
4. Verma, S.C. (1980). Direct Attack on Rural Poverty, Ministry of Rural Development, Delhi.
5. Desai, Vasant (2009). Rural Development in India, Himalaya Publishing House, Mumbai.
6. Mahajan, R.K. (1991). Integrated Rural Development Programme, Concept Publishing Company, New Delhi.
7. Mehta, Shiv R. (1984). Rural Development Policies and Programmes, Sage Publications.
8. Singh Katar (1986). Rural Development-Principles, Policies and Management, Sage Publications (India) Pvt. Ltd. New Delhi.
9. Annamalai, V. (2000). Role of Gram Panchayat in managing common property resources for the benefit of the rural poor: a study in Karnataka and Haryana, NIRD, Hyderabad.

16

Important Rural Development Programmes

1. Intensive Agriculture District Programme (IADP)
2. Intensive Agricultural Area Programme (IAAP)
3. High Yielding Varieties Programme (HYVP)
4. Green Revolution
   a) History and Development of the Green Revolution
   b) Role of Dr. Swaminathan
   c) What is the Green Revolution?
   d) Elements of Green Revolution
   e) Components of Green Revolution
   f) Results of the Green Revolution
   g) Problems with Green Revolution
5. Training and Visit System (T&V System)
   a) Salient features of T & V System
   b) Organizational Pattern of the T & V System of Agriculture Extension
   c) Strengths of T & V System
   d) Merits of T & V System
   e) Constraints of T & V System
6. Small Farmers Development Agency (SFDA)
7. Marginal Farmers and Agricultural Labourers (MFAL) Scheme
8. Drought Prone Area Programme (DPAP)
9. Tribal Area Development Programme / Integrated Tribal Development Agency (ITDA)

10. Hill Area Development Programme (HADP)
11. Desert Development programme (DDP)
12. National Rural Employment Programme (NREP)
13. Integrated Rural Development Programme (IRDP)
    a) Approaches of IRDP
    b) Salient features of the Programme
    c) Criteria for Allocation of Funds to the States
    d) Implementing Agency
14. Training of Rural Youth for Self Employment (TRYSEM)
15. Development of women and children in Rural Areas (DWCRA)
16. Agricultural Human Resource Development Programme (AHRDP)
    a) Salient features of AHRDP:
17. Important Rural Development Programmes and Schemes launched under different Five Year Plans
18. Suggested Readings and References

There are four major organizational system involved in the country for implementation of rural development and agriculture programmes in the county, and they are:

1. Ministry of Rural Development of Government of India and State Rural Development Departments
2. Ministry of Agriculture of Government of India and State Agriculture Departments
3. Indian Council of Agriculture Research (ICAR) and State Agriculture Universities (SAUs)
4. Private bodies like voluntary Organizations, Corporate houses, International agencies etc.

Various rural and agriculture development programmes have been launched and implemented in different five year plans for the socio-economic development of the rural poor. Some of the important programmes relevant to agriculture and animal husbandry are discussed in brief.

Intensive Agriculture District Programme (IADP)

The Intensive Agriculture District Programme, popularly known as "Package Programme" which employed the concentration of resources principles, was launched in 1960 to meet the food grain requirement of 110 million tones.

The programme was launched in three districts in 1960 - 61 and four districts in 1962 - 63. The seven districts were:

1. Thanjavur (Tamil Nadu)
2. West Godavari (Andhra Pradesh)
3. Shahabad (Bihar)
4. Raipur (Madhya Pradesh)
5. Aligarh (Uttar Pradesh)
6. Ludhiana (Punjab)
7. Pali (Rajasthan)

   In the second phase the programme was extended to nine more districts by 1963 64.

8. Allepy (Kerala)
9. Palghat (Kerala)
10. Mandya (Karnataka)
11. Surat (Gujarat)
12. Sambalpur (Orissa)

13. Burdwan (West Bengal)
14. Cachar (Assam)
15. Bhandara (Maharashtra)
16. Six blocks (Jammu and Kashmir)

The immediate objective of the programme was to achieve rapid increase in food grain production to meet the food grain requirement of the country. The programme was implemented in the district having potential irrigation facilities with less prone to natural hazards. Integrated and intensive approaches were adopted to solve the problems of agriculture production in the areas which were more responsive to such production effort. The programme sought to achieve rapid increase in the level of agricultural production through a concentration of financial technical, extension and administrative resources. In the long run it aimed at a self - generating break through in productivity and raising the production potential by stimulating the human and physical process of change.

IADP was a demonstrational programme which showed how to increase production more rapidly on one hand and a path finding experimental programme which facilitated the development of new innovations, new ideas and procedures for wider adoption in agriculture development.

One of the major drawbacks of IADP was its neglect of the equity aspect of the development. Even though this drawback, the spectacular results in improved production yield obtained in IADP, prompted Government to extending the benefit of the programme to other districts of the country with less cost and reduced staff strength. This resulted in launching of the Intensive Agriculture Area Programme (IAAP) in 1964.

Intensive Agricultural Area Programme (IAAP) (1964)

The favourable experiences with IADP had led to the consideration of the possibilities of extending the concept of IADP to other promising districts in India. The Agricultural Production Board (1964) agreed with the observations of mid-term appraisal of third five-year plan and recommended Intensive Agricultural Area Programme (IAAP) for 20 to 25 per cent of the cultivated area of the country. Thus, IAAP was started in 114 districts in March 1964 and later it was extended to 150 districts (Adivireddy, 1997).

Criteria for selection of districts: These criteria included the following. The IAAP was taken up in areas having assured irrigation. Selection of districts and blocks was made on the basis of predominant crops (entire crop economy of the area was kept in view). Area was selected based on the use of various intensive and coordinated aids for production (infrastructure facilities).

The staffing pattern of the IAAP districts was less intensive than in the IADP districts. However, the mode of operation was similar. In general, the Village Level Workers (VLWs) were increased from 10 per block to 15 or 20 per block, from one to two Agricultural Extension Officers (AEOs) and districts staff from 2 to 3 Subject-Matter Specialists.

Achievements of IAAP

Achieved the increased production by exploiting the land resources. Package approach was covered in 1410 community blocks spread over 114 districts in India. Increased production in 20-25 per cent of the cultivated area was achieved. Effective coordination between officials and non-officials was achieved. Multiplication of improved seed and its distribution to all cultivable land. Minor irrigation was undertaken in the villages, both through community participation and on an individual basis.

High Yielding Varieties Programme (HYVP)

The IADP and IAAP were concerned with the promotion of intensive agriculture with existing crop varieties which have low fertilizer response. In the year 1963 – 64, a few Mexican dwarf wheat varieties were tried out on selected basis and in 1964 - 65 an exotic variety of paddy, namely, Taichung native - 1 was tried and the results were found quite. The traditional varieties experienced a moderate increase in yields as a result of the package of practices emphasized by IADP and IAAP, but it also highlighted the inadequacy of the traditional varieties for optimum production even if provision of essential inputs. The real breakthrough in increasing crop yield came with the introduction of the HYVP in 1966 which helped the country in attending self sufficiency in food. The introduction of high yielding crop varieties and the increased use of chemical fertiliser and irrigation in the potential areas of production resulted 'Green Revolution" in India. High-yielding wheat was first introduced to India in 1968 by American agronomist Norman Borlaug who has been hailed as the Father of the Green Revolution but in India, M.S. Swaminathan is known as the "Father of the Green Revolution in India". M.S. Swaminathan and his team contributed significantly in mobilising the farmers in adoption of improved varieties of crop seeds leading to green revolution in India.

The influence of high yielding technology spread to other areas of farm production such as animal production, fishery, horticulture, sericulture etc. The high yielding technologies in these production enterprises also have some common characteristics such as shorter gestation period, improved management practices and higher investment in comparison to traditional technologies.

Green Revolution

History and Development of the Green Revolution

The history of Green Revolution is traced back to the 1940s when Daniels, the U S Ambassador to Mexico and Henry Wallace, Vice President of the USA set up a scientific mission to help the development of agricultural technology in Mexico. The Mexican government and the Rockefeller Foundation started a joint venture to introduce plant breeding programme in Mexico by introducing High Yielding Varieties (HYVs) or the 'miracle seeds' of dwarf varieties of high-yielding wheat to increase production. The success of the Green Revolution is often attributed to Norman Borlaug, the Norway-born, U.S-based agricultural scientist interested in agriculture. In the 1940s, he began conducting research in Mexico and developed new disease resistance 'miracle seeds' of dwarf varieties of high-yielding wheat. By combining Borlaug's wheat varieties with new mechanized agricultural technologies, Mexico was able to produce more wheat than was needed by its own citizens, leading to its becoming an exporter of wheat by the 1960s. Mexico was importing half of its wheat supply prior to use of this verieties. Due to the success of the Green Revolution in Mexico, its technologies spread worldwide in the 1950s and 1960s. In connection with the 'miracle seed' programme, two international agricultural research stations International Maize and Wheat Improvement Centre (CIMMYT) and the International Rice Research Institute (IRRI) were set up. These centres grew out of the Rockefeller Foundation's country programme to launch the new seeds, known as the New Agricultural strategy, by the mid-1960s. By 1966, IRRI started producing 'miracle' rice, in succession to the 'miracle' wheat from CIMMYT. The Green Revolution was given support in Mexico, Philippines and India from the 1940s through to the1960s by the Rockefeller, the Ford Foundation and the U S Government. The Rockefeller Foundation and the Ford Foundation, as well as many government agencies around the world funded research to increase food grain production to produce more food for the growing human population. In 1963 with the help of this funding, Mexico formed an international research institution called The International Maize and Wheat Improvement Center. Countries all over the world in turn benefited from the Green Revolution work conducted by Borlaug and this research institution. Borlaug and the Ford Foundation implemented in India a new variety of rice, IR8, that produced more The history of Green Revolution is traced back to the 1940s when Daniels, the U S Ambassador to Mexico and Henry Wallace, Vice President of the USA set up a scientific mission to help the development of agricultural technology in Mexico. The Mexican government and the Rockefeller Foundation started a joint venture to introduce plant breeding programme in Mexico by introducing High Yielding Varieties (HYVs) or the 'miracle seeds' of dwarf varieties of high-yielding wheat to increase production. The success of the Green Revolution is often attributed to Norman Borlaug, the Norway-born, U.S-based agricultural scientist interested in agriculture. In the 1940s, he began conducting research in Mexico and developed new disease resistance 'miracle seeds' of dwarf varieties of high-yielding wheat. By combining Borlaug's wheat varieties with new mechanized agricultural technologies, Mexico was able to produce more wheat than was needed by its own citizens, leading to its becoming an exporter of wheat by the 1960s. Mexico was importing half of its wheat supply prior to use of this verieties. Due to the success of the Green Revolution in Mexico, its technologies spread worldwide in the 1950s and 1960s. In connection with the 'miracle seed' programme, two international agricultural research stations International Maize and Wheat Improvement Centre (CIMMYT) and the International Rice Research Institute (IRRI) were set up. These centres grew out of the Rockefeller Foundation's country programme to launch the new seeds, known as the New Agricultural strategy, by the mid-1960s. By 1966, IRRI started producing 'miracle' rice, in succession to the 'miracle' wheat from CIMMYT. The Green Revolution was given support in Mexico, Philippines and India from the 1940s through to the1960s by the Rockefeller, the Ford Foundation and the U S Government. The Rockefeller Foundation and the Ford Foundation, as well as many government agencies around the world funded research to increase food grain production to produce more food for the growing human population. In 1963 with the help of this funding, Mexico formed an international research institution called The International Maize and Wheat Improvement Center. Countries all over the world in turn benefited from the Green Revolution work conducted by Borlaug and this research institution. Borlaug and the Ford Foundation implemented in India a new variety of rice, IR8, that produced more grain per plant when grown with irrigation and fertilizers. Today, India is one of the world's leading rice producers and IR8 rice usage spread throughout Asia in the decades following the rice's development in India.

Role of Dr. Swaminathan

Dr. M. S. Swaminathan was the adviser of the Minister of Agriculture and he invited Dr. Borlaug to India. Swaminathan is known for having lobbied with then Prime Minister Lal Bahadur Shastri to import 18000 tons of Mexican seed. He established National Bureau of Plant, Animal and Fish Genetic Resources of India and International Plant Genetic Resources Institute. Swaminathan is known as "Indian Father of Green Revolution" for his leadership and success in introducing and further developing high-yielding varieties of wheat in India.

What is the Green Revolution?

The dramatic transformation in agriculture practices that involves the use of new methods of cultivation and inputs refers to as Green Revolution. It was a period when the productivity of global agriculture increased drastically as a result of new advances. During this time period, agriculture technological advances in the field of seed, fertiliser, pesticides, etc. were used efficiently by the farming community to increase the production. In India, the green revolution occurs as a result of adoption of new agriculture strategy during mid 60's by Government of India to achieve self-sufficiency in the food grains production.

Elements of Green Revolution

Main elements of the Green Revolution:

1. Expansion of farming areas
2. Double-cropping
3. Use of improved seeds

a) Expansion of farming areas

As mentioned above, the area of land under cultivation was being increased right from 1947. But this was not enough in meeting with rising demand. Other methods were required. Yet, the expansion of cultivable land also had to continue. So, the Green Revolution continued with this quantitative expansion of farmlands. However, this was not the most striking feature of the Revolution.

b) Double-cropping

Increased irrigation facilities supported the farmers to go for double cropping which resulted more production from the same piece of land. Dams were built to arrest large volumes of natural monsoon water which were earlier being wasted. Simple irrigation techniques were also adopted.

c) Using seeds with superior genetics

This was the scientific aspect of the Green Revolution. The Indian Council for Agricultural Research developed new strains of high yield value (HYV) seeds, mainly wheat and rice but also millet and corn which were used to produce more. The most noteworthy HYV seed was the K68 variety for wheat. The credit for developing this strain goes to Dr. M.P. Singh who is also regarded as the hero of India's Green revolution.

Components of Green Revolution

The core components of new agriculture strategy are

i) **Use of High-Yielding Variety(HYV) seeds** that matures in short span of time.

ii) **Application of fertilizers, manures and chemicals** in the agriculture production.

iii) **Multiple Cropping Patterns** that allows farmers to grow two or more crops on the same land.

iv) **Mechanization of farming** with the use of machines like tractors, harvesters pump sets etc. in the agriculture occur in a big way.

v) **Creation of Infrastructure facilities** to provide better transportation, irrigation, warehousing, marketing facilities, rural electrification

vi) **Price Incentives** involving provision of the minimum support prices for various crops so as to allow reasonable price to farmers for their produce.

vi) **Better financial assistance** through spread of credit facilities with the development of wide network of commercial banks, cooperative banks and establishment of National Bank for Agriculture and Rural Development (NABARD) as an apex bank to coordinate the rural finance in India.

Results of the Green Revolution

Statistical Results of the Green Revolution

a) The Green Revolution resulted in a record grain output of 131 million tons in 1978-79. This established India as one of the world's biggest agricultural producers. No other country in the world which attempted the Green Revolution recorded such level of success. India also became an exporter of food grains around that time.

b) Yield per unit of farmland improved by more than 30 per cent between 1947 (when India gained political independence) and 1979 when the Green Revolution was considered to have delivered its goods

c) The crop area under HYV varieties grew from seven per cent to 22 per cent of the total cultivated area during the 10 years of the Green Revolution. More than 70 per cent of the wheat crop area, 35 per cent of the rice crop area and 20 per cent of the millet and corn crop area, used the HYV seeds.

Economic results of the Green Revolution

a) Crop areas under high-yield varieties needed more water, more fertilizer, more pesticides, fungicides and certain other chemicals. This spurred the growth of the local manufacturing sector. Such industrial growth created new jobs and contributed to the country's GDP,

b) The increase in irrigation created need for new dams to harness monsoon water. The water stored was used to create hydro-electric power. This in turn boosted industrial growth, created jobs and improved the quality of life of the people in villages

c) India paid back all loans it had taken from the World Bank and its affiliates for the purpose of the Green Revolution. This improved India's creditworthiness in the eyes of the lending agencies.

d) Some developed countries, especially Canada, which were facing a shortage in agricultural labour, were so impressed by the results of India's Green Revolution that they asked the Indian government to supply them with farmers experienced in the methods of the Green Revolution. Many farmers from Punjab and Haryana states in northern India were thus sent to Canada where they settled (That's why Canada today has many Punjabi-speaking citizens of Indian origin). These people remitted part of their incomes to their relatives in India. This not only helped the relatives but also added, albeit modestly, to India's foreign exchange earnings.

Sociological results of the Green Revolution

The Green Revolution created plenty of jobs not only for agricultural workers but also industrial workers by the creation of lateral facilities such as factories and hydro-electric power stations as explained above.

Political results of the Green Revolution

a) India transformed itself from a starving nation to an exporter of food. This earned admiration for India in the comity of nations, especially in the Third World.

b) The Green Revolution was one factor that made Mrs. Indira Gandhi (1917-84) and her party, the Indian National Congress, a very powerful political force in India.

Problems with Green Revolution

The new agriculture strategy has resulted into increased productivity and returns for farmers. This has resulted in decline in rural poverty to an extent. However, the revolution resulted into increased income, wide interpersonal and regional inequality and inequitable asset distribution. The major problems associated with green revolution are as follows:

1. Increase in personal inequalities in rural areas

The income inequality between rich and poor increases due to:

i) The owners of large farms were the main adopters of new technology because of their better access to irrigation water, fertilizers, seeds and credit. In other words, given the need for complex agricultural techniques and inputs, the green revolution benefits the large farmers. The small farmers lagged behind the larger farmer as small farmers had to depend upon traditional production method. Since the rich farmers were already better equipped, the green revolution accentuate the income inequalities between rich and poor.

ii) Green revolution resulted into lower product price and higher input prices which also encouraged landlords to increase rents or force tenants to evict the land.

iii) The mechanization pushed down the wages of and employment opportunities for unskilled labour in the rural areas thereby further widening the income disparities.

2. Increased Regional disparities

The states like Punjab, Haryana, Western UP etc. having good irrigation facilities used HYV seeds and got windfall profit. The states or regions without the access of sufficient water were left out that widened the regional disparities between states. The states who were able to derive the benefits of green revolution, achieved faster economic development while other states have recorded slow growth in agriculture production.

3. Environmental Damage

The rampant irrigation practices have led to soil degradation. It has caused over-use of soil and rapidly depleted its nutrients. Groundwater practices have fallen dramatically. Excessive and inappropriate use of fertilizers and pesticides has polluted waterway, killed beneficial insects and wild life. Further, heavy dependence on few major crops has led to loss of biodiversity of farmers. These problems were aggravated due to absence of training to use modern technology and vast illiteracy leading to excessive use of chemicals.

4. Restrictive Crop Coverage

The main reason for non-spread of green revolution to other crops than wheat, maize, bajra and rice was that in the early 1960's there was severe shortage of food grains and imports were resorted to overcame the shortage. Government initiated green revolution to increase food grain productivity and non-food grain crops were not covered. The new agriculture strategy involving use of HYV seeds was initially limited to wheat, maize and bajra. The other major crop i.e. rice responded much later. The progress of developing and application of HYV seeds in other crops especially commercial crops like oilseeds, jute etc has been very slow. In fact, in certain period a decline in the output of commercial crops is witnessed because of diversion of area under commercial crop to food crop production.

It can be concluded that green revolution is a major achievement for India which has given it a food-security. It has involved the adaptation of scientific practices in the agriculture to improve its production and productivity. It has provided benefits to poor in the form of lower food prices, increased migration opportunities and greater employment in the rural non-farm economy. However, the inequalities between region and individuals that adopted green revolution and those who failed to adopt has worsened. Further, green revolution has led to many negative environmental impacts. The policy makers and scientists are urged to develop and encourage the new technologies that are environmentally and socially sustainable.

Training and Visit System (T&V System)

The reorganized agriculture extension system popularly known as Training and Visit System was developed by the World Bank expert Daniel Benor. He implemented this system of extension first in Turkey in 1967. The gradually this system was introduced in Thailand, Burma, Sri Lanka, Indonesia, Nepal and Bangladesh. It is also known as Benor system as Mr. Benor was instrumental in introducing this new concept in agricultural extension. In India, this system was evolved on the basis of experience gained in the command areas of Andhra Pradesh, Madhya Pradesh and Rajasthan under World Bank Assistance. The main objective this system to remove shortcomings in the then existing agricultural extension system. This system gave the country a new vision bringing farm scientists and field extension functionaries closer with sole intention of improving production and income of farmers. The introduction of the Training-and-Visit (T&V) extension system was an important milestone in the history of extension in India. The basic premise of T&V was that there was enough technology available awaiting diffusion to and adoption by farmers. The T&V extension system was first introduced in 1974-75 on a pilot basis in the Chambal Command area of Rajasthan and Madhya Pradesh. Based on positive feedback, the project was further extended to 17 other states in 1978-79 and there after it was implemented in all states by 1985. The methodology of T and V system provides for a management system which can ensure delivery of expert know-how in every field on a state wide basis on every week or fort-night basis. Transfer of know-how from Subject Matter Specialists to the farmer is ensured in two stages , through :

- Training: Transfer of know-how from Subject Matter Specialist to the extension worker
- Visits : Transfer of know-how obtained during the training from extension workers to farmers.

Salient features of T & V System: The key features of the T & V system according to Benor and Baxter (1984) are as follows:

i) **Professionalism:** The extension staff must keep in close touch with relevant scientific developments and research in order to formulate specific recommendations that will be useful to farmers in all kinds of resource situations. This can be achieved only if each extension worker is fully and continuously trained to handle his particular responsibilities in a professional manner.

ii) **Single line of command:** The extension service must be under a single line of technical and administrative command within the Department of Agriculture. Support is required from teaching and research institutions, input supply and other agricultural support organizations and local government bodies, but all extension workers should be responsible administratively and technically to a unit within only one department.

iii) **Concentration of efforts:** All extension staff work only in agricultural extension. Staffs are not responsible for the supply of inputs, data collection, distribution subsidies, processing of loans, or any other activity not directly related to extension. It is assumed that the effective span of control for supervision or guidance is about eight. Similarly, extension-oriented research concentrates on key constraints to increase production and income that are faced by the farmers.

iv) **Time-bound work:** Messages and skills are taught to farmers in a regular, timely fashion, so that they will make best use of the resources at their commend. The Village Extension Worker (VEW) must visit his farmers regularly on a fixed day, usually once each fortnight. All other extension staff must make timely and regular visits to the field.

v) **Field and Farmers Orientation:** The contact of extension staff must be on a regular basis, on a schedule known to farmers and with a large number of farmers representing all major farming and socio- economic types. While spending all must all of their time in the field meetings with farmers, extension worker must attempt to understand farmers' production recommendations are formulated.

vi) **Regular and Continuous Training:** Regular and continuous training of extension staff is required both to teach and discuss with them the specific production recommendations needed by farmers for the coming fortnight and to up-date and upgrade their professional skills. Moreover, the basic training sessions, fortnightly training and monthly workshops are the key means of bringing actual farmers problems to the attention of research, identifying research findings of immediate relevance to farmers, and of developing the production recommendations that fit to specific local conditions.

vii) **Linkages with Researches:** Effective extension depends on close linkage with research. Linkages are two ways. Problems faced by farmers that cannot be resolved by extension workers are passed on to researchers for either an immediate solution or investigation. During seasonal and monthly workshops and joint field trips, extension and research staff formulates production recommendations that will be adopted by extension workers as necessary to make best use of the specific local environment and actual farmers 'resources.

The Organizational Pattern of the T & V System of Agriculture Extension evolved by Benor

The entire organization is based on the total number of farm families which one VAE or Village Extension Officer (VEO) or Village Level Worker (VLW) can reasonable cover. It is organized in such a manner that the Agricultural Extension Officer (AEO) guides, trains and supervise about 6 to 8 AEOs are in turn guided and supervised by a Sub-Divisional Extension Officer (SDEO). The SDEOs are supported by a team of Subject –Matter Specialists. 4 to 8 SDEOs are supervised by Divisional Extension Officer (DEO) who is also supported by SMSs depending upon the number of districts the DEO is supervising, either directly or through an intermediate superior, Zonal Extension Officer (ZEO)

Coverage of Various Extension Personnel

Level	Extension Personnel	Coverage
Field level	Village Extension Worker (VEW)	800-1200 farm families
Block level	Agriculture Extension Officer (AEO)	8 VEWs
Sub-Divisional Level	Sub-Divisional Extension Officer (SDEO)	5-8 AEOs
District level	District Extension Officer or District Agricultural Officer (DAOs)	4-8 SDEOs in a district

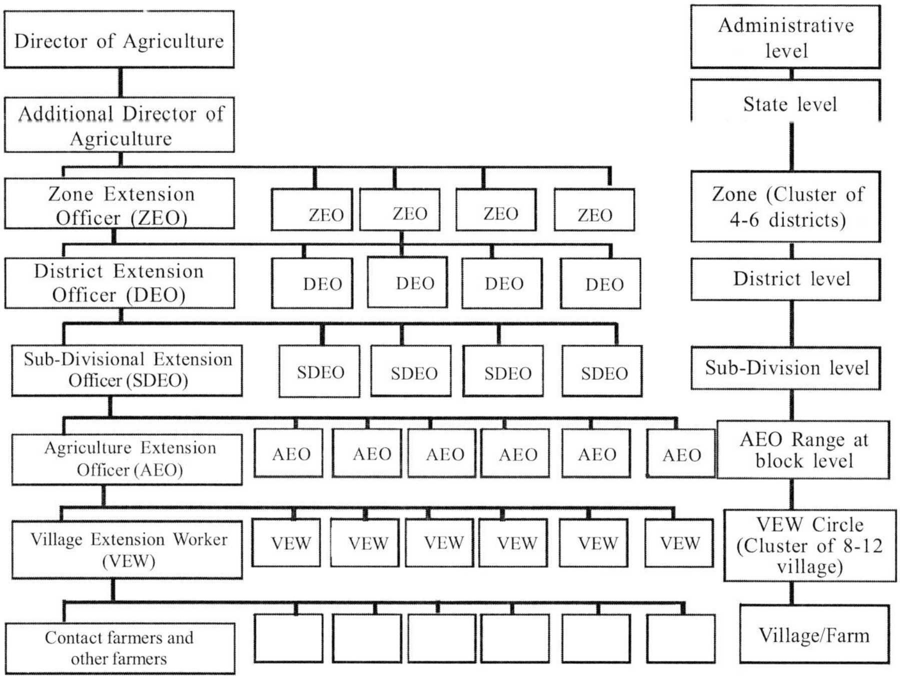

Organizational Pattern of the T & V System of Agricultural Extension

All farm families under a VAE jurisdiction are divided into eight groups of about equal size. From each group the VEW in consultation with village leaders will select about 10 per cent of the farmers as contact farmers on whom he will concentrate his efforts. The key point here is a fixed schedule of VEW visits, known to all under a fortnightly programme of visits. The VEW visits each of the eight groups on his cycle for a full day once each fortnight. An alternative is to visits two groups a day. In this case he will visit each group for one-half of a say only but once every week. Each week the VEW will devote four days to visits so that he covers his entire circle of eight groups in a week of a fortnight. One of the two remaining working days in each week will be devoted to in-service training which is crucial to this programme and the other day for unscheduled visits. One of the training sessions each fortnight will be conducted by the team of Subject Matter Specialist (SMS) responsible to the area. This will be the most important training session. The session is scheduled so that the VEWs are trained doe a full day in groups of 30-40. The other weekly training session during the fortnight will be conducted by the AEO who is the immediate supervisor of the VEWs, for the groups of VES under his charge. The schedule of the visits and training takes up 10 to 12 working days in the fortnight. Each VEW will maintain a table showing his fixed days for visiting each group and the time and place of the 'to meeting'.

The AEO will spend two days in training sessions for VEWs and eight days in the field supervising the VEWs and assisting them. The Sub-Divisional Extension Officer (SDEO) supervises VEWs under his jurisdiction and is in overall charge of the extension programme. THE SDEO would have with him a team of SMSs. The SMSs would devote one-third of their time to VEW training sessions, one-third to field and remaining one-third time visiting research facilities and conducting some research. In a fortnight, a team of SMSs has four days available for VEW and AEO training sessions. The DEO would be involved in regular training sessions of the VEWs and AEO training sessions as and when needed. At zonal level, the Zonal Extension Officer will be responsible for all extension activities in his/her districts and will be assisted by a few administrative staff only. The headquarters level may be different from state to state. It would be best if the headquarters unit dealt with agricultural extension exclusively and were called Extension Service, rather than Department of Agriculture. The Director of Extension or Additional Director of Agriculture (Extension) would be assisted by three deputies in-charge of administration, technical aspects, and execution and implementation of work.

Strengths of T & V System

The main strengths of the Training and Visit (T&V) System were the close Research and Extension linkage which provided an opportunity for the Subject Matter Specialists (SMSs) and the extension staff at Sub-divisional and Block level to interact regularly through monthly workshops. The main purpose was to build-up technical skills of Subject Matter Specialists (SMSs) regularly so that they can meet effectively the actual technological needs of farmers and adapt the recommendations suitably. The other purpose was that researchers and SMSs discuss and formulate relevant production recommendations for subsequent transfer to Agricultural Extension Officers and Village Extension Workers in the next fortnightly training sessions and ultimately reaching farmers through Contact farmer. The other strengths of the T&V system was the continuous trainings of field level functionaries by SMSs. This was made possible due to the availability of adequate manpower at all levels. The other important feature of T&V was, the Village Extension Worker (VEW), visiting farmers' field through contact farmers regularly on a scheduled day, to advise and train farmers on recommendations of relevant agricultural technology and to encourage them to adopt.

Merits of T & V System

1. Systematic and intensive training of extension workers
2. Effective supervision and guidance

3. Better linkage with researcher.
4. Systematic and continuous monitoring and evaluation
5. Quick mobility of extension functionaries
6. Minimum distortion of information
7. Absenteeism of extension workers will be minimum
8. Single line of command.

Constraints of T & V System

The research studies have revealed that T&V system had not created uniform impact. It achieved success mainly in irrigated areas for the selected crops like Rice and wheat. The system did not give due emphasis to other enterprises such as animal husbandry, fisheries, horticulture etc. Even within the agriculture, no visible impact was created on the crops, which are grown under rainfed agriculture like millets, pulses and oil seeds. The large increase in staff from district to village level put a heavy burden on state resources, with most funds being spent in meeting the salary component. The large contingent of village level workers were educated up to secondary school level and therefore were not able to transfer the technology as intended due to their poor absorption of the know-how.

The other constraints observed were :

i) Multiplicity of Public Extension System
ii) Narrow focus of the Agricultural Extension System
iii) Lack of farmer involvement in Extension programme planning
iv) Lack of local capacity to validate and refine technologies
v) Absence of public sector linkages with private sector
vi) Lack of gender concern
vii) Lack of involvement and coordination among line department functionaries

Even though, the project came to an end in early 1990s, the T & V System was continued in some states. Over a period of time, the states also modified the system due to lack of resources to fund basic extension activities. However, the following constraints were also observed in the post T&V extension systems across the states in the country in addition to above constraints:

i) Lack of transparency and accountability
ii) Inadequate technical capacity among the extension functionaries
iii) Supply driven rather than market driven extension
iv) Lack of emphasis on farmers' trainings
v) Inadequate operating resources and financial sustainability

Small Farmers Development Agency (SFDA)

The All India Rural Credit Review Committee appointed by Reserve Bank of India (RBI) in 1969 recommended in their report to establish an agency for the assistance of the small farmers who had not benefitted from the gains of green revolution. Accordingly, SFDA agency was started during 1971-72 in selected districts of the country. Each SFDA project was expected to cover during the five year period (fourth plan) approximately 50,000 families of identified small farmers defined as those who owned land holdings ranging from 2.50 to 5.0 acres. SFDA was the first programme in the country in which there was a proper linkage of the central government, state government and financial institutions.

The main functions of SFDA were:

- Indentifying small farmers and investigating their problems;
- Developing economic programmes for them;
- Developing institutional, financial and administrative arrangement for them;
- Strengthening cooperative mechanism;
- Promoting rural industries.

Marginal Farmers and Agricultural Labourers (MFAL) Scheme

Marginal Farmers and Agricultural Labourers Development Agency (MFALDA) was launched along with SFDA as per the recommendation of the All India Rural Credit Review Committee in 1971-72 to assist the marginal farmers and agricultural labourers to improve their productivity and income through variety of activities of agriculture, animal husbandry, fisheries etc. Marginal farmers were those having land holding of less than 2.5 acres of dry land and agriculture labourers are those who had more than 50 percent of their income from agriculture wages. MFAL scheme covered about 1500 marginal farmers and 5000 agricultural labourers in each project. During the Fifth plan, based on the recommendation of the National Commission of Agriculture, the SFDA and MFAL schemes were merged in to one composite scheme called the Small Farmers, Marginal Farmers and Agricultural Labourers Project. Later in 1980, this project was merged with Integrated Rural Development Programme (IRDP).

Drought Prone Area Programme (DPAP)

The Rural Works Programme was started in the 1970-71 with the focus on execution of rural works and employment generation in order to mitigate the condition of scarcity in draught prone areas . But, later on it was realized that the rural works programme alone was not sufficient in attaining these goals, hence the programme was reoriented on the basis of area development approach and was redesignated as the Draught Prone Area Programme (DPAP) in the midterm appraisal of Fourth Five Year Plan. It was the first area specific programme launched in 1973-74 with the objectives to reduce to reduce the severity of impact of drought, i.e. to minimize the adverse effects of drought on the production of crops and livestock and productivity of land, water and human resources thereby ultimately leading to the drought proofing of the affected areas. Restoration of ecological balance i.e. the programme aimed at promoting overall economic development and improving the socio-economic condition of the resource poor and disadvantaged section inhabiting in the programme areas through creation, widening and equitable distribution of the resource base and increased employment opportunities. It was a people's programme with Government assistance. There was specific arrangement for maintenance of assets and social audit by Panchayat Raj Institutions. Allocation to the project was equally shared by the Centre and State Government on 50:50 basis.

Tribal Area Development Programme /Integrated Tribal Development Agency (ITDA)

A special programme for the development of tribal areas was started in 1971-72. Under this programme, six pilot tribal development projects in (i) Srikakulam district of Andhra Pradesh, (ii) Singhbhum district of Bihar, (iii) Danteweda and (iv) Konta tehsils of Bastar district of Madhya Pradesh and (v) Ganjam and (vi) Koraput district of Orissa, were sanctioned by the Government of India for economic development of these areas. Two more projects in Orissa (Keonjhar and Phulbani) were sanctioned as part of the programme in the Fifth Plan. The main objectives of the programme were to minimize the gaps between the level of development among non-tribal and tribal areas and also to improve the quality of life of tribal communities. A separate agency named as Integrated Tribal Development Agency (ITDA) was set up in the year 1971-72 to sensitize administration to the basic problems and needs of the tribes and to enforce the existing laws concerning to debt relief, poverty relief/alleviation(lessening), and protection of tribal lands. The special features of ITDA are:

- Narrowing down the gap between the levels of development of tribal areas and other areas;
- Revision of excise and forest policies
- Organizing training programmes in agro and forest-based industries;
- Setting –up of tribal development cooperation;
- Starting special programmes for tribal development
- Providing subsidy to the tribal
- Restructuring administration of tribal areas

Hill Area Development Programme (HADP)

The strategies of rural development adopted in the past had lead to an uneven distribution of the benefits of development to the people between different geographical areas and also between the different socio-economic groups of the country. In response to that realization, certain area specific programmes like SFDA and MFAL were launched in the Fourth Five Year Plan. After reviewing SFDA and MFAL, a third programme named as Hill Area Development Programme (HADP) was launched in 1975. The programme emphasized the effective utilization of indigenous resources and generation of employment through development of horticulture, plantations, animal husbandry, agriculture, bee keeping, sericulture, forestry, cottage industries etc. for the development of hilly regions.

Desert Development Programme (DDP)

The Desert Development Programme (DDP) was started both in hot desert areas of Rajasthan, Gujarat and Haryana and the cold deserts of Jammu & Kashmir and Himachal Pradesh in 1977-78 with aims at checking desertification of the desert and enhancing productivity of local resources to raise the income and employment level of local people. From 1995-96, the coverage has been extended to a few more districts in Andhra Pradesh and Karnataka. In hot sandy desert areas, sand dune stabilization and shelterbelt plantations were given greater weightage. On the other hand, in cold desert areas, since rainfall is negligible, crop cultivation and afforestation were taken up only through assured irrigation. In these areas, the main activity was water resources development by construction of channels for diversion of water flow from glaciers and springs to the fields and lift irrigation works in the valleys.The programme was reviewed in 1994-95 by a Technical Committee. The main reason identified by the Committee for below satisfactory results under the programme was that area development was not taken up on watershed basis and the involvement of the local people was virtually non-existent, both in planning and execution of the programme. Besides inadequacy of funds, non-availability of trained personnel and taking up of too many activities, which were neither properly integrated nor necessarily related to the objectives of the programme, were also identified as contributory factors towards reducing the impact of the programme.

National Rural Employment Programme (NREP)

To meet the problems of rural unemployment and under employment, various programmes and schemes rural employment generation were taken up in the country from time to time. The first of such programme was "Rural Manpower Programme" started in 1960-61 to provide employment of 100 days to 2.5 million people of the country by the end of Third Plan Period. However, due to resource constraints the programme came to an end in 1968-69.

This programme was followed by Rural Works Programme in 1971 for providing supplementary employment opportunities to the rural people especially in the lean season. However, due its limited scope and various organizational and administrative deficiencies, it did not make any significant dent on the problem of unemployment.

Another programme named as "Crash Scheme of Rural Employment (CSRE) was initiated in 1971 for a period of three years to create employment opportunities for 1000 persons in a district. The targets of mandays generation were achieved through this programme but the employment and assets creation were found to be widely scattered due to poor planning and lack of durability of assets.

Along with CSRE, a "Pilot Intensive Rural employment Programme (PIREP) was started in November 1972 for a period of three years. The objectives of the PIREP were: provision of additional employment opportunities for unskilled labourers, creation of durable assets which would help create new job, creation of new job skills on the field site etc. The programme review committee on PIREP did not rate it as successful and pointed that due to organizational problem, it could not make much headway.

The State Government of Maharashtra during that time introduced "Employment Guarantee Scheme (EGS)' to provide guaranteed employment within 15 days of the demand of work to all the adults above eighteen years of age in the field of unskilled manual works. The programme aimed to create durable assets which would increase growth as well as employment potentiality in the state.

To utilize surplus food grains available with the Government of India during that period, the Food For Work Programme (FFWP) was launched in 1977 as an employment programme in which part wage payment was made by subsidized food grains. Through this employment programme, Government intended to meet the minimum nutritional requirement of the beneficiaries by making provision of food grains. The Programme Evaluation Organisation (PEO) wing of Planning Commission on his evaluation report on FFWP pointed out that the reasons of the programme failure were pertained to its administrative and implementation problems. The Programme continued up to 1980.

The lessons learnt from the implementation of all the past employment generation related programmes suggested that the benefits were spread very thinly and the impacts in term of overall employment was not substantial. It was realized that the public works should be planned systematically and should be implemented by the concerned department and not by the labour contractor. On the basis of these lessons, the 'National Rural Employment Programme' was launched during Sixth Five Year Plan. The main objectives of the programme were: (a) generation of additional employment opportunities for the unskilled man and women in the rural areas, (b) creation of durable community assets to strengthen the rural infrastructure which would help in rising the living standard of the rural people.

Integrated Rural Development Programme (IRDP)

Poverty reduction occupied the centre stage of India's economic policy since the beginning of Fifth Plan. But, the employment generation oriented programmes as well as area specific programmes launched during Fourth and Fifth Plan Periods could not make much dent in to the poverty and employment in the country. The major cause of the persistent poverty in the rural India was the paucity of productive assets which could generate adequate income to raise people above the poverty line. For the purpose of alleviation of rural poverty, the concept of integrated Programme for Rural Development was first introduced by the Finance Minister, Government of India, in his Budget Speech in 1976, and the Programme was initially started in 20 selected districts of the Country. The programme was reviewed in 1978-79 to integrate the methodology and approach of the three major special programmes of SFDA, Command Area Development (CAD) and Drought Prone Area Programme (DPAP). All the principal contents of these three major programmes were integrated into a new programme called Integrated Rural Development Programme (IRDP) and taken up in 2300 blocks of the country in 1978-79. Upto 1978-79, IRDP was a central sector scheme and 100% funds were provided by the Centre Government. During 1979-80 this programme was made a centrally sponsored scheme in which funding was shared on 50:50 basis between the Centre and the States. In case of UTs, however, 100% funds were provided by the central government. IRPD was extended to all the Blocks in the country with effect from 2nd October, 1980.

The main aim of the IRDP was to assist the selected families of target group in rural areas to help them to cross above the poverty line once and for ever by providing them income generating assets and access to credit and other inputs. The programme covered small and marginal farmers, agricultural workers and landless labourers and rural craftsmen and artisans and other families whose family income was below the poverty line.

Approaches of IRDP

In order to achieve the objectives of the IRDP, three types of approaches were employed.

1. The Cluster approach: To select the villages which are having supporting infrastructure or can be made available at relatively lower cost.
2. The *Antyodaya* approach: Selection of the poorest of the poor for the programme to get the benefit first.
3. The Package approach: Provision of inputs and other services required for the beneficiary.

Financial assistance was given to the beneficiary through viable bank projects which has subsidy and loan. The loan amount is subsidized to the extent of 25 per cent for small farmers, 33.33 per cent for marginal farmers, agricultural and non agricultural labourers and rural artisans, 50 per cent for the tribals.

Salient features of the Programme

- The programme targeted the people remaining below poverty line and mostly they were small farmers, marginal farmers, agriculture laboureres, rural artisans and others.
- Family was considered as the unit of development
- It provided institutional credit with subsidies to create income generating assets.
- At least 30 per cent of the assisted families were from SC and ST
- A minimum of 30 per cent of total beneficiaries were women
- Emphasis was given on Block planning- 3000 families for each block covering 600 families per year for five years
- Selection of the scheme was done keeping the infrastructure facilities in the area.

Criteria for Allocation of Funds to the States

Allocation of funds to states is being made by the central government in proportion to the poverty levels in each state on the basis of official estimates of the Planning Commission. These official estimates of poverty are arrived at by the Planning Commission based on the National Sample Survey Organisation, Consumer Expenditure Surveys conducted every five years.

Implementing Agency

District Rural Development Agency / Zilla Parishad is the implementing agency for this programme. The Government Body at the district level provides guidance and directions to DRDAs. It includes local MPs, MLAs, and Chairman of Zilla Parishad, Heads of District Development Departments and representative of

SCs/STs, women and NGOs. At the grassroots level, the programme is carried out by Block Development Officer, and the other block staff with the help of the village level functionaries.

Training of Rural Youth for Self Employment (TRYSEM)

The national scheme of Training of Rural Youth for Self Employment (TRYSEM), as a special component of IRDP, was initiated in August 1979, aimed at providing basic technical and entrepreneurial skill to the rural poor in the age group of 18-35 years to enable them take up income generating activities (self/wage employment). The scheme proposed to train about 2 lakh rural youth every year in various skills. The strategy adopted for the training included institutional training, training in industrial units, training under master-craftsmen, artisans and skilled workers. There was provision of covering at least of 50 per cent of SC/ST youth under this programme and 50 per cent of beneficiaries should be women. Later, this programme was merged with Swarnajayanti Gram Swarojgar Yojana (SGSY) along with IRDP, DWCRA etc. from April, 1999.

Development of Women and Children in Rural Areas (DWCRA)

The DWCRA programme was launched in 1982, as a part of the Integrated Rural Development Programme. The programme aimed to improve the socio-economic status of the poor women in the rural areas through creation of groups of women for income-generating activities on a self-sustaining basis. The main strategy adopted under the programme was to facilitate access for poor women to employment, skill up gradation training, credit and other support services so that the DWCRA women as a group could take up income-generating activities for supplementing their incomes. It sought to encourage collective action in the form of group activities which were known to work better and were more sustainable than the individual effort. It encouraged the habit of thrift and credit among poor rural women to make them self-reliant. It was first programme of its kind that specifically focused on improving the quality of life of rural women.

Objectives: The objectives of DWCRA included the following.

i) To help and promote self-employment among the rural women, who were below poverty line, by providing skill training in vocations which were acceptable to the beneficiaries by encouraging productivity and introducing new activities;

ii) To organize the beneficiaries into groups and promote economic and social

iii) To generate income for the rural poor by creating avenues for production of goods and services;

iv) To organize production-enhancing programmes in rural areas; and

v) To provide for care of children of the working women by providing an improved environment, care and food by establishing Balwadis.

DWCRA was designed to facilitatrator women to: i) improve their earning; ii) acquire new skills; iii) reduce their daily work; iv) have better access to credit facilities; and v) participate in social service.

The Scheme was later merged with Swarnajayanti Gram Swarojgar Yojana (SGSY) along with IRDP, TRYSEM etc. from April, 1999.

Agricultural Human Resource Development Programme (AHRDP)

The world bank –aided AHRDP project was launched in the year 1995 for the purpose of assisting financially the Indian Agricultural education sector. The project aimed at improving the quality and relevance of higher agricultural education through in-service training programmes and effective management of agricultural human resources.

In India, Andhra Pradesh, Haryana and Tamil Nadu being the three states and ANGRAU (Acharya N.G. Ranga Agriculture University), HAU (Haryana Agricultural University), TNAU (Tamil Nadu Agricultural University and TANUVAS(Tamil Nadu University of Animal Sciences) were the four agricultural universities selected under this project.

Salient features of AHRDP

i) AHRDP was initiated to fulfill its objective of financing to equip laboratories and class rooms for better teaching programmes. Staff training for better faculty teaching skills, library modernization for effective services and computerization for better management and administration.

ii) SAUS were provided with financial assistance for purchase of modern equipments and furniture needed for improvement of classroom, laboratory and farms.

iii) The project financed to depute teachers of SAUs for training inadvanced studies in reputed institutions of India and abroad.

iv) Lack of adequate resources severely affected the usefulness of libraries in SAUs, and to overcome this deficiency, the project financed the purchase of needed equipment, latest text books, journals, etc. for the library.

v) The project also financed the SAUS for effective computer systems and establishing computer networks.

Important Rural Development Programmes and Schemes Launched under Different Five Year Plans

S.No.	Programme	Year of Introduction
I	**First five year plan (1951-56)**	
	Community Development Programme (CDP)	1952
	National Extension Service (NES)	1953
	Community Development Block(CDB)	1954
II	**Second Five Year (1956-61)**	
	Khadi and Village Industries Programme (KVIP)	1957
	Village Housing Scheme	1957
	Multi –Purpose Tribal Development	1959
	Package Programme	1960
	Intensive Agriculture District Programme (IADP)	1960
III	**Third Five Year Plan (1961-66)**	
	Applied Nutrition Programme (ANP)	1962
	Rural Industries Projects	1962
	Intensive Agricultural Area Programme (IAAP)	1964
	Intensive Cattle Development Programme (ICDP)	1964-65
	High Yielding Variety Programme (HYVP)	1966
	National Family Welfare Programme	1966
	Annual Plan (1966-67)	
	Farmer's Training and Education Programme	1966
	Well Construction Programme	1966
	Annual Plan (1967-68)	
	Rural Works Programme (RWP)	1967
	Annual Plan (1968-69)	
	Tribal Development Block	1968
	Rural Manpower Programme	1969
	Composite Programme for Women and Pre-school Children	1969
IV	**Fourth Five Year Plan (1969-74)**	
	Drought Prone Area Programme (DPAP)	1970
	Crash Scheme for Rural Development (CSRD)	1971
	Small Farmer's Development Agency (SFDA)	1971
	Marginal Farmers' and Agricultural Labourers Programme(MFAL)	1971
	Tribal Area Development Programme (TADP)	1972
	Pilot Project for Tribal Development	1972
	Pilot Intensive Rural Employment Programme (PIREP)	1972
	Minimum Needs Programme (MNP)	1972
	Command Area Development Programme	1974
	Training and Visit Programme (T&V)	1974
V	**Fifth Five Year Plan (1974-79)**	
	Hill Area Development Programme (HADP)	1975
	Special Livestock Production Programme	1975
	Food for Work Programme (FWP)	1977
	Desert Development Programme (DDP)	1977
	Whole Village Development Programme	1979

	Training of Rural Youth for Self-Employment (TRYSEM)	1979
	Integrated Rural Development Programme (IRDP)	1978-79
VI	**Sixth Five Year Plan (1980-85)**	
	National Rural Employment Programme (NREP)	1980
	Prime Minister's Twenty -Point Programme	1980
	New Twenty -Point Programme	1982
	Development of Women and Children in Rural Areas (DWCRA)	1983
	Nutrition Noon Meal Scheme	1982
	Rural Landless Employment Guarantee Programme (RLEGP)	1983
	National Agricultural Extension Project (NAEP)	1984
VII	**Seventh Five Year Plan (1985-90)**	
	Indira Awas Yojana (IAY)	1985
	Reclamation and Development of Alkali and Acid Soils (RADAS)	1985-86
	New Twenty -Point Economic Programme	1986
	Technology Mission on oilseeds (TMO)	1986
	Jawahar Rozgar Yojana (JRY)	1989
	Annual Plans 1990-91 and 1991-92	
	National Watershed Development Project for Rainfed Areas (NWDPRA)	1990-91
VIII	**Eighth Five Year Plan (1992–1997)**	
	Milk and Milk Products Order	1992
	Rashtriya Mahila Kosh	1992
	Mahila Samridhi Yojana	1993
	Prime Minister's Rozgar Yojana	1993
	Integrated Dairy Development Scheme	1993-94
	Indian Mahila Yojana	1995
	Mid-day Meal Scheme	1995
	National Social Assistance Programme	1995
	The Rural Group Life Insurance Scheme	1995
IX	**Ninth Five Year Plan (1997–2002)**	
	Experimental Crop Insurance Scheme (ESIS)	1997-98
	Jawahar Gram Samridhi Yojana (JGSY)	1998
	Rural Housing	1998
	Swarnajayanthi Gram Swarozgar Yojana (SGSY)	1999
	Employment Assurance Scheme (EAS)	1999
	National Agricultural Insurance Scheme (NAIS)	1999-2000
	Pilot Scheme on Seed Crop Insurance (PSSCI)	1999-2000
	National Project on Cattle and Buffalo Breeding (NPCBB)	2000
	Pradhan Mantri Gram Sadak Yojana (PMGSY)	2000
	Grameen Bhandaran Yojana	2001
X	**Tenth Five Year Plan (2002–2007)**	
	Agriclinics and Agribusiness Centres (AABC) Scheme	2002
	Farm Income Insurance Scheme (FIIS)	2003-04
	Kissan Call Centre (KCC) Scheme	2004
	Agricultural Marketing Infrastructure, Grading & Standardization (AMIGS)	2004
	Providing Urban Amenities in Rural Areas (PURA)	2004
	Intensive Dairy Development Programme (IDDP)	2005

	Bharat Nirman	2005
	National Rural Health Mission	2005
	Agricultural Technology Management Agency (ATMA) Scheme	2005-06
	National Horticulture Mission (NHM)	2005-06
	MGNREGS	2006
	National Bamboo Mission	2006-07
XI	**Eleventh Five Year Plan (2007–2012)**	
	Pilot Weather Based Crop Insurance Scheme (WBCIS)	2007
	National Food Security Mission	2007-08
	Rashtriya Krishi Vikas Yojana (RKVY)	2007-08
	National Land Records Modernization Programme (NLRMP)	2008
	Agricultural Debt Waiver & Debt Relief (ADWDR) Scheme	2008
	Integrated Watershed Management Programme (IWMP).	2009-10
	National Mission on Micro Irrigation (NMMI)	2010
	Dairy Entrepreneur Development Scheme (DEDS)	2010
	National Rural Livelihood Mission (NRLM)	2011
	Rainfed Area Development Programme (RADP)	2011-12
	Accelerated Fodder Development Programme (AFDP)	2011-12
	National Mission for Protein Supplements	2011-12
	National Dairy Plan	2012
XII	**Twelve Five Year Plan (2012–2017)**	
	National Mission for Sustainable Agriculture (NMSA)	2014-15
	National Livestock Mission(NLM)	2014-15
	National Mission on Oil Seeds and Oil Palm (NMOOP)	2014-15
	Mission for Integrated Development of Horticulture (MIDH)	2014-15

The 12th FYP is the last FYP of India. NITI Aayog has come in to existence from 1st January 2015. NITI: National Institution for Transforming India.

Suggested Readings and References

1. Reddy, A.A. (1993). Extension Education, Sree lakshmi Press, Bapatla
2. Dhama, O.P. and Bhatnagar, O.P. (2007). Education and Communication for Development. Oxford and IBH Pub. Co. Pvt. Ltd.
3. Sagar Mondal and Ray G.K. (2006). Entrepreneurship and Rural Development, Mumbai,Oxford and IBH Publishing Co.
4. Mathialagan, P. (2007). Textbook of Animal Husbandry and Livestock Extension, International Book Distributing Co. 7, Meerabai Marg, Lucknow, India.
5. Singh, Katar (1999). Rural Development: Principles, Policies and Management, Second Edition, New Delhi, Sage Publications.
6. Kelsey, L.D. and Hearne, C.C. (1949). Cooperative Extension Work, Vail-Ballou, Inc, Binghamton, New York, U.S.A.
7. Ray, G.L. (2006). Extension Communication and Management, New Delhi, Kalyani Publishers.

8. Sanders, H.C. (1968). The Cooperative Extension Services, New Jersey, US, Prentice Hall Inc.
9. Dey, S.K. (1964). Community Development: A Bird's Eye View, Asia Publishing House, New Delhi.
10. Rural Development - Some Facets, (ed.) NIRD, Hyderabad – 1979.
11. Five Year Plans (1st -10th), Planning Commission, Government of India, New Delhi.
12. Verma, S.C. (1980). Direct Attack on Rural Poverty, Ministry of Rural Development, Delhi.
13. NIRD, Fifty Years of Rural Development in India (1998). NIRD, Hyderabad.
14. Desai, Vasant (2009). Rural Development in India, Himalaya Publishing House, Mumbai.
15. Mahajan, R.K. (1991). Integrated Rural Development Programme, Concept Publishing Company, New Delhi.
16. Mehta, Shiv R. (1984). Rural Development Policies and Programmes, Sage Publications.
17. Arora, R.C. (1979). Integrated Rural Development, New Delhi: S.Chand and Company Limited.
18. Lawania, Vinod Kumar (1992). Rural Development in India. New Delhi: Ashish Publishing.
19. Ray, G.L. (2001). Extension, Communication and Management, 4th Edition, Naya Prokash, Calcutta.
20. B.S.Mathur (1977). Cooperation in India, Sahitya Bhavan, Agra.
21. Ensminger, Douglas (1957). A guide to Community Development, Ministry of Community Development, Government of India, Coronation Printing Works, Fatehpuri, Delhi-6.
22. Ministry of Agriculture, Government of India (2009). Report of the High Powered Committee on Cooperative.
23. Sharma, K.R.G. (2008). Veterinary Extension Education, BSPBS Publications, Hyderabad, Hyderabad,
24. Supe S.V. (1987). An Introduction to Extension Education, Oxford and IBH Publishing Co. Pvt. Ltd. New Delhi.

17

Swarnajayanti Gram Swarozgar Yojana (SGSY) and National Rural Livelihood Mission/Ajeveeka

Swarnjayanti Gram Swarozgar Yojana (SGSY)

The Swarnjayanti Gram Swarozgar Yojana (SGSY), a programme for the self employment of rural poor was started from 01.04.1999 after restructuring the six erstwhile Integrated Rural Development Programme (IRDP) and its allied programmes, These were : IRDP, Training of Rural Youth for Self Employment (TRYSEM), Development of Women and Children in Rural Areas (DWCRA), Supply of Toolkits in Rural Areas (SITRA) and Ganga Kalyan Yojana (GKY), and Million Wells Scheme (MWS). The basic objective of the SGSY was to bring the assisted poor families (Swarozgaris) above the Poverty Line by providing them income-generating assets through a mix of bank credit and governmental subsidy. The programme aimed at establishing a large number of micro enterprises in rural areas based on the ability of the poor and potential of each area.

Main Features of the Programme

i) Emphasis was laid on mobilization of rural poor to enable them to organize into Self Help Groups(SHG).

ii) It was a credit-cum-subsidy scheme where credit was critical component and subsidy was only an enabling element and was linked with credit.

iii) Emphasis was on participatory approach in selection of key activities.

iv) Project approach for each key activity.

v) Emphasis was on development of activity clusters to ensure proper forward and backward linkages.

vi) Strengthening of groups through Revolving Fund Assistance(RFA)

vii) Training of beneficiaries in group dynamics and skill development for taking up micro enterprises.

viii) Marketing support with emphasis on market research, up gradation/ diversification of products, packaging, creation of market facilities, etc.

ix) Provision for development of infrastructure to provide missing critical link. 20% fund (in case of North Eastern States 25%) was earmarked for infrastructure development.

x) Active role of NGOs in formation and capacity building of SHGs.

xi) Focus on vulnerable groups i.e. SC, ST, Women, minorities and disabled

xii) 15% fund earmarked for Special Projects to ensure a time-bound programme for bringing a specific number of Below Poverty Line (BPL) families above the poverty line though self employment generation.

Funding Pattern

Funds under Swarnjayanti Gram Swarojgar Yojana (SGSY) were shared between the Centre and the States (except NE States including Sikkim) in the ratio of 75:25. The ratio of sharing of funds between the Centre and the North Eastern States including Sikkim was 90:10.

Strategy

The SGSY is different from earlier programmes, in terms of the strategy envisaged for its implementation. It was conceived as a holistic programme of self-employment. It covered all aspects of self-employment of the rural poor viz. organisation of the poor in to Self Help Groups (SHGs), their capacity building and training, credit linkages and subsidy, selection of key activities, planning of activity clusters, infrastructure build up, technology and marketing support.

Implementing Agencies

The SGSY was implemented by the District Rural Development Agencies (DRDAs), with the active involvement of Panchayati Raj Institutions (PRIs), the Banks, the Line Departments and the Non Government Organizations (NGOs).

Social Mobilization of the poor

A major shift in the SGSY compared to the erstwhile programmes was in terms of its emphasis on social mobilization of the poor.The programme focused on organization of the poor at grassroots level through a process of social mobilization for poverty eradication. Social mobilization enabled the poor to build their own organizations, the Self-Help Groups (SHGs), in which they participated fully and directly and through internal credit and thrift, they were able to meet small emergent expenditures through loans from group savings.

SGSY - Main Criteria for SHG Formation

i) SHG is a group of rural poor who volunteer to organize themselves in a group.

ii) Group consists of 10-20 members (5-20 members in case of minor irrigation project, disabled persons and in difficult areas like desert hills and areas with scattered and sparse population).

iii) Members of group to be from BPL family, however maximum of 20% and in exceptional case 30% of the group members can be from families marginally above poverty line.

iv) Only one member from a family is eligible for membership of group.

Role of NGOs/Banks in Group Formation

i) NGOs or Community Based Organization (CBOs)/ Community Coordinators/ facilitators/Self Help Groups Promoting Institutions (SHPIs) /animators were involved in Group Formation and even for SHG's capacity building.

ii) Rs.10, 000 per group was paid to NGOs/CBOs / SHPI / facilitators etc. for formation and development of SHG in four instalment.

Selection of Key Activities

The SGSY emphasized assistance to the Swarozgaris for those activities which were identified and selected as key activities in terms of their economic viability in the area. Each block was asked to select about 10 key activities but focus was concentrated only on 4-5 Key Activities based on local resources, occupational skills of the people and availability of markets so that the Swarozgaris could draw sustainable incomes from their investments.

Block Level SGSY Committees were mainly responsible for selection of key activities. Selection of key activity was done in consultation with Banks, industrial/ technical organizations, local Khadi & Village Industries officials and District Industry Centre.

Target Group

Families living below the Poverty Line (BPL) in rural areas were the target group of the SGSY. Within the target group, special safeguards had been provided to vulnerable sections of the society , by way of reserving 50% benefits for SCs/STs, 40% for women, 15% for minorities and 3% for disabled persons.

Financial Assistance

Assistance under the SGSY, to individual Swarozgaries or Self Help Groups, was given in the form of subsidy by the government linked to credit by the banks. Credit was critical components of the SGSY, subsidy being a minor and enabling element. Accordingly, the SGSY envisaged greater involvement of the banks. The banks were involved closely in the planning and preparation of project reports, identification of activity clusters, infrastructure planning as well as capacity building and choice of activities of the SHGs, selection of individual Swarozgaries, pre-credit activities and post-credit activities and post-credit monitoring including loan recovery.

Revolving Fund Assistance under SGSY

Assistance in terms of Revolving Fund was given by DRDA and Banks to SHGs after passing of the groups on different gradings.

Subsidy under SGSY

- Subsidy was only an enabling element of the Scheme
- Subsidy was back ended and it was kept by Bank in Subsidy Reserve Fund Account.

Quantum of subsidy

a) For individual Swarozgaris 30% of Project cost subject to a maximum of Rs.7500. In case of SC/ST & disabled 50% of Project cost or Rs.10,000 whichever was less.

b) For Self Help Groups 50% of project cost subject to Rs.1.25 lakhs or Rs.10,000 per SHG Member whichever was less.

Training under SGSY

SGSY was a process-oriented scheme which involved organization of rural poor into Self Help Groups (SHGs), their training and capacity building to enable them to evolve into a self managed organization. Provision of capacity building of the SHG members and implementers of the programme at all levels were given much emphasis. Under this programme 10 per cent of the budget provision was earmarked for training and skill development of Swarojgaries. Ministry of Rural Development in the year 2008-09 took a decision to establish Rural Self Employment Training Institutes in (RSETIs) in each district of the country in partnership with Public Sector Banks (PSBs) and State Governments to train rural youth on various income generating activities.

Monitoring

A comprehensive system of monitoring was adopted under the SGSY. At the Central level, the Central Level Coordination Committee (CLCC) on SGSY was set up and assigned the responsibility to formulate various broad guidelines of SGSY. The CLCC also monitored and reviewed the implementation of the programme in different states. At the State level, a State Level Coordination Committee (SLCC) monitored the Programme. At the district and block level, the programme was monitored by District level SGSY Committee and Block Level SGSY Committees. In addition, the progress under the SGSY was monitored periodically through reports and returns submitted by DRDAs/States including the on-line Monthly Progress Reports (MPRs). Issues related to implementation of the programme were discussed in Project Directors' workshops and periodic meetings with the State Secretaries with the objective of bringing out improvement in implementation of the programme at the Block/ DRDA level. Monitoring was also done through field visits and physical verification of assets. The Ministry of Rural Development constituted the

Vigilance and Monitoring Committees with a view to fulfilling the objective of ensuring quality of expenditure under SGSY. These Committees kept a close watch on the implementation of the Programmes as per the prescribed procedures and Guidelines.

Progress of the Programme

a) **Physical Progress :** The physical progress under the SGSY since inception (1.4.99) up to March 2013 at all India level was as follows:

Physical Progress under SGSY since Inception in India

Years	SHG Formed	Women SHGs formed	% of Women SHGs	Total Swarozgaris Assisted	%age of SC/STs Assisted	%age of Women Assisted	%age of Disabled Assisted	%age of Minorities assisted
1999-2000	292426	176263	60.28	933868	44.32	44.62	0.91	
2000-2001	223265	153285	68.66	1006152	44.60	40.73	0.67	
2001-2002	434387	296175	68.18	937468	45.62	41.16	0.65	
2002-2003	398873	221085	55.43	826267	45.97	46.31	0.74	
2003-2004	392136	233136	59.45	896895	46.14	52.49	0.95	
2004-2005	266230	191666	71.99	1115928	44.98	54.32	1.14	
2005-2006	276414	213213	77.14	1151116	47.65	57.58	1.29	
2006-2007	246309	176712	71.74	1691926	49.75	73.71	1.88	3.58
2007-2008	306688	231670	75.54	1699295	47.83	63.79	2.13	8.38
2008-2009	563530	404972	71.86	1861875	47.04	64.80	2.27	14.78
2009-2010	389259	292788	75.22	2085177	51.59	72.05	2.20	11.60
2010-2011	311314	207280	66.58	2109986	51.98	67.49	1.94	11.57
2011-2012	233713	153558	65.70	1677117	47.05	65.80	1.46	16.30
2012-2013	128445	97002	75.52	1144199	42.41	81.38	1.31	9.28
Total	**4334544**	**2951803**	**68.10**	**17993070**	**47.27**	**60.59**	**1.58**	**11.12**

Source: Ministry of Rural Development (MoRD), Government of India, Annual Report 2013-14

b) i) **Financial Progress :** The Financial progress under the SGSY since inception (1.4.99) up to November 2012-13 at all India level is as follows:

Financial Progress under SGSY since Inception in India (Rs. Crore)

Years	Total Funds Utilised	Credit Disbursed to SHGs	Credit Disbursed to Individual Swarozgaris	Total Credit Mobilised	Subsidy Disbursed to SHGs	Subsidy Disbursed to Individual Swarozgaris	Total Subsidy Disbursed
1999-2000	959.86	187.30	869.16	1056.46	124.58	417.11	541.69
2000-2001	1117.94	256.64	1202.80	1459.44	167.93	533.92	701.85
2001-2002	970.32	318.34	1011.34	1329.68	209.94	455.68	665.62
2002-2003	921.11	459.08	725.21	1184.30	282.53	323.35	605.89
2003-2004	1043.43	707.82	594.28	1302.10	444.36	269.01	713.38
2004-2005	1290.83	1027.66	630.52	1658.18	586.08	272.73	858.81
2005-2006	1338.78	1275.41	547.75	1823.16	671.22	233.61	904.83
2006-2007	1424.20	1803.34	487.87	2291.21	771.46	199.59	971.05
2007-2008	1965.97	2090.70	669.60	2760.31	990.97	298.14	1289.10
2008-2009	2285.40	2513.38	1016.69	3530.07	1150.94	591.33	1742.27
2009-2010	2779.19	3475.21	971.82	4447.03	1477.21	484.92	1962.13
2010-2011	2804.04	3753.02	832.95	4585.98	1499.17	314.94	1814.11
2011-2012	2318.17	3568.07	830.93	4399.00	1310.81	365.09	1675.90
2012-2013	1012.33	3280.20	4461.58	4461.58	586.72	106.37	693.09
Total	**21219.23**	21435.98	10390.94	31826.91	9687.21	4759.42	14446.63

Source: Ministry of Rural Development (MoRD), Government of India, Annual Report 2013-14

ii) **Savings and Loan status of SHGs under SGSY :** More than 22.5 lakh SGSY-SHGs had savings bank accounts with different banks with saving amount of Rs 2477 crore by the end of March, 2014.

Status of SGSY-SHGs savings and loans from 2009-10 to 2013-14 (Amount Rs. in crore / Number in Lakh)

Particulars	2009-10		2010-11		2011-12		2012-13		2013-14	
	No of SHG	Amount	No of SHG	Amount	No of SHG	Amount	No of SHG	Amount	No of SHG	Amount
Savings of SHG with Banks as on 31st March	16.94	1292.62	20.23	1817.12	21.23	1395.25	20.47	1821.65	22.62	2477.58
Bank loan disbursed to SHG during the year	2.67	2198	2.41	2480.37	2.10	2643.56	1.81	2207.47	2.26	3480.60
Bank loan outstanding with the SHGs as on 31st March	12.45	6251.08	12.86	7829.39	12.16	8054.83	11.93	8597.09	13.07	10177.42

Source: Status of Microfinance in India 2012-13 and 2013-14, NABARD

A Critical Appraisal of SGSY

- The choice of activity under SGSY must be governed by the resources and skills available in the area and also the market.
- The process of technology identification should be closely interlinked with the identification of key activity itself.
- The technology identified for each activity should be such that it can be managed comfortably by the Swarozgaries, and at the same time leads to quality products.
- The DRDA could not effectively implement IRDP. As such, it will not be successful in monitoring and grading the assisted SHGs.

Factors Responsible for slow progress of SGSY

The Working Group for the Tenth Plan identified the following factors as responsible for slow progress of SGSY.

i) Delayed start of the programme during 1999-2000 and initial preparatory works;

ii) Time involved in sensitization of different stake holders;

iii) DRDA continued to assist individual swarozgaries more than the SHGs with the resource available with them under the scheme.

iv) Flow of bank credit was also not as desired during the period;

v) Inadequate delegation of powers to bank branches to sanction beyond a certain limit.

vi) Demand by bank to collateral security for loan beyond Rs.50, 000.

Also, inadequate availability of credit has adversely affected average per family investment and credit subsidy ratio during the first two years of the programme.

The national conference of the state ministers of rural development. NGOs, Field level functionaries, banks, SHG members held at the National Institute of Rural development (NIRD), Hyderabad, in 2001 made some **suggestions** to strengthen SGSY.

These include:

- Relaxation in the number of key activities per block/district.
- Relaxation in the size of the self help group.
- Relaxation in minimum time involved for gradation of groups first for revolving funds and then for assistance to take up economic activities;
- Increasing the loan limit for collateral security both for individual and groups;
- Bankers accountability in implementation of the scheme.
- Active involvement of voluntary sector in social mobilization of the poor;
- Continues sensitization of all concerned and
- Gradual shift from individual finance to group finance and ultimately making group finance 100 percent under the scheme.

National Rural Livelihood Mission/Aajeeveka

During 1980's, programmes like Integrated Rural Development Programme (IRDP), Training of Rural Youth for Self Employment (TRYSEM), Development of Women and Children in Rural Areas (DWCRA), Supply of Improved Toolkits to Rural Artisans (SITRA), Ganga KalyanYojana (GKY), and the Million Wells Scheme (MWS), etc., were the major programmes implemented in the country with the basic objective of alleviating rural poverty. On account of multiplicity poverty alleviation programmes, the desired linkage among the programmes were not established effectively. These programmes were more concerned with achieving individual programme targets rather than focusing on the substantive issue of sustainable income generation. The Planning Commission set up a committee under the chairmanship of Prof S R Hashim in 1997, to review and rationalize various Centrally Sponsored Schemes for Poverty Alleviation and

Employment Generation. The Committee recommended the integration of allied programmes with IRDP for better linkages. The report formed the base for shifting from an individual beneficiary approach to a group approach for poverty alleviation. Based on the recommendations of the Planning Commission, the schemes of TRYSEM, SITRA, GKY, DWCRA and MWS were merged into a single self-employment programme namely Swarnjayanti Gram Swarozgar Yojana (SGSY), which was implemented by the States, with effect from April, 1999.

SGSY had the objective of improving the family incomes of the rural poor while at the same time, providing for a flexibility of design at the grassroots level to suit local needs and resources. The objective of the restructuring was to provide sustainable income generation through micro-enterprise development, both land-based and otherwise. SGSY moved from the individual oriented approach of the earlier programmes like the IRDP, TRYSEM etc. to a group based approach with Self Help Groups (SHG) of rural BPL as the unit of assistance. The cornerstone of the SGSY strategy was that the poor need to be organized and their capacities built up systematically so that they can access self employment opportunities. This restructuring also helped in establishing effective linkages between the various components of the programme, such as capacity building of the poor, credit availability, technology transfer/up gradation, marketing and infrastructure development.

Evaluation of the SGSY by National Institute of Rural Development (NIRD), Bankers Institute of Rural Development (BIRD) and several others institutions showed mixed results. Out of estimated 25 million households organized into SHGs until 2010, only 22% succeeded in accessing bank credit. The studies showed that there were significant variations in the extent of mobilization of poor SHGs and the quality of their operation. The one-off assetization programme focusing on single livelihood activity did not meet multiple livelihood requirements of the poor. Often, the capital investment was provided up-front as a subsidy, without adequate investment in social mobilization or group formation. Furthermore, uneven geographical spread of SHGs, high attrition rates among members of SHGs, and lack of adequate banking sector response impeded the program performance. Several states did not fully invest the funds received under SGSY. This fact indicated a lack of proper delivery systems and dedicated efforts for skill training and building capacity for resource absorption among the rural poor. There was a considerable mismatch between program capacity and program requirements. Absence of collective institutions in the form of SHG federations precluded the poor from accessing higher order support services for productivity enhancement, marketing linkages or risk management.

Performance of SGSY was assessed through concurrent evaluations, various studies and reports. Prof. Radhakrishna Committee on Credit Related Issues Related to SGSY, set up by the Ministry of Rural Development in April, 2008 reported the shortcomings in the implementation of SGSY like uneven mobilisation of rural poor and formation of SHGs across the States, insufficient capacity building of beneficiaries, low credit mobilization and lack of professionals to implement the programme. Based on the findings of the report, SGSY was restructured as National Rural Livelihoods Mission (NRLM), subsequently renamed as *"Aajeevika"*, and implemented it in a mission mode across the country. The programme was formally launched on 3rd June, 2011. The name of the mission has been renamed as 'Deendayal Antyodaya Yojana-National Rural Livelihood Mission(DAY-NRLM)'. It aims at creating efficient and effective institutional platforms of the rural poor enabling them to increase household income through sustainable livelihood enhancements and improved access to financial services. The mission has set out an agenda to cover 70 to 80 million rural poor households, across 646 districts, 6910 blocks, 2.38 lakh Gram Panchayats and 6.40 lakh villages across 28 states and 7 Union Territories of the country through self-managed Self Help Groups (SHGs) and federated institutions and support them for livelihoods collectives in a period of 8-10 years. In addition, the poor would be facilitated to achieve increased access to their rights, entitlements and public services. The Mission seeks to reach out to all rural poor households in a phased manner and impact their livelihoods significantly by 2022-23. The Mission seeks to achieve its objective through investing in four core components and they are :

a) Social mobilisation and promotion of sustainable community institutions of the rural poor (SHGs, VOs, CLFs, etc.)
b) Financial inclusion of the rural poor;
c) Sustainable livelihoods; and
d) Convergence and entitlement.

NRLM Mission Statement

"To reduce poverty by enabling the poor households to access gainful self-employment and skilled wage employment opportunities, resulting in appreciable improvement in their livelihoods on a sustainable basis, through building strong grassroots institutions of the poor."

NRLM Guiding Principles

- Poor have a strong desire to come out of poverty, and they have innate capabilities

- Social mobilization and building strong institutions of the poor is critical for unleashing the innate capabilities of the poor.
- An external dedicated and sensitive support structure is required to induce the social mobilization, institution building and empowerment process.
- Facilitating knowledge dissemination, skill building, access to credit, access to marketing, and access to other livelihoods services underpins this upward mobility.

NRLM Values

The core values which guide all the activities under NRLM are as follows:

- Inclusion of the poorest, and meaningful role to the poorest in all the processes
- Transparency and accountability of all processes and institutions
- Ownership and key role of the poor and their institutions in all stages – planning, implementation and monitoring
- Community self-reliance and self-dependence

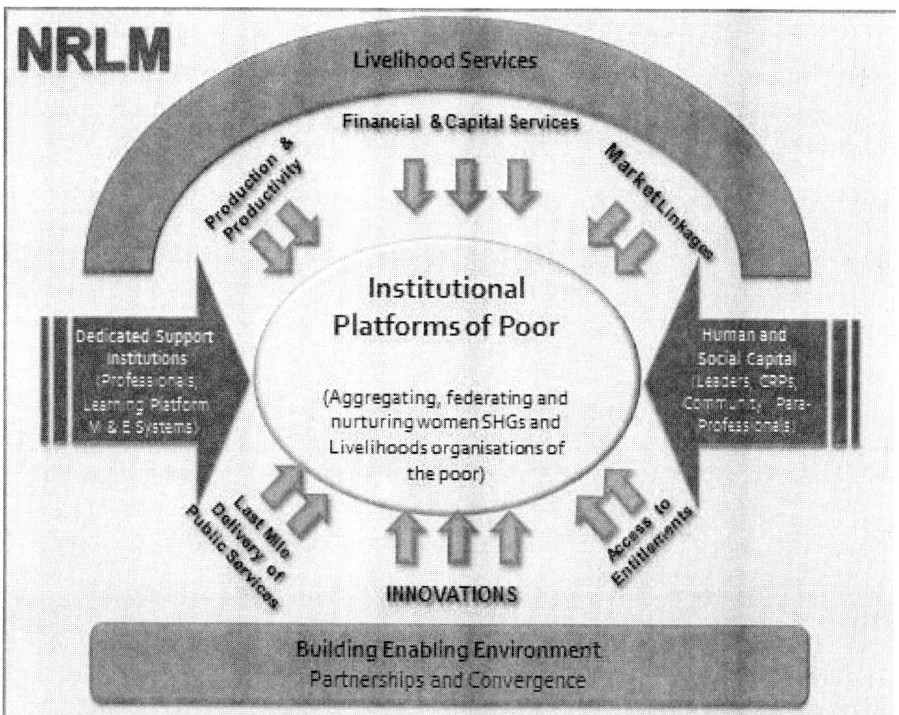

Source: NRLM Website

Support Structure

NRLM has set up dedicated sensitive support units at the National, State, district and sub-district levels, to catalyze social mobilization, build institutions, capacities and skills, facilitate financial inclusion and access to financial services, support livelihoods and convergence and partnerships with various programmes and stakeholders. These units are staffed with professionally competent and dedicated human resources.

a) At the National Level

i) NRLM Advisory Committee (NRLM-AC) ,chaired by the Union Minster of Rural Development. It is a policy making body which gives direction and set priorities, and also reviews the overall progress.

ii) NRLM Coordination Committee (NRLM-CC), chaired by Secretary, Rural Development, MoRD, oversees NRLM to ensure that its objectives are achieved in time.

iii) NRLM Empowered Committee (NRLM-EC) reviews and approves the State Perspective and Implementation Plans and Annual Action Plans and releases the funds to SRLMs.

iv) National Mission Management Unit (NMMU), is headed by the Joint Secretary/ Additional Secretary, NRLM, MoRD designated as Mission Director. The NMMU is staffed with the personnel from multidisciplinary profession.

b) At the State Level

i) **State Rural Livelihoods Mission (SRLM)** : SRLM is constituted by State Government which oversees the implementation of all NRLM related activities in the state. It is an autonomous body under the State Government, and incorporated as a society, trust or company.

ii) **State Mission Management Unit (SMMU):** SRLM implements the NRLM activities in the state through an SMMU. At the state level SRLM is headed by a full-time State Mission Director (SMD). A multidisciplinary SMMU team comprising of experts in Social Inclusion, Financial Inclusion, Livelihoods, Programme Management, Programme Support etc., supports the SMD in implementing NRLM in the state.

The major responsibilities of the SMMU include:

i) Lead all NRLM activities in the state;

ii) Drafting policies and implementation guidelines of the mission at the state level;

iii) Handholding support to district and sub-district implementation/support structures;

iv) Ensuring quality implementation of different components/thematic interventions;

v) Ensuring proper linkages with the DRDAs;

vi) Managing convergence and partnerships; and

vii) Any other function, as required.

c) At the District Level

District Mission Management Unit (DMMU): The DMMU of the SRLM is responsible for meeting NRLM objectives and implementation of NRLM activities in the district. DMMU is a multidisciplinary team which is led by District Mission Manager (DMM).

d) At the Sub-district level

Block Mission Management Unit (BMMU): The BMMU is led by a Block Mission Manager (BMM) and consisting of 3-5 spearhead teams; or a Project Facilitation Team at cluster (sub-block) level.

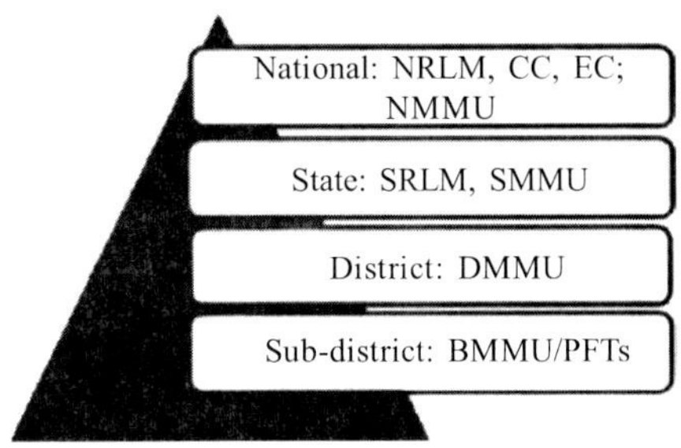

Fig: NRLM Support Structure

Implementation Phase

Year wise break up in terms of coverage of districts and blocks as envisaged by NRLM:

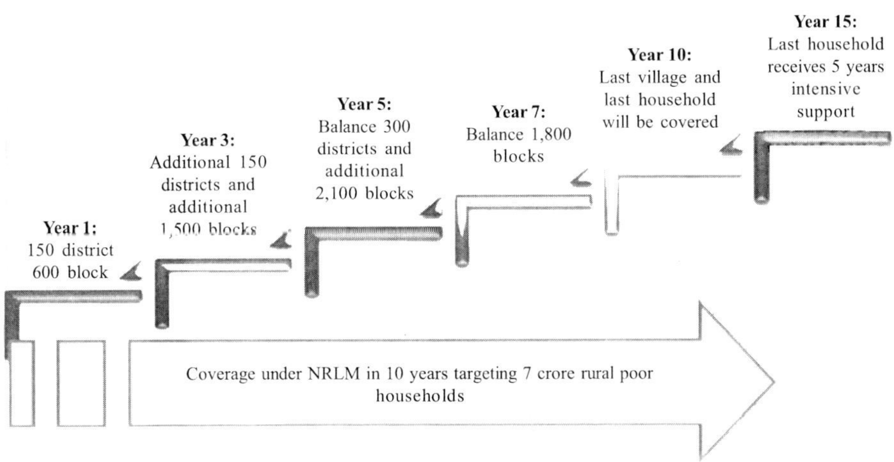

Key Features of NRLM

i) Universal Social Mobilization

NRLM will ensure that states adopt saturation approach, where at least one member from each identified rural poor household, preferably a woman, is brought under the Self Help Group (SHG) network in a time bound manner. The Mission will adopt differential strategies for social inclusion and mobilisation of all identified BPL households into functionally effective and self-managed institutions, with particular focus on inclusion of vulnerable sections like scheduled castes, scheduled tribes, disabled, landless, migrant labour, manual scavengers, victims of human trafficking, Particularly Vulnerable Tribal Groups (PVTGs), Persons with Disabilities (PwDs) and bonded labour, isolated communities and communities living in disturbed areas.

ii) Participatory Identification of Poor (PIP)

The target group under NRLM is determined by a well-defined, transparent and equitable process of participatory identification of poor, at the level of the community. All households identified as poor through the PIP process are part of NRLM Target Group and are eligible for all the benefits under the programme. The NRLM Target Group derived through the PIP is de-linked from the BPL list. The PIP exercise is carried out by the primary federation, i.e. at least 6-12 months after village entry. The list of poor identified through the PIP is vetted by the Gram Sabha and approved by the Gram Panchayat.

iii) Funds to the community as Resources in Perpetuity

NRLM provides Revolving Fund and Community Investment Fund (CIF) as Resources in Perpetuity to the institutions of the poor to strengthen their institutional and financial management capacity and build their track record to attract mainstream bank finance. The funds provided to community institutions are based on micro-planning process and it is treated as loans to individual SHG members but it is a grant to the Community institutions. Funds are disbursed to these institutions in multiple tranches based on triggers and milestones achieved and not merely their chronological age and time-period.

iv) Universal Financial Inclusion

NRLM works on both demand and supply sides of financial inclusion. On the demand side, it promotes financial literacy among the poor and provides catalytic capital to the SHGs and their federations. On the supply side, it coordinates with the financial sector and encourages use of business correspondents (and community facilitators like 'Bank Mitras') Information, Communication &

Technology (ICT) based financial technologies, business correspondents and community facilitators like 'Bank Mitras'. It also works towards universal coverage of rural poor against loss of life, health and assets.

v) Mission Mode Implementation

NRLM is designed to be implemented in a Mission mode. This implies:

a. a shift from allocation based strategy to a demand driven strategy, enabling the States to formulate their own livelihoods based poverty reduction action plans;
b. focusing on targets and time bound delivery of outputs/ outcomes;
c. continuous capacity building, imparting of requisite skills and creating linkages with livelihood sectors including the organized sectors, for the poor; and
d. close monitoring of outputs and outcomes.

vi) Implementation by the Poor

Mission is designed to mainstream the role of poor in its implementation. Key processes of NRLM are driven by the institutions of rural poor women, especially by women who have come out of poverty and whose lives have been transformed by this very process. Thus, it is a programme for the poor, of the poor and by the poor.

vii) Convergence

NRLM places a high emphasis on convergence with other programmes of the Ministry of Rural Development and other Central Ministries and programmes of State Governments for developing synergies directly and through the institutions of the poor.

viii) Partnerships with NGOs and other CSOs

NRLM has been proactively seeking partnership with Non-Governmental Organizations (NGOs) and other Civil Society Organizations (CSOs), at two levels – strategic and implementation. The partnerships are guided by NRLM's core belief and values, and mutual agreement on processes and outcomes.

ix) Linkages with PRIs

In view of the important roles of Panchayat Raj Institutions (PRIs) in local governance and development, NRLM envisages to establish formal platforms for regular consultations between Community Based Institutions (CBOs) and

PRIs, particularly at the level of Village Panchayats for exchange of mutual advice, support and sharing of resources.

x) Exit Strategy

The Mission has a clear exit strategy. It is expected that after 10 years in a block, women SHG federations take over management of their own affairs entirely and external support structure in the form of Block Mission Management Unit (BMMU) would be taken over by the internal support structure of Cluster and Block level federations supported by community professionals.

Key Components of NRLM

i) Promoting Institutions of the Poor

Strong, affinity based and quality institutions of poor starting from SHGs at village level would be the primary building block of the NRLM institutional design. NRLM would promote SHGs with exclusive women membership. The idea is to reach out to all family members through women. Strong quality institutions of the poor such as SHGs and their federations are set up on a priority basis. In addition to generic thrift and credit based community institutions and their federations, Aajeevika promotes specialized institutions like livelihoods collectives, producers' cooperatives/companies for livelihoods promotion through deriving economies of scale, backward and forward linkages. The institutions of the poor empower their members and act as instruments of knowledge and technology dissemination, and hubs of production, collectivization and commerce.

ii) Training, Capacity Building and Skill Building

A multi-pronged approach is adopted for providing continuous capacity building of the targeted families, SHGs, their federations, government functionaries, bankers, NGOs and other key stakeholders. The capacity building is aimed at providing the poor with skills to manage their institutions, link up with markets, manage their existing livelihoods and enhance their credit absorption capacity and credit worthiness. Focus is on developing and engaging community professionals and community resource persons (CRP) for capacity building of SHGs and their federations and other collectives.

iii) Revolving Fund

A Revolving Fund (of Rs. 15,000/SHG) is provided to the SHGs (where more than 70% members are from NRLM Target Group households) as an incentive to inculcate the habit of thrift and accumulation of own corpus funds to meet their small credit needs.

iv) Vulnerability Reduction Fund (VRF) and Community Investment Support Fund (CIF)

Vulnerability Reduction Fund (VRF) and Community Investment support Fund (CIF) is routed to SHGs through federations (primary and secondary levels) to support the livelihoods of the members and initiate collective activities for the members. The VRF and CIF are disbursed against Micro Credit Plans (MCP) developed by the institutions. The institutions prioritise the needs of the poorest of the poor members (or SHGs with high concentration of poorest of poor) while preparing their micro credit plan. The institutions fund these micro credit plans either through their own resources or through the Revolving Fund/ Community Investment support Fund (CIF) or through bank loans.

v) Interest Subvention

NRLM has a provision for interest subvention to all women SHGs. The districts have been classified as Category I and Category II Districts, according to the modality of interest subvention being provided.

In Category I Districts (including 82 Integrated Action Plan districts and 8 Northeast districts under the World Bank Supported NERLP) all women SHGs can avail loans up to Rs. 3 lakh per SHG at 7% rate per annum. Further, these SHGs are eligible for an additional interest subvention of 3% on prompt repayment of loan, reducing the effective rate to 4%. In the Category II districts (remaining districts), all women SHGs meeting the NRLM eligibility norms can avail loans up to 3 lakh per SHG at a 7% rate per annum.

vi) Mahila Kisan Sashaktikaran Pariyojana (MKSP)

Mahila Kisan Sashaktikaran Pariyojana (MKSP), launched in 2010-11, is a special programme for livelihood enhancement under NRLM. It is a concerted effort to recognize the role of women in agriculture and an investment is being made to enhance their capacities and increase their income to take lead role in agriculture and allied activities. It aims at ensuring household food and nutrition security of poor and poorest of poor, by securing and strengthening the primary livelihood baskets of poorest of poor households. The primary objective of MKSP is to empower women in agriculture by making systematic investments to enhance their participation and productivity in agriculture based livelihoods.

vii) Infrastructure creation and Marketing support

NRLM provides support for marketing to the institutions of the poor. The range of activities in marketing support includes market research, market intelligence, technology extension, developing backward and forward linkages, building livelihoods collectives and supporting their business plans. About 20% of the state's program outlay (25% in case of North-Eastern States and Sikkim) is earmarked for this purpose.

viii) Skills and Placement Projects

For strengthening the existing skills and creating environment for placement of rural youth in jobs, various models of partnerships with public, private, nongovernment and community organizations would be developed. A strong relationship would also be developed with industry associations and sector specific employers' associations. 25% of the central allocation under NRLM is earmarked for this purpose.

ix) Rural Self Employment Training Institutes (RSETIs)

NRLM encourages public sector banks to set up RSETIs in all districts of the country. RSETIs transform unemployed rural youth in the district into confident self–employed entrepreneurs through need-based experiential training program followed by systematic handholding support and bank linkage. Banks are involved in selection, training and post training follow-up stages. RSETIs partner with others, including the institutions of the poor, to achieve their mandate and agenda. RSETIs core offering includes its free, unique and intensive short-term residential self-employment training programs with free food and accommodation, designed specifically for rural youth. As on 31st March, 2014, 580 RSETIs were established across the country out of which 570 were functional. They have reached out to 3.39 lakh beneficiaries through their training programmes. Of the 3.39 lakh beneficiaries, 2.92 lakh have set up enterprises.

x) Innovations

Aajeevika believes that successful innovations can reduce the learning curve for poverty eradication by showing a different pathway out of poverty. 5% of the Central allocation is therefore, earmarked for innovations. Those innovations, which have the potential for reaching out specifically to the poorest or for reaching out to the largest number of poor and having maximum impact with limited resources, would be preferred and supported.

xi) Sensitive Support Structures

NRLM has set up sensitive and dedicated support structures at the National, State, district and sub-district levels. These support structures are staffed with dedicated professionals. The support structures form and nurture the institutions of the poor. NRLM has earmarked 5% of the allocation as administrative costs.

Only the costs of national, state and district support structures are covered in this provision. The costs incurred on professional support costs at the block and sub-block levels are considered as programme costs and not as administrative costs. NRLM is implementing World Bank supported National Rural Livelihoods Project (NRLP) to professionalize NRLM; to provide technical support to States; and to develop large sized proof of concept of NRLM processes in 400 select blocks across 13 States.

Implementation Strategy

NRLM is a process-intensive community driven large scale poverty reduction program. It has adopted a phased implementation approach for reaching out to all villages in all blocks of the country.

Implementation at Block Level

NRLM intends to work in a block for a period of ten years till community federations take responsibility of implementation. A typical block having about 13,500 (90% of total poor) mobilisable poor households spread over 100-120 villages is divided into 4 clusters of 30 villages each. In a typical intensive block, the first 3 years are spent in building the organisations of the poor by mobilising them into SHGs, Federations at Village, Cluster level and Block level. Funds flow to the community institutions over the first 4-5 years. The middle years, years 3-6, are invested in deepening the activities and addition of various layers such as health, nutrition, interventions for Persons with Disability (PwD), etc. Last 4 years is essentially a maintenance and withdrawal phase where the community institutions graduate to self reliance and self-sustainability. Implementation in the blocks is being done in four ways - a) Resource Blocks with the support from National Resource Organization(s) (NRO) [5-6% blocks in a state]; b) Intensive Blocks implemented with SRLM staff and internal community resource persons and the CRPs generated in resource blocks; c) Partnership Blocks with the support from local community federations and NGO partners; and d) Non-intensive Blocks are the remaining blocks in the state which are not taken up for implementation in the initial phase.

i) **Resource Blocks:** It is envisaged that about 5- 6% of the blocks in a state would be taken up as resource blocks. These blocks would be model blocks where all the key strategies of NRLM would be piloted. These blocks would create a 'proof of concept' for other blocks to adopt and replicate. The social capital expected to be generated in the resource blocks would support the intensive blocks in implementation. A National Resource Organisation (NRO) supports the states in implementation in the resource blocks. A NRO is a SRLM which has experience in successfully implementing NRLM protocols on a large scale. The NRO deputes a State Anchor Person to SRLM to anchor implementation. A Project Resource Person (PRP) is seconded to each cluster in the resource block to facilitate implementation on the ground. External Community Resource Persons in teams of 5 each from NRO take-up mobilisation, formation of institutions of the poor and train the institutions in the block. NRO also nurtures social capital–active women, internal CRPs, bookkeepers and other community activists from the resource blocks to support the institutions in the resource block as well as other blocks. NRO also implements livelihood promotion and layering activities in the block.

ii) **Intensive Blocks:** SRLMs directly implement in other intensive blocks where they enter with their own staff at block level, and take support of the internal resources from the resource blocks. CRPs are chosen from the resource blocks to accelerate implementation in these blocks. The protocols of implementation followed in the resource blocks would be adopted in these blocks as well.

iii) **Partnership Blocks:** SRLMs take up implementation in blocks where there is pre-existing significant mobilization of poor women into SHGs as partnership blocks in partnership with Community Federations and the NGOs working in these blocks. NRLM has developed Partnership Guidelines to identify and work with NGOs and CBOs. NGOs that have significant presence (done 80% mobilization or promoted a SHG federation) in a block are identified as partner NGOs. These NGOs are expected to follow NRLM's implementing protocols and processes in the blocks.

iv) **Non-intensive Blocks:** The remaining blocks in a state (other than resource, intensive and partnership blocks) are non-intensive blocks. NRLM strengthens existing SHGs in these blocks with some capacity building and limited financial assistance. No new mobilisation would be done in these blocks. Over time, as NRLM implementation progresses, these blocks also would come into the intensive-fold.

Aajeevika Skills

Aajeevika Skills is the skill and placement initiative of the Ministry of Rural development, Government of India (MoRD). It is a part of the National Rural Livelihood Mission (NRLM). It evolved out of the need to diversify incomes of the rural poor and to cater to the occupational aspirations of their youth. It aims to skill rural youth who are poor and provide them with jobs with regular monthly wages at or above the minimum wages. Aajeevika Skills is critical to the national skill agenda and to the 430 million (Census 2011) young people in the country in the age group of 15-35 which is closed to 70% of whom live in rural areas. Aajeevika Skills has its origin in the 'Special Project' component of the Swarnajayanti Gram Swarozgar Yojana (SGSY). The programme was revisited in the light of the new skills framework of the country and restructured under NRLM as 'Aajeevika Skills'.

National Rural Livelihoods Mission
Cumulative Progress up to Februrary, 2014 (since inception of NRLM)

S.No.	States	Intensive blocks Covered	Villages Covered	SHGs Covered	VOS Formed	Revolving Fund Provided		Community Investment Fund Period	
						No of SHGs	(Amount in Rs. Lakh)	No. of SHGs	Rs. Lakh (Amount in Rs. Lakh)
1.	Assam	44	7762	41412	2474	6437	958.8	0	0
2.	Bihar	179	9434	117504	7039	70988	10223.5	71455	15461
3.	Chattisgarh	17	2468	12735	173	3742	561.3	629	345.95
4.	Gujarat	20	1112	15092	198	6154	437.69	39	19.5
5.	Jharkhand	23	1117	7343	126	2997	449.5	2152	1075.9
6.	Karnataka	20	500	192	0	2400	360	0	0
7.	Madhya Pradesh	98	10154	57174	5322	41153	5709.95	27817	27488
8.	Maharashtra	36	1882	10067	424	2950	348.08	365	202.05
9.	Odisha	58	9347	93249	1098	9604	1049.49	28738	10502.2
10.	Rajasthan	32	3074	18161	870	9585	1344.15	3189	3206.19
11.	Tamil Nadu	180	6903	305395	8276	0	0	1782	891
12.	Uttar Pradesh	5	0	2502	0	190	11.4	0	0
13.	West Bengal	32	3243	46796	729	21533	2584	0	0
14.	Andhra Pradesh	326	44055	1060459	44055	516699	45775	219156	97350
15.	Kerala	152	1453	223883	19477	0	0	0	0
16.	Haryana	4	117	733	6	291	43.8	0	0
17.	Himachal Pradesh	0	0	0	0	0	0	0	0
18.	Jammu & Kashmir	4	170	1808	179	1271	188.36	0	0
19.	Punjab	8	144	395	0	167	22.94	45	0
20.	Uttarakhand	0	274	162	0	0	0	0	0
21.	Arunachal Pradesh	0	9	0	0	0	0	0	0
22.	Meghalaya	0	0	0	0	0	0	0	0
23.	Mizoram	0	0	0	0	0	0	0	0
24.	Nagaland	ft	143	870	17	0	0	0	0
25.	Tripura	6	45	300	0	0	0	0	0
	Total	1253	103397	2017112	90564	696161	54603	355367	156542

Source: Ministry of Rural Development (MoRD), Government of India, Annual Report 2013-14

Key Features of Aajeevika Skills

i) Placement linked, market driven training for 3 months to 12 months to rural poor youth between the age of 18-35 with 75% assured placement with facility for providing customized residential and non-residential training.

ii) Social Inclusion through Mandatory 33% candidates to be women in every project. 50% of target candidates from SC / ST families (nationally, in each

State it will vary depending on their percentage share in population). 15%to belong to Minorities and 3% may be allotted to differently-abled persons.

iii) Regional inclusion through:

- **Himayat:** A special scheme for the youth (rural & urban) of Jammu & Kashmir.
- **Roshni:** A special initiative for the rural youth of poor families in 27 Left-wing Extremist (LWE) districts across nine States of Northeast Region.

iv) Separate modules on trade specific skills, English, Soft skills, Information Technology (IT), onthe job training (OJT) as well as Finishing and work readiness Certificates given to Trainees on completion of training.

v) Food, uniform and transport support given to candidates during training.

vi) Mandatory placement in job with salary above minimum wages. Post Placement Support given to candidates in the form of financial assistance, migration support centre and alumni support.

vii) Transparency and accountability through:

a) Geo-tagged, time-stamped, biometric attendance based on unique ID for trainers and trainees.

b) Online check of inventory available for training in every Training Centre.

c) CCTV and audio recording of all classroom and lab sessions.

d) Mapping of Project Implementing Agencies on the Public Financial Management System for tracking payments.

e) Reporting of performance on real-time basis.

viii) Concurrent monitoring process for reliability and validity of the monitoring process.

ix) Independent mechanisms for project appraisal and project monitoring, apart from State level monitoring, through designated Technical Support Agencies, i.e. the National Institute of Rural Development and Panchayat Raj and the NABCONS.

Programme Funding

Aajeevika Skills is a Centrally Sponsored Scheme (CSS) and follows the funding pattern as given below:

i) For all States (excluding North-east States) - 75% by Central Government 25% by State Government

ii) North-east States - 90% by Central Government 10% by State Government.

Aajeevika Skills mandates two types of training in every course, i.e. a Generic Training on Soft Skills, English and Information Technology, and Trade Specific Skills. Such training can be structured for different duration, i.e. for 3 months, 6 months, 9 months, and 12 months. The training plan can also provide On-the-Job Training (OJT) as part of the training module, which cannot exceed 30 days for a 3-month course, 60 days for a 6-month course, 90 days for a 9-month course. The training content is currently required to be aligned with National Council for Vocational Training (NCVT) or Sector Skill Council (SSC) Standards. Aajeevika Skills mandates independent third party certification of every trainee to assess the skill, knowledge and attitude of each trainee. Such third party certification shall be undertaken by the PIAs only through those agencies empanelled by NCVT or Sector Skill Councils.

Progress of NRLM during Financial Year 2019-20

Physical Progress

DAY-NRLM have reached all 28 States and 7 Union Territories. As of October, 2019, a total of 5894 blocks were covered under intensive block strategy and out of which 646 blocks were taken up in during FY 2019-20. More than 6.47 crore households are mobilised in to 58.66 lakh SHGs and out of which 6.66 lakh SHGs are formed during this financial year. The SHGs have federated into 3.33 lakh Village Organisations (VOs), which are in turn federated into 29,653 Cluster Level Federation (CLFs). Revolving Fund @ Rs10,000 to Rs.15,000/- per SHG) to the tune Rs. 2839.99 crore have been provided to 20.28 lakh SHGs and out of which 3 lakh SHGs to the tune of Rs.480 crore have received RF during this financial year. Also, the Mission has provided a total of Rs. 5495 crore as Community Investment Fund (CIF) to 10.34 lakh SHGs and out of which Rs. 1019.81 crore was provided to 1.22 lakh SHGs during the financial year. The of physical progress of DAY-NRLM is presented below in the tables.

Table : NRLM Footprint : Progress in All Intesive Blocks

S. No	Particulars	Progress up to Mar* 19	Progress During 2019-20 (Upto Oct* 19)	Cummulative Progress (Up to Oct* 10)
1.	States	28	-	28
2.	Union Territories transited	7	-	7
3.	Districts entered	622	24	646
4.	Intensive block under implementation	5246	648	5894
5.	Househoulds covered (in lakhs)	592.35	54.73	647.08
6.	SHGs promoted (in lakhs)	52.00	6.66	58.66
7.	VOs promoted (in lakhs)	2.95	0.38	3.33
8.	CLF promoted	27150	2503	29653
9.	SHGs provided RF (in lakhs)	17.28	3.00	20.28
10.	SHGs provided CIF (in lakh)	9.12	1.22	10.34
11.	Amount of RF disbursed (in lakh)	2359.06	480.93	2839.99
12.	Amount of CIF disbursed (in lakh)	4474.91	1019.81	5494.72

Source: Annual Report (2019-20), Ministry Development, Government of India

Table : Deendayal Antyodaya Yojana - National Rural Livelihoods Mission (DAY-NRLM) Physical Progress under DAY-NRLM during 2019-20 till October, 2019

S. No.	States	Households Group	Self Help Organisation	Village SHGs provided RF	No. of provided CIF	No. of SHGs
1.	Andhra Pradesh	0	0	0	0	0
2.	Assam	324549	30633	5047	35879	14148
3.	Bihar	180272	15134	0	613	120
4.	Chhattisgarh	209320	18951	909	11722	3928
5.	Gujarat	114826	11079	433	2800	1129
6.	Jharkhand	447097	31121	3247	11457	205
7.	Karnataka	266535	18944	1840	385	3358
8.	Kerala	15847	1220	0	31	0
9.	Madhya Pradesh	275253	25536	2352	15134	1403
10.	Maharashtra	1000368	113585	3292	24571	4495
11.	Odisha	265331	25338	1924	62	6972
12.	Rajasthan	331361	29987	1020	10650	5592
13.	Tamil Nadu	81248	7326	2	784	2409
14.	Telangana	0	0	0	0	0
15.	Uttar Pradesh	1157580	104167	2712	20646	14348
16.	West Bengal	1833831	184514	6290	29856	9128
17.	Haryana	84244	7830	365	5102	1818
18.	Himachal Pradesh	16184	2019	20	692	121
19.	Jammu & Kashmir	12480	1424	333	2679	2407
20.	Punjab	46257	4388	218	1618	457
21.	Uttarakhand	45640	5849	410	2893	1006
22.	Arunachal Pradesh	2679	303	87	359	210
23.	Manipur	3926	351	30	372	202
24.	Meghalaya	43673	4460	287	2744	594

25.	Mizoram	4450	495	39	434	553
26.	Nagaland	14977	1710	36	579	37
27.	Sikim	147	15	16	73	46
28.	Tripura	19969	2368	116	1439	465
29	Andaman	448	46	0	4	0
30.	Dada & Nagar Haveli	0	0	0	0	0
31.	Daman & DIU	257	27	0	0	0
32.	Goa	851	66	0	22	0
33.	Lakshadweep	0	0	0	0	0
34.	Puducherry	688	52	0	0	0

Source : Annual Report (2019-20), Ministry of Rural Development, Government of India

Financial Progress

The financial inclusion is a key component of the Mission. The objective is to make rural women and their households the preferred clients of the banking system. Up to October, 2019, 21.43 lakh SHGs have been credit linked and bank have disbursed more than Rs.33,855 crore to SHGs. The performance of SHG bank linkage in the last 6 years has been presented below.

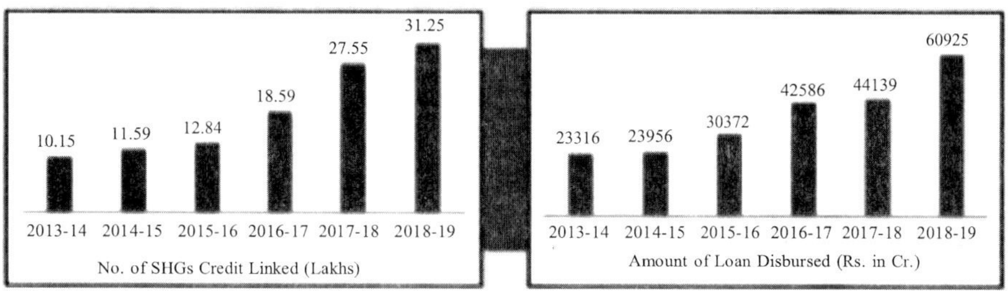

A snapshot of performance in SHG bank linkage over last 6 years

Suggested Readings and References

1. Annual Reports (2008 to 2011). Ministry of Rural Development, Government of India.
2. Annual Reports (2006-20014). National Institute of Rural Development and Panchayat Raj, Governent of India.
3. Reddy, A.A. (1993). Extension Education, Sree lakshmi Press, Bapatla.
4. Dhama, O.P. and Bhatnagar, O.P. (2007). Education and Communication forDevelopment. Oxford and IBH Pub.Co.Pvt. Ltd.
5. Mathialagan, P. (2007). Textbook of Animal Husbandry and Livestock Extension, International Book Distributing Co. 7, Meerabai Marg, Lucknow, India.
6. Singh, Katar (1999). Rural Development: Principles, Policies and Management, Second Edition, New Delhi, Sage Publications.

7. Ray, G.L. (2006). Extension Communication and Management, New Delhi, Kalyani Publishers.
8. Dey, S.K. (1964). Community Development: A Bird's Eye View, Asia Publishing House, New Delhi.
9. Rural Development - Some Facets, (ed.) NIRD, Hyderabad – 1979.
10. Five Year Plans (1st -10th), Planning Commission, Government of India, New Delhi.
11. NIRD, Fifty Years of Rural Development in India (1998). NIRD, Hyderabad.
12. Desai, Vasant (2009). Rural Development in India, Himalaya Publishing House, Mumbai.
13. Mahajan, R.K. (1991). Integrated Rural Development Programme, Concept Publishing Company, New Delhi.
14. Sharma, K.R.G. (2008). Veterinary Extension Education, BSPBS Publications, Hyderabad, Hyderabad.
15. Mehta, Shiv R. (1984). Rural Development Policies and Programmes, Sage Publications.
16. Arora, R.C. (1979). Integrated Rural Development, New Delhi: S.Chand and Company Limited.
17. Lawania, Vinod Kumar (1992). Rural Development in India. New Delhi: Ashish Publishing.
18. Ray, G.L. (2001). Extension, Communication and Management, 4th Edition, Naya Prokash, Calcutta.
19. Supe S.V. (1987). An Introduction to Extension Education, Oxford and IBH Publishing Co. Pvt. Ltd. New Delhi.

18

Mahatma Gandhi National Rural Employment Guarantee Act (MGNREGA)

1. Rationale of the Programme
2. History of Rural Wage Employment Programmes in India
3. Objectives of the Programme
4. Salient features of the Act
5. Key Achievements since inception
6. Suggested Readings and References

Mahatma Gandhi National Rural Employment Guarantee Act (MGNREGA)

Rationale of the Programme

A vast majority of the poor people in rural areas of the country depend mainly on the wages they earn through unskilled labour. They are often on threshold levels of subsistence and are vulnerable to the possibility of sinking from transient to chronic poverty, in the event of inadequate labour demand or in the face of unpredictable crises that may be general in nature like natural disaster or personal like ill-health, all of which adversely impact their employment opportunities. In a context of poverty & unemployment, wage employment programmes provide unskilled manual workers with short-term employment. The wage employment programmes provide income transfers to poor households during critical times and so also enable consumption smoothing specially during slack agricultural seasons or years. Durable assets created under these programmes have the potential to generate sustainable livelihood.

History of Rural Wage Employment Programmes in India

The need to evolve a mechanism to supplement existing livelihood sources in rural areas was recognised early in development planning in India. The Government has implemented wage employment programmes that offered wage employment on public works on minimum wages. The wage employment programmes started as pilot projects in the form of Rural Manpower Programme (RMP) [1960-61], Crash Scheme for Rural employment (CRSE) [1971-72], Drought Prone Area Programme was started as Rural work Programme (RWP)[1972], Small Farmers Development Agency (SFDA), Marginal Farmers & Agricultural Labour Scheme (MF&AL) to the poorest of the poor. These experiments were translated into a full-fledged wage-employment programme in 1977 in the form of Food for Work Programme (FWP). In 1980's this programme was further streamlined into the National Rural Employment Programme (NREP) and Rural Landless Employment Guarantee Programme (RLEGP), Jawahar Rozgar Yojana (JRY1993-94) and Employment Assurance Scheme (EAS). The Jawahar Rozgar Yojana (JRY) was merged with Jawahar Gram Samridhi Yojana (JGSY) from 1999-2000 and was made a rural infrastructure programme. The programme was merged with Sampoorna Grameen Rozgar Yojana during the year 2001-02 and National Food for Work (NFFWP, 2005). These wage employment programmes implemented by State Governments with Central assistance were self-targeting and the objective was to provide enhance livelihood security, specially of those dependent on casual manual labour. At the State Level, the Govt. of Maharashtra formulated the

Maharashtra Employment Guarantee Scheme and Maharashtra Employment Guarantee Act, 1977 to provide wage employment to those who demanded it.

Based on the experience of these programmes, National Rural Employment Guarantee Act(NREGA) was enacted on 5th September, 2005 and came into force w.e.f. 2nd February, 2006. On 31st December, 2009, the Act was renamed by an Amendment as the Mahatma Gandhi National Rural Employment Guarantee Act, 2005. It is now commonly referred as MGNREGA.

In the first phase, NREGA was implemented in 200 most backward districts with effect from February 2, 2006 and was extended subsequently to additional 113 and 17 districts with effect from April 1st 2007 and May 15th 2007, respectively. The remaining districts were included under the Act with effect from April 1, 2008. Thus, the Act now covers all the rural districts (644) of the country. The MGNREGA was enacted to reinforce the commitment towards livelihood security in rural areas. This Employment Guarantee Act is the most significant legislation in many ways. For the first time, rural communities have been given not just a development programme but a regime of rights. The MGNREGA is a legal guarantee that people can use to secure their entitlement of wage employment. It holds the Government responsible for making this employment available to the people. It is a legal instrument in the hands of the poor based on the demand of the workers. The Rights-based design of MGNREGA has a genesis in the preceding wage employment programmes. Almost all the rights related features of MGNREGA are inherited from previous wage employment programme launched by Government of India and from the rights based programme of Maharashtra Employment Guarantee Act 1977.

Objectives of the Programme

The core objectives of the programme are:

i) Providing not less than one hundred days of unskilled manual work as a guaranteed employment in a financial year to every household in rural areas as per demand, resulting in creation of productive assets of prescribed quality and durability.

ii) Strengthening the livelihood resource base of the poor;

iii) Proactively ensuring social inclusion and

iv) Strengthening Panchayati Raj Institutions

Salient Features of the Act

i) **Rights based Framework:** For adult members of a rural household willing to do unskilled manual work.

ii) **Time bound Guarantee:** 15 days for provision of employment, else unemployment allowance to be paid. Upto 100 days of work in a financial year per household, depending on the actual demand.

iii) **Labour Intensive Works:** 60:40 wage and material ratio for permissible works at the Gram Panchayat; no contractors/machinery

iv) **Decentralized Planning:** Gram Sabhas to recommend works
At least 50% of works by Gram Panchayats for execution
Principal role of PRIs in planning, implementation and monitoring

v) **Work site facilities:** Crèche, drinking water, first aid and shade provided at worksites

vi) **Women empowerment:** At least one-third of beneficiaries should be women

vii) **Transparency & Accountability:** Proactive disclosure through wall writings, citizen information boards and MIS and Social Audits

viii) **Funding:** 100% cost towards unskilled wages and 75% towards skilled, semi-skilled and material is borne by Central Government and 25 % of skilled, semi-skilled and material costs is contributed by States. In addition 6% administrative expenses are borne by the Centre for effective implementation of the Act.

ix) **Permissible work:** Water conservation, Drought proofing (including plantation and afforestation) Irrigation canals, Minor irrigation, horticulture and land development on the land of SC/ST/-BPL/IAY and land reform beneficiaries, Renovation of traditional water bodies, Flood protection, Land development, Rural connectivity, Any other work that may be notified by the Central Government in consultation with the State Government.

Performance during the financial year 2019-20 (till 17th December, 2019)

The outcomes of the programme implementation in the financial year 2019-20 (till 17th December, 2019) are as follows:

Employment Generated : in 2019-20, 4.51 crore households were provided employment and 177.47 crore person-days of employment generated.

Increasing outreach to the poor and marginalised: Self targeting in nature, the programme had high work participation from the marginalised groups like SC/ST (38%), women (56%).

Strengthening Natural Resource Base: In 2019-20, 17 lakh works related to natural resources management costing approximately Rs. 27, 206.96 crore (67% of the total cost) was taken up.

Financial Inclusion of the Poor: With a view to universalize the system of wage payments through institutional accounts, it has been recommended to all States to disburse wages through post office and Bank Accounts. Around 11.54 crore banks and post office accounts have been reopened on NREGASoft for disbursement of wages.

The Mahatma Gandhi National Rural Employment Guarantee Act (MGNREGA) Employment generated during 2019-20 as on 17-12-2019

S.No	State	HH Issued job cards	No. of HH Provided Employment	No of Person days generated					Hills completed 100 days of employment
				SCs	STs	Others	Total	Women	
1.	Andhra Pradesh	89.06	37.93	340.18	172.36	1064.98	1577.52	393.74	1.65
2.	Arunachal Pradesh	2.29	1.31	0.04	37.97	5.55	43.56	18.02	0.00
3.	Assam	46.88	14.67	18.76	72.68	295.10	386.54	159.62	0.06
4.	Bihar	157.68	23.43	149.91	12.91	708.75	871.57	485.58	0.06
5.	Chhattisgarh	37.71	19.34	76.57	262.02	445.11	783.70	397.81	0.73
6.	Goa	0.33	0.00	0.00	0.01	0.02	0.03	0.02	0.00
7.	Gujarat	37.58	6.33	13.83	82.40	138.81	235.04	105.82	0.07
8.	Haryana	9.46	1.86	23.09	0.00	27.39	50.48	25.92	0.01
9.	Himachal Pradesh	12.53	4.34	46.16	20.80	104.09	171.06	106.30	0.23
10.	Jammu and Kashmir	12.07	2.71	5.44	25.28	64.90	95.62	32.60	0.01
11.	Jharkhand	44.33	11.78	50.09	119.71	305.91	475.70	195.14	0.16
12.	Karnataka	61.64	19.83	128.11	83.92	630.88	842.90	414.13	0.31
13.	Kerala	36.06	13.24	79.93	35.97	393.26	509.16	454.79	0.28
14.	Madhya Pradesh	68.29	29.77	194.88	442.98	712.81	1350.66	509.17	0.43
15.	Maharashtra	85.12	12.18	48.46	76.88	301.77	427.11	188.87	0.74
16.	Manipur	5.70	5.24	5.03	66.07	88.56	159.66	77.26	0.00
17.	Meghalaya	5.74	4.20	0.79	178.29	7.31	186.39	91.10	0.24
18.	Mizoram	1.98	2.02	0.03	149.14	0.94	150.11	57.74	0.00
19.	Nagaland	4.34	3.72	0.54	79.10	3.09	82.73	29.19	0.00
20.	Odisha	66.70	18.27	97.90	227.63	304.47	630.00	269.15	0.34
21.	Punjab	16.59	6.56	118.82	0.08	51.29	170.19	100.20	0.03
22.	Rajasthan	102.16	50.15	529.30	574.96	1387.77	2492.03	1666.45	2.45
23.	Sikkim	0.83	0.51	0.73	6.83	10.58	18.14	9.31	0.01
24.	Tamil Nadu	82.38	53.52	550.42	22.23	1433.44	2006.08	1726.75	0.45
25.	Telangana	55.35	23.47	214.10	174.64	586.67	975.41	604.80	1.14
26.	Tripura	6.26	5.50	34.83	129.39	75.55	239.76	111.75	0.18
27.	Uttar Pradesh	163.27	44.67	495.61	16.23	1166.76	1678.59	572.12	0.37
28.	Uttarakhand	10.62	3.28	18.15	4.08	83.97	106.20	57.39	0.07
29.	West Bengal	120.89	32.35	316.56	100.18	687.63	1104.36	533.55	0.52
30.	Andaman and Nicobar	0.35	0.05	0.00	0.00	1.41	1.41	0.86	0.00
31.	Dadra & Nagar Haveli	0.04	0.00	0.00	0.00	0.00	0.00	0.00	0.00
32.	Daman & Diu	0.00	0.00	0.00	0.00	0.00	0.00	0.00	0.00
33.	Lakshadweep	0.08	0.00	0.00	0.02	0.00	0.02	0.00	0.00
34.	Puducherry	0.07	0.36	2.02	0.01	3.94	5.97	5.18	0.00
	Total	1344.96	452.59	3560.26	3174.74	11092.68	17827.69	9946.33	10.52

Source : Annual Report, 2019-20, Ministry of Rural Development

Suggested Readings and References

1. Annual Reports (2005-2011). Ministry of Rural Development, Government of India,
2. Annual Reports (2005-2014). National Institute of Rural Development and Panchayat Raj, Governent of India.
3. Dhama, O.P. and Bhatnagar, O.P. (2007). Education and Communication forDevelopment. Oxford and IBH Pub.Co.Pvt. Ltd.
4. Mathialagan, P. (2007). Textbook of Animal Husbandry and Livestock Extension, International Book Distributing Co. 7, Meerabai Marg, Lucknow, India.
5. Ray, G.L. (2006). Extension Communication and Management, New Delhi, Kalyani Publishers.
6. Five Year Plans (1st -10th), Planning Commission, Government of India, New Delhi.
7. Desai, Vasant (2009). Rural Development in India, Himalaya Publishing House, Mumbai.
8. Sharma, K.R.G. (2008). Veterinary Extension Education, BSPBS Publications, Hyderabad, Hyderabad.
9. Ambily, A.S. (2016). A study on Mahatma Gandhi National Rural Employment Guarantee Act and Women Empowerment.

19

Agricultural Technology Management Agency (ATMA)

1. Salient Features of ATMA
2. Organizational Structure of ATMA
3. Governing Body (GB) and Management Committee (MC)
   a) Composition of ATMA Governing Board (GB)
   b) Functions of ATMA Governing Board
   c) ATMA Management Committee (MC)
   d) Functions of Management Committee (MC)
4. Farm Information and Advisory Centre (FIAC) at Block Level
5. Block Technology Team (BTT)
   a) Composition of BTT
   b) Functions of Block Technology Team (BTT)
6. Farmer Advisory Committee (FAC)
   a) Functions of FACs
7. State Agricultural Management and Extension Training Institute (SAMETI)
   a) Functions of SAMETI
   b) State Level Inter -Departmental Working Group (IDWG)
   c) Composition:
   d) Functions of IDWG
8. Process Intervention
   a) Strategic Research and Extension Plan (SREP)
   b) State Extension Work Plan (SEWP)
   c) Cafeteria of Activities
9. Suggested Readings and References

Agriculture Technology Management Agency (ATMA)

Extension Reforms were introduced during 2005-06 by the Department of Agriculture & Cooperation (DAC), Ministry of Agriculture, Government of India as a major intervention in addressing the constraints as observed in T & V and post T & V system by making the extension system farmer driven and farmer accountable through process and institutional reforms mechanism. The institutional mechanism in the form of Agricultural Technology Management Agency (ATMA) at district level was pilot tested under Innovations in Technology Dissemination (ITD) component of National Agricultural

Technology Project (NATP) in seven states viz. Andhra Pradesh, Bihar, Himachal Pradesh, Jharkhand, Maharashtra, Orissa and Punjab covering 4 districts in each State from 1998 to 2004. The key features of reforms are:

i) New institutional arrangements – Decentralized decision making
ii) Convergence of line departments – gap filling mode
iii) Multi agency extension strategies – encourage private sector (minimum 10% allocation)
iv) Broad-based extension delivery through Farming Systems Approach (FSA)
v) Group approach to extension through Farmers Organizations(FOs) and Commodity Interest Groups (CIGs)
vi) Gender concerns-Minimum 30% allocation
vii) Sustainability of extension services – Minimum 10% beneficiary contribution
viii) Bottom-up planning

Salient Features of ATMA

ATMA is registered body under the "Societies Registration Act of 1860" that has considerable operational flexibility. It represents various stakeholders, including farmers, in project planning and implementation under the guidance of the National Institute of Agricultural Extension Management (MANAGE), Hyderabad. ATMA involves in agricultural activities for sustainable agricultural development in the district. It is a focal point for integrating Research and Extension activities and decentralizing day-to-day management of Agricultural Extension System. It operates under the guidance of a Governing Board (GB) that determines program priorities and assesses program impact. The executive head of ATMA is known as the Project Director (PD) and reports directly to the ATMA Governing Board. One of the most important activities undertaken by ATMA is to prepare Strategic Research and Extension Plan (SREP), which consist of detailed information about agriculture and allied sectors in the district. The purpose of preparation of

SREP is to identify research and extension needs of the district. This helps in undertaking only those extension activities which are needed by farmers in the district. SREP is prepared with full participation of farmers and their representatives at different level. Technical officers of agriculture and allied departments as well as from KVKs and other research institutions fully participate in preparation of SREPs.

The ATMA at district level would be increasingly responsible for all the technology dissemination activities at the district level. It would have linkage with all the line departments, research organizations, non-governmental organizations and agencies associated with agricultural development in the district. Research and Extension units within the districts such as Zonal Research Stations (ZRS) or substations, Krishi Vigyan Kendras (KVKs) and the key line Departments of Agriculture, Animal Husbandry, Horticulture and Fisheries etc. would become constituent members of ATMA. Each Research-Extension (R-E) unit would retain its institutional identity and affiliation but programmes and procedures concerning district-wise R-E activities would be determined by ATMA Governing Board to be implemented by its Management Committee (AMC). As a society, it would be able to receive and expend funds, entering into contracts & agreements and maintaining revolving accounts that can be used to collect fees and thereby recovering operating cost.

Illustration of Organizational Structure of ATMA

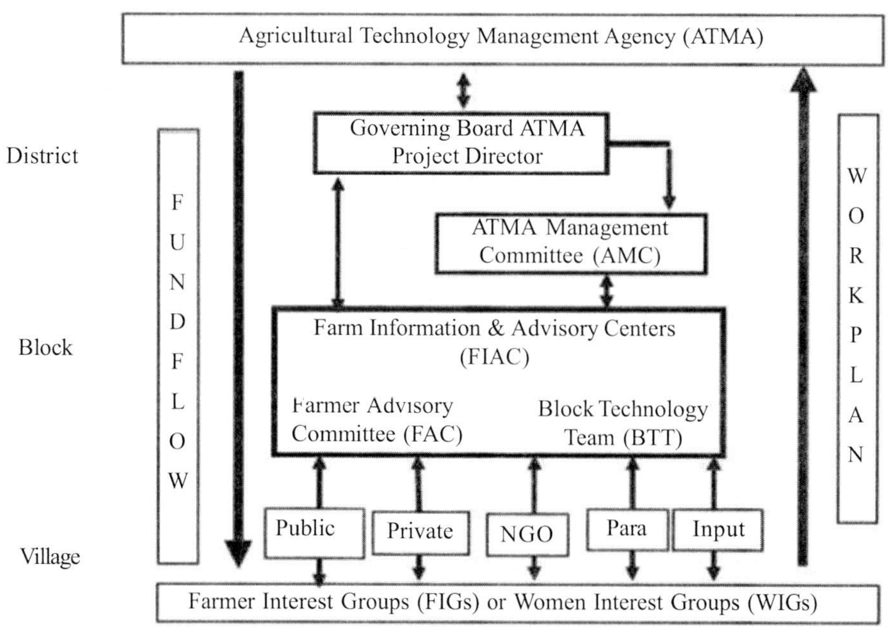

ATMA is a unique district level institution, which caters to activities in agriculture and allied departments adopting a Farming Systems Approach. It can receive funds directly from Government of India/States, Membership fees, beneficiaries contribution etc. Local research and extension priorities are set through Strategic Research and Extension Plans (SREPs) which are developed by using participatory methodologies such as Participatory Rural Appraisal (PRA). In order to manage programme implementation at block level and below, ATMA has established a Farm Information and Advisory Centre (FIAC) at each block in the district. In effect, the FIACs act as extension planning and operational arm of ATMA. These are supported by two groups; one is a group of technical officers at block derived from different functional areas termed as Block Technology Team (BTT) whereas another is a Farmers Advisory Committee (FAC) which is a body exclusively of farmers. While BTT develops the Block Action Plans (BAPs) in light of the SREP and is responsible for its implementation, the FAC plays a more proactive role by scrutinizing, improving and approving BAPs, before these are referred to the ATMA GB for its final approval. Commodity Interest Groups (CIGs) are promoted at block/village level to make the technology generation/dissemination farmer driven and farmer accountable. These Village level CIGs are ultimately federated at block/district level and represented in FACs and GB. In order to address the extension needs of these groups, ATMA will establish close linkages with various players operating at cutting edge level viz. public, private, NGOs, Para extension workers, input dealers, etc. In order to provide needed Human Resource Development support (HRD) in innovative areas of extension delivery a State Agricultural Management and Extension Training Institute (SAMETI) has been established either by strengthening one of the existing apex training institute in the state or by creating a new SAMETI in a State Agricultural University (SAU). Project activities, at state level are closely monitored by an Inter-Departmental Working Group (IDWG) functioning under the Chairmanship of Agriculture Production Commissioner or Secretary (Agriculture) of the state. A Project Implementation Cell with State Nodal Officer (SNO) is created at the State Headquarter in the Department of Agriculture to provide support to the IDWG.

Governing Body (GB) and Management Committee (MC)

ATMA is supported by Governing Board (GB) and Management Committee (MC). The Governing Board is a policy making body and provide guidance as well as review the progress and functioning of the ATMA. The Management Committee would be responsible for planning and executing the day-to-day activities of ATMA.

Composition of ATMA Governing Board (GB)

Composition of ATMA Governing Body is as follows:

1.	District Magistrate / Collector	Chairman
2.	Chief Executive Officer (CEO) Chief Development Officer (CDO)	Vice-Chairman
3.	Joint Director / Deputy Director (Agri.) & allied departments	Member
4.	A representative from ZRS/ Krishi Vigyan Kendra	Member
5.	One Farmer representative	Member
6.	One Livestock Producer	Member
7.	One Horticulture Farmer	Member
8.	Representative of Women Farmers Interest Group	Member
9.	One SC / ST farmer representative	Member
10.	A representative of NGO	Member
11.	Lead Bank Officer of the District	Member
12.	A representative of District Industrial Center	Member
13.	Representative of Agriculture Marketing Board	Member
14.	Representative of input supplying Associations	Member
15.	One Fisheries / Sericulture representative	Member
16.	Project Director ATMA	Member Secretary-cum-Treasurer (Ex-officio)

Non-official members of GB will be appointed for a period of 2 years by APC on the recommendation of the Chairman of GB. Thirty per cent of the farmer representatives on the GB would be reserved for women farmers to ensure their interests are fully represented.

Functions of ATMA Governing Board

The key functions of ATMA Governing Board would be to:

1. Review and approve Strategic Research and Extension Plan (SREP) and annual action plans that are prepared and submitted by the participating units.
2. Receive and review annual reports presented by the participating units, providing feedback and direction to them as needed, for various research and extension activities being carried out within the district.
3. Receive and allocate funds to carry out priority research, extension and related activities within the district.

4. Foster the organization and development of Commodity Interest Groups (CIGs) and Farmers' Interest Groups (FIGs) to their federation within the district.
5. Facilitate the greater involvement of private sector, firms and organizations in providing inputs, technical support, agro-processing and marketing services to farmers.
6. Encourage agriculture lending institutions to increase the availability of capital to resource poor and marginal farmers, especially SC, ST and women farmers.
7. Encourage line departments, the KVK and ZRS, to establish farmer advisory committees to provide feedback and input into their respective R-E Programmes.
8. Enter into contracts and agreements as appropriate to promote and support agricultural development activities within the district.
9. Identify other sources of financial support that would help ensure the financial sustainability of the ATMA and its participating units.
10. Establish revolving funds / accounts for each participating unit, and encourage each unit to make available technical services, such as artificial insemination or soil testing, on a cost recovery basis moving towards full cost recovery in a phased manner.
11. Arrange for the periodic audit of ATMAs financial accounts; and
12. Adopt and amend the rules and bye-laws for the ATMA.

ATMA Management Committee (MC)

The Management Committee would be responsible for planning and executing the day-to-day activities of ATMA.

Composition

1.	Project Director of Agriculture Technology Management Agency	Chairman
2.	District Head of Dept., Agri.	Member
3.	District Head of Dept., Horticulture	Member
4.	District Head of Dept., Animal Husbandry	Member
5.	District Head of dept. Fisheries	Member
6.	District Head of Dept. Sericulture	Member
7.	District Head of other appropriate line departments.	Member
8.	Head, Krishi Vigyan Kendra	Member
9.	Head, Zonal Research Station	Member

10.	One representative of NGO in-charge of Farmers' Organization	Member
11.	Two representatives of Farmer's Organizations (one year rotation basis)	Member

Functions of Management Committee (MC)

1. Carryout periodic Participatory Rural Appraisal (PRA) to identify the problems and constraints faced by different socio-economic groups and farmers within the district.
2. Prepare an integrated, Strategic Research and Extension Plan (SREP) for the district that would specify short and medium term adaptive research as well as technology validation and refinement and extension priorities for the district: these priorities should reflect during the PRA.
3. Prepare annual action plans that would be submitted to the ATMA Governing Board for review, possible modification and approval.
4. Maintain appropriate project accounts for submission to Ministry of Agriculture, Govt. of India.
5. Coordinate the execution of these annual action plans through participation of line departments, ZRSs, KVKs, NGOs, CIGs / FOs and allied institutions, including private sector firms.
6. Establish coordinating mechanisms at the Block level, such as Farm Information & Advisory Centres (FIACs) that would integrate extension and technology transfer activities at the block and village levels.
7. Provide annual performance reports to the Governing Board outlining the various research extension and related targets that were actually carried out.
8. Provide secretariat to Governing Board and initiate action on policy direction, investment decisions and other guidance received from the Governing Board.

Farm Information and Advisory Centre (FIAC) at Block Level

Under each ATMA, FIACs are created at the block level. It consists of two bodies namely Farmer Advisory Committee (FAC) and Block Technology Team (BTT). The FAC is a body of farmer representatives (11-15 members representing various Enterprises and socio economic strata). The BTT on the other hand is a group of technical advisors operating at block level representing agriculture and allied sectors.

Block Technology Team (BTT)

It is an Inter-Departmental Team of Agriculture and line departments operating at block level.

An indicative composition of BTT is given below, however, the composition would change from place to place depending on the critical areas pertaining to different states.

Composition of BTT

Block level officers of Agriculture, Horticulture, Animal Husbandry, Fisheries, Plant Protection, Veterinary Science, Soil Conservation, Extension, Sericulture, Cooperative, Marketing etc. The senior most officials irrespective of the participating departments heads the Block Technology Team as BTT convener.

Functions of Block Technology Team (BTT)

- Operationalize the SREP in each block and move towards single window extension system.
- Help district core team in up gradation of SREP.
- Prepare Block Action Plan detailing extension activities to be undertaken.
- Coordinate the implementation of extension programmes detailed in the Block Action Plan.
- Facilitate formation of CIGs/ FIGs at the block level and below.

Farmer Advisory Committee (FAC)

The Farmer Advisory Committee consists of 11 to 15 members covering different categories of farmers under the given block, with due representation to women farmers and weaker sections of the society. Typical composition of FAC which is given below may be suitably modified as per the agro-ecological situations.

Composition

1	Farmer	Agriculture
2	Farm Women	Agriculture (SC)
3	Farmer	Horticulture
4	Farm Women	Horticulture
5	Farmer Live Stock	Producer
6	Farm Women Live Stock	Producer (SC)
7	Farm Women	Mahila Mandal
8	Farmer	Yuvak Mandal
9	Farmer	Input Dealer
10	Farmer	Farmer Group
11	Farmer	BDC Member (Block Development Council)

Chairman shall be elected out of the above members on rotation basis. BTT Convenor also acts as Member Secretary to FAC.

Functions of FACs

- Act as an agency for providing farmer feedback mechanism.
- Help set block extension priorities and recommend resource allocation across programme areas.
- Recommend Block Action Plan for approval of ATMA GB.
- Review and provide advise to each implementation unit at block level.
- FAC shall meet once in a month during the season and quarterly in lean season.
- Help in formation of Farmer Interest Groups at block level and below.

State Agricultural Management and Extension Training Institute (SAMETI)

The State Agricultural Extension Management and Training Institutes (SAMETIs) would be strengthened by way of providing support to training, communication, programs and equipments. SAMETIs are proposed to be autonomous institutes with greater flexibility in structural and operational aspects.

Functions of SAMETI

- To provide capacity building support in Extension Management related areas to the extension functionaries both from public and private sector.
- To provide consultancy in the areas like project planning, appraisal, implementation etc:
- Develop and promote the application of management tools for improving the effectiveness of Agricultural Extension services through better management of human and material resources.
- Organize need based training programmes for middle level and grassroots level agricultural extension functionaries,: and
- Develop modules on Management, Communication, Participatory Methodologies etc, as a sequel to the feedback from training programmes.

State Level Inter -Departmental Working Group (IDWG)

In pursuance of the number of mechanisms built into the project design and to ensure effective coordination among the departments like agriculture, animal husbandry, fisheries, horticulture, soil conservation etc. it is proposed to constitute a state level Inter-Departmental Working Group under the chairmanship of the Agriculture Production Commissioner/ Secretary agriculture with the following composition:

Composition

1.	Agriculture Production Commissioner/Secretary Agriculture	Chairman
2.	Secretary (Finance)	Member
3.	Secretary (Fisheries)	Member
4.	Secretary (Horticulture)	Member
5.	Secretary (Rural Development)	Member
6.	Secretary (Animal Husbandry)	Member
7.	Secretary (Soil Conservation)	Member
8.	Secretary (Women Development)	Member
9.	Secretaries of related departments (wherever necessary)	Member
10.	Vice Chancellor (s) of SAU(s)	Member
11.	Secretary (Agri.)/ Deputy Secretary (Agri.) / State Nodal Officer (SNO)	Member Secretary

In departments like horticulture, soil conservation etc, where separate secretaries do not exist, Director of the concerned departments may act as a member on the interdepartmental group.

Functions of IDWG

- To provide a mechanism for interactions with the Technology Dissemination Management Committee (TDMC) of the DAC, GOI, guide the human resource development activity andto monitor the district level technology dissemination programme.
- To oversee and support Agricultural Extension Research activities being undertaken by ATMA and to make policy interventions on inter departmental matters including issues related to Women in Agriculture and co-ordination thereof.

Process Intervention

(i) Strategic Research and Extension Plan (SREP)

One of the first tasks of ATMA like institutions is to facilitate the preparation of Strategic Research and Extension Plan (SREP) of the district. The SREP is prepared through participatory methodologies such as Participatory Rural Appraisal (PRA) involving all the stakeholders and farmers. The SREP contains detailed analysis of all the information on existing farming systems in the district and research – extension gaps required to be filled-up. It also prioritizes the research – extension strategies within the district. It becomes the basis for development of work plans at block / district level.

(ii) State Extension Work Plan (SEWP)

Based on the research-extension strategies given in the SREPs, block/ district level plans shall be developed by each ATMA like institutions. The State Extension Work Plan developed at state level shall contain a consolidated activity-wise plan incorporating all the District Agriculture Action Plans (DAAPs) in the state and state level activities to be carried out with activity-wise budgetary requirement as per the norms prescribed in the cafeteria. It will also indicate all other extension activities that may be undertaken from out of resources provided under any other scheme of the Centre/ State Governments. The DAAPs developed under the scheme should be processed consistent with Article 243 ZD of the Constitution.

(iii) Cafeteria of Activities

The Cafeteria includes cost norms and ceilings applicable for each activity. Under the Cafeteria, activities to be undertaken at State and District level are categorized separately. The state level activities include support for upgrading state level training institutions such as SAMETI, HRD of extension functionaries, organization of state level Agri-Exhibitions and Monitoring and Evaluation of the Scheme.

The district level activities are further categorized in four groups namely, farmer oriented activities, farm information dissemination, research-extension-farmer-market (R-E-F-M) linkages and administrative expenses. Farmer oriented activities include development of SREP, mobilization of farmer groups, training/ exposure visit of farmers, field demonstrations, all aimed at empowering the farmers and improving their participation in technology dissemination process. Under the category of farm information dissemination, local level agricultural exhibitions, information dissemination through printed materials and development of technology packages in electronic form are covered. The R-E-FM linkages based activities include organization of Farmer-Scientist Interaction at local level, organization of Field-days and Kisan Goshties and support for local level researchable issues emanated from the SREP. The administrative expenses under district level activities provide support for running ATMA like Institutions and a few block level Farm Information and Advisory Centres. It has been specified in the Cafeteria that funds for 'Farm-Information Dissemination' category can't exceed 20% of total resources available for district level activities under the Scheme. These percentage for 'REFM Linkage' and 'Administrative Expenses' categories are 15% and 20% respectively. Any savings in any of these three categories could be utilized for 'Farmer-Oriented Activities'. The cost norms and ceilings may be exceeded by a maximum of 10% of the specified amount in exceptional circumstances by a local decision. All such cases shall have to be reported in the next year's Work Plan and shall be subject to ex-post guidance. Any other deviation from the prescribed norms/ ceilings or any new activity not specified in the Cafeteria could be taken up by States with prior approval of the DAC. The sum total of all activities specified in the cafeteria is more than the funds likely to be available for State/district level activities. States will have to prioritize their proposed activities based on gaps identified in the SREP.

Source: Department of Agriculture and Cooperation (DAC), Ministry of Agriculture – Guidelines circulated vide letters dated 20th April, 2005.

Suggested Readings and References

1. Annual Reports (2005-2010). Department of Agriculture and Cooperation (DAC), Ministry of Agriculture
2. Five Year Plans (9th -12th), Planning Commission, Government of India, New Delhi.
3. Dhama, O.P. and Bhatnagar, O.P. (2007). Education and Communication for Development. Oxford and IBH Pub. Co. Pvt. Ltd.
4. Mathialagan, P. (2007). Textbook of Animal Husbandry and Livestock Extension, International Book Distributing Co. 7, Meerabai Marg, Lucknow, India.
5. Ray, G.L. (2006). Extension Communication and Management, New Delhi, Kalyani Publishers.
6. Sharma, K.R.G. (2008). Veterinary Extension Education, BSPBS Publications, Hyderabad, Hyderabad.
7. Ray, G.L. (2001). Extension, Communication and Management, 4th Edition, Naya Prokash, Calcutta.

20

National Agriculture Development Programme/ Rashtriya Krishi Vikas Yojana (RKVY)

1. Objective of RKVY
2. Eligibility Criteria
3. District and State Agriculture Plans
4. Programme Components of RKVY (Streams)
5. RKVY (Production and Growth)
6. Broad Areas of focus under the RKVY
7. RKVY (Infrastructure and Assets)
8. Illustrative List of Projects that can be funded under RKVY (infrastructure & Assets) Stream
9. RKVY (Special Schemes)
10. Illustrative List of Projects that should not be funded under RKVY
11. State Level Project Screening Committee (SLPSC)
12. State Level Sanctioning Committee (SLSC)
13. Composition of State Level Sanctioning Committee (SLSC)
14. Planning & Implementation of RKVY
15. Release of Funds
16. Monitoring & Evaluation
17. Convergence
18. Sub-Schemes launched under RKVY
    a) Bringing Green Revolution to Eastern Region (BGREI)
    b) Vegetable Initiative for Urban Clusters (VIUC)
    c) National Mission for Protein Supplements (NMPS)
    d) Saffron Mission
    e) Vidarbha Intensive Irrigation Development Programme (VIIDP)
    f) Crop Diversification Programme (CDP) in Original Green Revolution States
19. Funds Release and Utilization
20. Suggested Readings and References

National Agriculture Development Programme/Rashtriya Krishi Vikas Yojana (RKVY)

Economic reforms initiated since 1991 have put the Indian economy on a higher growth trajectory. Annual growth rate in the total Gross Domestic Product (GDP) has accelerated from below 6 per cent during the initial years of reforms to more than 8 per cent in recent years. The Planning Commission in its approach paper to the Eleventh Five-Year-plan has stated that 9 per cent growth rate in GDP would be feasible during the Eleventh Plan period. However, Agriculture that accounted for more than 30 per cent of total GDP at the beginning of reforms failed to maintain its pre-reform growth. On the contrary, it witnessed a sharp deceleration in growth after the mid-1990s. This happened despite the fact that agricultural productivity in most of the states was quite low as it were, and the potential for the growth of agriculture was high. The GDP of agriculture increased annually at more than 3 per cent during the 1980s.

Since the Ninth Five-Year Plan (1996 to 2001-02), India has been targeting a growth rate of more than 4 per cent in agriculture, but the actual achievement has been much below the target. More than 50 per cent of the workforce of the country depends upon agriculture for it's livelihood and slow growth in Agriculture and allied sectors can lead to acute stress in the economy because a large proportion of population depend on this sector. A major cause behind the slow growth in agriculture is the consistent decrease in investments in the sector by the state governments. While public and private investments are increasing manifold in sectors such as infrastructure, similar investments are not forthcoming in Agriculture and allied sectors, leading to distress in the community of farmers, especially that of the small and marginal segment. Hence, the need for incentivising states that increase their investments in the Agriculture and allied sectors has been felt.

Concerned by the slow growth in the Agriculture and allied sectors, the National Development Council (NDC), in its meeting held on 29th May, 2007 resolved that a special Additional Central Assistance Scheme (RKVY) to be launched. The NDC resolved that agricultural development strategies must be reoriented to meet the needs of farmers and called upon the Central and State governments to evolve a strategy to rejuvenate agriculture. The NDC reaffirmed its commitment to achieve 4 per cent annual growth in the agricultural sector during the 11th plan. The Resolution with respect to the Additional Central Assistance scheme reads as below:

Introduce a new Additional Central Assistance scheme to incentivise States to draw up plans for their agriculture sector more comprehensively, taking agro-climatic conditions, natural resource issues and technology into account, and integrating livestock, poultry and fisheries more fully. This will involve a new scheme for Additional Central Assistance to State Plans, administered by the Union Ministry of Agriculture over and above its existing Centrally Sponsored schemes, to supplement the State-specific strategies including special schemes for beneficiaries of land reforms. The newly created National Rainfed Area Authority will on request assist States in planning for rainfed areas.

In pursuance to aforesaid observation and in consultation with the Planning Commission, Department of Agriculture and Cooperation(DAC), Ministry of Agriculture, Government of India launched Rashtriya Krishi Vikas Yojana (RKVY) from 2007-2008, which has been operational since then.

During XI Plan, Rs.22,408.76 crore was released to States, out of which Rs.21,586.6 crore was utilized in implementing 5768 projects in certain broad categories namely: crop development, horticulture, agricultural mechanization, natural resource management, marketing and post-harvest management, animal husbandry, dairy development, fisheries, extension, etc.

By virtue of these enhanced investments, agriculture and allied sectors could achieve an annual growth rate of 3.64 % during XI plan period against a growth rate of 2.46 % per annum in the X plan period.

Based on feedback received from States, experiences garnered during implementation in XI pan and inputs provided by Stakeholders; Operational Guidelines of RKVY have been revised to not only enhance efficiency and efficacy of the programme but also its inclusiveness during XII plan period.

Objective of RKVY

The RKVY aims at achieving and sustaining desired annual growth during XII Plan Period, by ensuring a holistic development of Agriculture and allied sectors.

The main objectives of the scheme are :

i) To incentivise the states so as to increase public investment in Agriculture and allied sectors.

ii) To provide flexibility and autonomy to states in the process of planning and executing Agriculture and allied sector schemes.

iii) To ensure the preparation of agriculture plans for the districts and the states based on agro-climatic conditions, availability of technology and natural resources.

iv) To ensure that the local needs/crops/priorities are better reflected in the agricultural plans of the states.

v) To achieve the goal of reducing the yield gaps in important crops, through focussed interventions.

vi) To maximize returns to the farmers in Agriculture and allied sectors.

vii) To bring about quantifiable changes in the production and productivity of various components of Agriculture and allied sectors by addressing them in a holistic manner.

These guidelines are applicable to all the States and Union Territories that fulfill the eligibility conditions. The RKVY will be a State Plan Scheme. The list of allied sectors as indicated by the Planning Commission will be the basis for determining the sectoral expenditure, i.e Crop Husbandry (including Horticulture), Animal Husbandry and Fisheries, Dairy Development, Agricultural Research and Education, Forestry and Wildlife, Plantation and Agricultural Marketing, Food Storage and Warehousing, Soil and Water Conservation, Agricultural Financial Institutions, other Agricultural Programmes and Cooperation.

Eligibility Criteria

A state will become eligible to receive RKVY allocation, if and only if :

i) The base line share of Agriculture and allied sectors in its total State Plan (excluding RKVY funds) expenditure is at least maintained; and

ii) District Agriculture Plans (DAP) and State Agriculture Plans (SAP) have been formulated.

District and State Agriculture Plans

District and State Agriculture Plans will remain as cornerstone of planning and implementation of this scheme. Each district will have a DAP after taking into consideration of resources that would be available during XII Plan from other ongoing schemes (both State and Central) like Mahatma Gandhi National Rural Employment Guarantee Scheme (MGNREGS), Swarnajayanti Gram Swarojgar Yojana (SGSY) and Backward Regions Grant Fund (BRGF), Integrated Watershed Management Programme (IWMP), Accelerated Irrigation Benefit Programme (AIBP), Bharat Nirman, etc.

The District Agricultural Plans shall not be the usual aggregation of the existing schemes but would aim at moving towards projecting the requirements for development of Agriculture and allied sectors of the district. These plans will present the vision for Agriculture and allied sectors within the overall development perspective of the district. The District Agriculture Plans would present the financial requirement and the sources of financing the agriculture development plans in a comprehensive way. Since achievement of RKVY's objective is sequel to proper District Planning, these requirements should be adhered to by the State as far as possible. The state will have to specify the institutional mechanisms evolved by them for District Planning and submit a status a status report at the stage of annual exercise. DAP will include animal husbandry and fishery development, minor irrigation projects, rural development woks, agricultural marketing schemes and schemes for water harvesting and conservation, etc, keeping in view the natural resources and technological possibilities in each district.

The district level potential linked credit plans (PLP) already prepared by the National Bank for Agriculture and Rural Development (NABARD) and Strategic Research and Extension Plans (SREPs) developed under the Agriculture Technology Management Agency (ATMA) may be referred for revision of DAP. It should also be ensured that the strategies for convergences with other programmes as well as the role assigned to the Panchyati Raj Institutions (PRIs) are appropriately incorporated in DAPs. Each State will also have a comprehensive State Agricultural Plan (SAP) for XII Plan by integrating the District Plans. SAPs will invariable have to indicate resources that can flow from the State to the districts. Each State will be required to prepare State Agriculture Infrastructure Development Programme (SAIDP) in similar manner to that of DAPs and SAPs for identifying shelf of projects for RKVY. State Planning Department will provide revised/ updated SAP and SAIDP to Department of Agriculture and Planning Commission as a part of State's annual State Plan exercise.

Programme Components of RKVY (Streams)

RKVY funds would be provided to the States as 100% grant by the Central Government in following streams.

a) RKVY (Production Growth) with 35% of annual outlay,
b) RKVY (Infrastructure and Assets) with 35% of annual outlay;
c) RKVY (Special Schemes) with 20% of annual outlay; and
d) RKVY (Flexi Fund) with 10% of annual outlay (States can undertake either Production Growth or Infrastructure & Assets projects with this allocation depending upon State specific needs/priorities).

RKVY (Production and Growth)

States can take up any project under this stream to raise production and productivity in agriculture and allied sectors. This will normally include all food crop activities, including distribution of agricultural inputs, extension, soil health, plant health & Integrated Pest Management(IPM), production & distribution of seeds, animal husbandry, dairying & fisheries, training and skill development of stakeholders, production specific research projects, information dissemination etc. Projects proposed under RKVY (Production Growth) shall normally emanate from the District and State Agriculture Plans. Broad areas of focus for this Stream are presented below.

Broad Areas of Focus under the RKVY

The components / activities which would be eligible for project based assistance under RKVY (Production and Growth) are elaborated below. This is an indicative list; the states may choose other components/activities, but ensure that they are reflected adequately in the SAP and the DAP.

a) **Integrated development of major food crops such as wheat, paddy, coarse cereals, minor millets, pulses, oilseeds:** Assistance can be provided for making available certified/HYV seeds to farmers; production of breeder seed; purchase of breeder seed from institutions such as ICAR, public sector seed corporations, production of foundation seed; production of certified seed; seed treatment; Farmers Field Schools at demonstration sites; training of farmers etc. Similar support would be provided for development of other crops such as sugarcane, cotton or any other crop/variety that may be of importance to the state.

b) **Agriculture mechanization**: Assistance would be provided for farm mechanization efforts especially for improved and gender friendly tools, implements and machinery. Specific agricultural mechanization projects oriented toward enhancing farm productivity can be considered under this scheme. However, tractors are not covered under the scheme.

c) **Activities related to enhancement of soil health:** This would include efficient quality control of inputs including strengthening of laboratories and enhancing soil health. Assistance can be provided to the farmers for distributing soil health cards; micro nutrient demonstration; training of farmers for promotion of organic farming including printing of publicity/ utility literature; assistance to the state government to strengthen existing soil testing and fertilizer testing laboratories and setting up new ones; amelioration of soils affected with conditions such as alkalinity and acidity.

d) **Development of rainfed farming systems in and outside watershed areas:** Assistance for development of land as also assistance for horticulture, generating livelihoods for farmers Below the Poverty Line (BPL).

e) **Integrated Pest Management schemes:** This would include training of farmers through Farm Field Schools etc. on pest management practices; printing of literature/ other awareness programmes.

f) **Promoting Extension Services:** This would include the new initiatives for skill development

g) **Promoting Extension Services:** This would include new initiatives for skill development and training in the farming community and to revamp the existing State agricultural extension systems.

h) **Activities relating to enhancement of horticultural production:** Assistance will be available for nursery development and other horticulture activities.

i) **Animal husbandry and fisheries development activities:** Assistance will be available for improvement in fodder production, genetic up-gradation of cattle and buffaloes, enhancement of milk production, enlarging raw material base for leather industry, improvement in livestock health, poultry development, development of small ruminants and enhanced fish production.

j) **Study tours of farmers:** Study tours of farmers within the country specially to research institutions, Model farms etc.

k) **Organic and bio-fertilizers:** Support for decentralized production at the village level and their marketing, etc. This will include vermicomposting and introduction of superior technologies for better production

l) **Sericulture:** Sericulture upto the stage of cocoon production along with extension system for cocoon and silk yarn production and marketing.

The above list is not exhaustive. Therefore, schemes that are important for agriculture, horticulture and allied sector development, but cannot be categorized under (a) to (l) can also be proposed under this stream.

RKVY (Infrastructure and Assets)

Projects under this stream will emanate from State Agriculture Infrastructure Development Programme (SAIDP). This will normally include projects selected on the basis of normative requirement of infrastructure, actual availability thereof and the gap in agriculture infrastructure in the State viz. setting up of laboratories and testing facilities, storage including cold-storages, mobile vans, agricultural marketing etc. An illustrative list of possible infrastructure and assets which can be funded under this stream is given below State Governments will also determine sectoral classification for investment requirements for infrastructure in public, public-private and private sectors and accordingly work out financial support for funding gaps in infrastructure taking into account viability gap which would be based on financial analysis. However, in any case, subsidy will be capped to 25% of total project cost. While a number of infrastructure items are covered under Rural Infrastructure Development Fund (RIDF) and Viability Gap Funding (VGF) of the Ministry of Finance, RKVY funds should supplement those sources and not replace them. In any case, quantum of assistance under RKVY should not exceed assistance under VGF.

Illustrative List of Projects that can be funded under RKVY (Infrastructure & Assets) Stream

S.No.	Sector	Description of Infrastructure
1	Horticulture	Nurseries Tissue Culture Labs Community tanks/Farm ponds/on farm water resources with plastic/RCC lining Green House/ Poly house/Shade net House structures Sanitary and phytosanitary infrastructure INM/IPM infrastructure such as Disease Forecasting Units, Plant Health Clinics, Leaf/Tissue Analysis labs, Bio-control laboratories Vermi compost units Controlled atmosphere storage Cold storage/pre cooling/refrigerated van, cold chain infrastructure Ripening/Curing chamber Primary/minimal processing units Terminal/wholesale/Rural market Functional infrastructure for collection, sorting, grading etc. Infrastructure related to Horticulture produce processing as per Ministry of Food Processing Industries (MoFPI) guidelines
2	Natural Resources Management	Soil & Water conservation activities (Terracing, Gully Control Measures, Spill Ways, Check Dams, Spurs, Diversion Drains, Protection Walls etc.) Reclamation of problem Soils (Acid/Alkali/Saline/ Ravine/Water logged).
3	Pest Management & Pesticide quality control	Labs for production of bio-control agents State Pesticide Residue Testing Labs State Pesticide Testing Labs Bio-Pesticide Testing Labs Seed Treatment drums & chemicals
4	Soil Nutrient Management Fertilizers Bio Fertilizers /Organic Farming	Setting up of new soil testing laboratories. Strengthening of existing soil test laboratories with micro-nutrient testing facilities. Setting up of new Fertilizer Quality Control Laboratories (FQCLs). Strengthening of existing FQCLs. Bio fertilizer Production Units. Fruit/Vegetables waste, compost production units.

5	Animal Husbandry	Semen collection and Artificial Insemination (AI) Units/Production Center
		Breeding farms
		Dispensaries/Hospitals for treatment of Animals
		Vaccine Production Unit
		Diagnosis Labs, including Mobile Units
		Animal Ambulance
		Cold Chain for storing and transportation of frozen Semen
		Tractor fitted with Fodder Block Machine
		Carcass rendering Plant to collect the fallen animals for processing/utilization in scientific manner
		Modernization of animal slaughter houses[1] and markets for livestock/livestock products
	Dairy	Milk Collection Centers and Infrastructure:
		Purchase of milking machines (single/double bucket)
		Setting up of milk chilling/bulk milk cooling centres (BMC)
		Along with automatic milk collection units (AMC)
		Setting up/modernization/strengthening of milk processing units
		Strengthening /expansion of cold storage facility for milk and milk product
		Purchase of insulated/refrigerated transport vehicles
		Setting up of milk parlor/milk booth
		Strengthening of lab facility in milk chilling/milk processing unit
		Establishment of cattle feed storage godown
		Establishment/strengthening of cattle feed plant
		Establishment of cattle shed for milch animals
		Setting/strengthening of ETP at milk chilling/milk processing unit
	Fisheries	Fish Ponds/Reservoirs
		Fish seed Hatcheries
		Marketing infrastructure
		Mobile Transport / Refrigerated vans
6	Marketing and Post- Harvest	Fruits & Vegetable Markets/Distribution Centres
		Market Infrastructural Facilities, including Agricultural Produce Market Committees (APMC)
		Construction of Specialized Storage Facilities like Onion Storage
		Godowns
		Electronic Trading including Spot and Futures Markets and E-auctioning

		Farmers Service Centres Food Grain Procurement Centres E-Kisan Bhawans/ Internet Kiosks Grading including grading line Quality Control Packing
7	Seeds	Seed Testing Labs Seed Processing Facilities Seed Storage Godowns including Dehumidified Refrigerated Seed Storage Godowns Seed Certification Agencies and Certification infrastructure Seed Multiplication Farms
8	Agriculture Mechanization	Custom Hiring Centers for Agricultural Equipment Agriculture Machines Testing Centers
9	Agricultural Extension	Kisan Call Centres ATMA Infrastructure Knowledge/Technology Resource Centres
10	Agriculture Research	Research Infrastructure Strengthening of Krishi Vigyan Kendras (KVKs)
11	Minor/Micro Irrigation	Shallow Wells & Dug Wells Tube Wells (except in dark/grey /critical zone Identified by Central Ground Water Board) Percolation & Minor Irrigation Tanks Farm Ponds Drip & Sprinkler Irrigation System Field Channels

RKVY (Special Schemes)

This will comprise of schemes based on national priorities as notified by Govt, of India from time to time. In the event of Government of India not declaring any special sub-scheme in a year (or not continuing sub-schemes of previous year) or the aggregate amount earmarked for such special sub-schemes falling short of 20% of the RKVY budgetary allocation for the year, the remaining amount will be allocated additionally to RKVY (Production Growth Stream) funds.

Under RKVY (Production Growth) & RKVY (Infrastructure & Assets) streams, States are free to choose appropriate components / activities, but it has to be ensured that these are reflected adequately in SAP and DAPs. Scheme(s) administered by the Departments of Agriculture and Cooperation, Animal Husbandry, Dairying and Fisheries, Dept. of Land Resources, Ministry of Water Resources, Ministry of Food Processing Industries etc., already have elaborate guidelines, which ought to be followed by the implementing Agencies for similar activities/project components. However, State must refrain from undertaking activities/components as illustrated below.

Illustrative List of Projects that should not be Funded under RKVY

1. Creation/topping up of any kind of revolving fund / corpus fund;
2. Expenditure towards maintenance of assets or any such recurring expenses;
3. Expenses towards Salary, Transport, Travelling Allowances (TA), Daily Allowances (DA) of permanent / semi-permanent employees. However, expenses towards hiring of manpower onoutsourcing/contractual basis can be met within 1% allocation earmarked for administrative expenses with approval of SLSC.
4. Expenses towards POL (Petrol, Oil, Lubricants);
5. FinancingState'sshareand/or topping up subsidy level in respect with other Central/ StateSchems;
6. Foreign Visits/Tours including study tours of farmers abroad;
7. Purchase of vehicles;
8. Financing any kind of debt waiver, interest subvention, payment of insurance premium, compensation to farmers and calamity relief expenditure; additional bonus over & above Minimum Support Price (MSP);
9. Creating/Strengthening assets in Private Sector/NGO's beyond what is permissible under any schemes/ program,,es of Govt. of India.

State Level Project Screening Committee (SLPSC)

A State Level Project Screening Committee (SLPSC) will be constituted by each State for screening RKVY project proposals, which will be headed by Agriculture Production Commissioner or any other officer nominated by Chief Secretary. Other members of SLPSC would be decided by the State Chief Secretary. SLPSC will screen all project proposals for ensuring conformity with RKVY guidelines and that they flow from SAP/DAPs besides being consistent with technical requirements / standards and financial norms (cost norms and pattern of assistance) etc. in respect of components that have been specified in relevant Central Government/State Government schemes. SLPSC will also screen all Detailed Project Reports (DPRs) prepared by various departments for its suitability, its linkage to DAP, SAIDP and SAP and its adherence to the RKVY guidelines. Before recommending projects to State Level Sanction Committee (SLSC), SLPSC will further examine and ensure that:

a) Funds available under other schemes of the State Government and / or Government of India for the proposed projects have been accessed and utilized before they are brought under the RKVY umbrella;

b) RKVY projects/activities should not create any duplication or overlapping of assistance /area coverage vis-à-vis other schemes/programmes of State/ Central Government:

c) RKVY funds are not being proposed as additional or 'top-up' subsidy to other ongoing schemes/programmes of State/Central Government:

d) State Agriculture Infrastructure Development Programme (SAIDP) has been prepared:

e) At least 25% of total value of projects including 'Production growth' and 'Assets & Infrastructure' Streams have emanated from comprehensive district agricultural plan (CDAP) and have been approved by the District level Panchayati Raj Institutions (PRIs) so that field level gaps are correctly addressed;

f) DPRs have included provision for monitoring and evaluation;

g) For Research Projects proposed under RKVY, clearance of Indian Council of Agriculture Research (ICAR) has been obtained;

h) Convergence with other State/Central Schemes has been attempted; and

i) Recommended projects ensure adequate allocation to allied sectors including Farmer Producer Organizations (FPO).

State Level Sanctioning Committee (SLSC)

A State Level Sanctioning Committee (SLSC) headed by the Chief Secretary of the State is vested with the authority to sanction specific projects recommended by the SLPSC under each stream of RKVY in a meeting attended by representatives of Government of India. The quorum for SLSC meetings would not be complete without the presence of at least one representative from the Government of India. SLSC shall meet as often as required but shall meet at least once in a quarter. Composition of SLSC is at presented in the table.

Chief Secretary	- Chairman
Agri. Prod. Commissioner/Principal Secretary (Agriculture)	- Vice-Chairman
Secretary, Finance	- Member
Secretary, Planning	- Member
Secretary, Fisheries	- Member
Secretary, Animal Husbandry	- Member
Secretary, Environment and Forests	- Member
Secretary, Panchayati Raj	- Member
Secretary, Rural Development	- Member
Secretary, Water Resources/Irrigation/Minor Irrigation	- Member
Director, Agriculture	- Member
Director, Horticulture	- Member
Director, Animal Husbandry	- Member

Director, Fisheries	- Member
Representative of Department of Agriculture & Cooperation, Govt, of India (Officer not below the rank of Joint Secretary)	- Member
Representatives of Departments of Animal Husbandry, Dairying & Fisheries, Govt, of India (Officer not below the rank of Joint Secretary)	- Member
Representative of State Agriculture University	- Member
Representative of Planning Commission	- Member
Secretary, Agriculture	- Member-Secretary

Composition of State Level Sanctioning Committee (SLSC)

SLSC may co-opt two more members from Agricultural Research Organizations, reputed NGOs working in the field of Agriculture, District Collectors/Deputy Commissioners of important districts, and leading farmers. The State Governments will notify the constitution of SLSC and consequent changes in its composition/incumbent. SLSC will, interalia, be responsible for

a) Sanctioning the projects under RKVY;

b) Monitoring progress of each project sanctioned by it under each stream of RKVY;

c) Reviewing implementation of the schemes' objectives and ensure that the projects / schemes are implemented in accordance with the guidelines laid down;

d) Ensuring that no duplication of efforts or resources takes place;

e) Commissioning/undertaking field studies to monitor the implementation of projects;

f) Initiating evaluation studies from time to time, as may be required;

g) Undertaking any other project of importance to the State's Agriculture and allied sectors;

h) Ensuring that there are no inter- district disparities with respect to the financial patterns / subsidy assistance in the projects; and

i) Ensuring that all extant procedures and instructions of Govt, of India in addition to RKVY guidelines are followed so that the expenditure incurred on implementation of the projects is barest minimum with due concern for economy in expenditure.

Planning & Implementation of RKVY

State Agriculture Department shall be the nodal department for the implementation of the scheme. For administrative convenience and ease of implementation, State governments may identify, or create an exclusive agency for implementing the scheme on a fast-track. Even where such an Agency is created/designated, the entire responsibility of ensuring proper implementation of RKVY rests with the State Agriculture Department. In a situation where the States notify a Nodal agency, the costs of running the agency, will have to be met from within the 1% limit of RKVY allocation.

The Agriculture department/nodal agency will be responsible for the following:-

i) Preparing State Agriculture Plan (SAP) & State Agriculture Infrastructure Development Programme (SAIDP) and ensuring the preparation of the District Agriculture Plans (DAPs).
ii) Effectively coordinating preparation and appraisal of projects, implementing, monitoring, and evaluation with various Departments and implementing Agencies.
iii) Management of funds received from the Central, and State Governments and disbursement of the funds to the implementing agencies.
iv) Furnishing of utilization certificates and quarterly physical & financial progress reports to the Department of Agriculture and Cooperation
v) Effectively utilizing and regularly updating web enabled IT based RKVY Management Information System (RKVY-MIS).

The State Level Nodal Agency will forward SLSC meeting notice along with sufficient number of copies (not less than 20) of agenda and project details to Department of Agriculture & Cooperation (DAC) so as to reach at least 15 days before the meeting of SLSC to enable Government of India's representatives to come prepared and to participate meaningfully in the SLSC meeting. Once SLSC sanctions the projects, DAC will release funds to State Government only. As envisaged in National Policy for Farmers (2007), Panchayati Raj Institutions (PRI) should be actively involved in implementation of RKVY especially in selection of beneficiaries, conducting social audit etc.

Release of Funds

50% of the RKVY annual allocation will be released as first installment to the State, upon the receipt of the minutes of SLSC approving implementation of new projects and/or continuation of ongoing projects during current financial year along with lists of projects approved and their entry in RKVY Database (RDMIS). In case, total cost of approved project is less than annual outlay, funds to the tune of 50% of approved project cost will be released. If a State fails to submit these documents within reasonable period of time, balance funds may be reallocated to better performing States.

Monitoring & Evaluation

RKVY-Management Information System (RKVY-MIS): DAC has put in place a web- based Management Information System (MIS) for RKVY to collect essential information related to each project. States will be responsible for timely submission/updating project data online in the system (preferably on a fortnightly basis), which has been designed to provide current and authenticated data on outputs, outcome and contribution of RKVY.

Convergence

RKVY is additional central assistance to the State Plan for Agriculture and allied sectors and thus it is essential to encourage convergence with schemes like Mahatma Gandhi National Rural Employment Guarantee Scheme (MGNREGS), Swarnajayanti Gram Swarojgar Yojana (SGSY) and Backward Regions Grant Fund (BRGF). States shall also ensure convergence with other Central Schemes of Ministry of Agriculture (e.g. Department of Agriculture & Cooperation & Department of Animal Husbandry, Dairying & Fisheries & Department of Agriculture Research & Education) and other relevant Ministries/ Departments viz., Ministry of Food Processing Industries, Ministry of New and Renewable Energy, Department of Land Resources, Ministry of Rural Development, Ministry of Water Resources etc. Ministry of Panchayati Raj shall also be appropriately consulted for ensuring that local/Panchayat level requirements are adequately addressed in District Development Plans. Planning Commission and the Ministry of Agriculture will together examine the States' overall Plan proposals for Agriculture and allied sectors as part of the Annual Plan approval exercise.

Sub-Schemes Launched under RKVY

RKVY has enabled launching of new schemes/programmes keeping States' flexibility and authority intact. Since 2010-11 several sub-schemes have been introduced under RKVY with focused objectives. Following six special Programme /schemes are being implemented as sub-schemes of RKVY with a total allocation of Rs.1,975 crore for 2014-15.

Bringing Green Revolution to Eastern Region (BGREI)

Initiated in 2010-11, BGREI has been targeting productivity improvement in the rice based cropping system of Assam, West Bengal, Odisha, Bihar, Jharkhand, Eastern Uttar Pradesh and Chhattisgarh. Allocation for this scheme in 2010-11 & 2011-12 was Rs. 400 crore each, which has been enhanced to Rs. 1,000 crore during 2012-13, 2013-14 & 2014-15.

Vegetable Initiative for Urban Clusters (VIUC)

Launched in 2011- 12, VIUC aims at meeting growing demand for vegetables by increasing productivity and improving market linkage. In addition, VIUC envisages establishing an efficient supply chain to provide quality vegetables at competitive prices. The allocation for this programme during 2014-15 is Rs.175 crore.

National Mission for Protein Supplements (NMPS)

National Mission for Protein Supplements was launched with an allocation of Rs.300 crore during 2011-12 to promote animal based protein production through livestock development, dairy farming, piggery, goat rearing and fisheries in selected blocks. The allocation for this programme for 2014-15 is Rs.300 crore.

Saffron Mission

The Scheme was initiated in 2010-11 for revival of Saffron cultivation in Jammu& Kashmir. Allocation for the scheme was Rs. 39.44 crore in 2010-11 and Rs. 50 crore each in 2011-12 & 2012-13. The allocation for this programme has been enhanced to Rs. 100 crore during 2013- 14& 2014-15.

Vidarbha Intensive Irrigation Development Programme (VIIDP)

The Scheme was initiated in 2012-13 with an allocation of Rs. 300 crore to bring in more farming areas in Vidarbha region under protective irrigation. The allocation for this programme for 2014- 15 is Rs.150 crore.

Crop Diversification Programme (CDP) in Original Green Revolution States

Pursuant to announcement in Union Budget (2013-14), this scheme has been launched in 2013- 14 with an allocation of Rs. 500 crore to promote technological innovation and encourage farmers to choose crop alternatives in original green revolution states of Punjab, Haryana and Uttar Pradesh. The allocation for this programme for 2014-15 is Rs.250 crore.

Funds Relsease and Utilisation

Status of year-wise funds released to the States & their expenditure & utilization status as on 31.12.2014 is given below:

Year	Funds Released	Expenditure Reported
2007-08	1246.89	1246.79
2008-09	2886.80	2880.89
2009-10	3760.93	3756.53
2010-11	6720.06	6719.02
2011-12	7794.09	7716.02
2012-13	8400.00	8353.30
2013-14	7052.51	6544.70
2014-15	7851.64	-

Source : Annual Report 2014-15, Department of Agriculture and Cooperation, Govt. of India

Suggested Readings and References

Annual Report (2008-2016). Department of Agriculture and Cooperation, Govt. of India.

21

Other Related Programmes

1. Integrated Watershed Management Programme (IWMP)
2. Providing Rural Amenities in Rural Areas (PURA)
3. National Rural Health Mission
4. National Food Security Mission (NFSM)
5. Mission for Integrated Development of Horticulture (MIDH)
6. National Horticulture Mission (NHM)
7. Horticulture Mission for North East and Himalayan States (HMNEH)
8. National Bamboo Mission (NBM)
9. Coconut Development Board (CDB)
10. National Horticulture Board (NHB)
11. National Mission on Oilseeds and Oil Palm (NMOOP)
12. National Mission for Sustainable Agriculture (NMSA)
13. National Mission on Agricultural Extension & Technology (NMAET)
    a) Sub Mission on Agricultural Extension
    b) Support to State Extension Programmes for Extension Reforms Scheme (ATMA Scheme)
    c) Mass Media Support to Agricultural Extension
    d) Establishment of the Agri-Clinics and Agri-Business Centres (ACABC)
    e) Kisan Call Centers (KCC)
    f) HRD Support
    g) National e-Governance Plan in Agriculture (NeGP-A)
14. Sub Mission on Seed and Planting Material (SMSP)
15. Sub Mission on Agricultural Mechanization (SMAM)
16. Sub Mission on Plant Protection and Plant Quarantine (SMPP)
17. National Crop Insurance Programme (NCIP)
    a) Salient features of NCIP
18. National Agricultural Insurance Scheme (NAIS)
19. Modified National Agricultural Insurance Scheme (MNAIS)
20. Weather Based Crop Insurance Scheme (WBCIS)
21. Coconut Palm Insurance Scheme (CPIS)
22. Suggested Readings and References

Integrated Watershed Management Programme (IWMP)

Integrated Watershed Management Programme (IWMP) is a modified programme of erstwhile Drought Prone Areas Programme (DPAP), Desert Development Programme (DDP) and Integrated Wastelands Development Programme (IWDP) of the Department of Land Resources. The scheme was launched during 2009-10. The programme is being implemented as per Common Guidelines for Watershed Development Projects 2008. The main objectives of the IWMP are to restore the ecological balance by harnessing, conserving and developing degraded natural resources such as soil, vegetative cover and water. The outcomes are prevention of soil erosion, regeneration of natural vegetation, rain water harvesting and recharging of the ground water table. This enables multi-cropping and the introduction of diverse agro-based activities, which help to provide sustainable livelihoods to the people residing in the watershed areas.

The salient features of IWMP are as below

i) Setting up of Dedicated Institutions with multi-disciplinary experts at State level - State Level Nodal Agency (SLNA), District level - Watershed Cell cum Data Centre (WCDC), Project level - Project Implementing Agency (PIA) and Village level - Watershed Committee (WC).

ii) Cluster Approach in selection and preparation of projects: Average size of project - about 5,000 ha.

iii) Enhanced Cost Norms from Rs. 6000 per ha. to Rs.12,000/ha. in plains; Rs.15,000/ ha in difficult/hilly areas

iv) Uniform Funding pattern of 90:10 between Centre & States.

v) Release of central assistance in three installments (20%, 50% & 30%) instead of five installments.

vi) Flexibility in the project period i.e. 4 to 7 years

vii) Scientific planning of the projects by using IT, remote sensing techniques, GIS facilities for planning and monitoring & evaluation

viii) Earmarking of project funds for DPR preparation (1%), Entry point activities (4%), Capacity building (5%), Monitoring (1%) and Evaluation (1%).

ix) Introduction of new livelihood component with earmarking of project fund under Watershed Projects i.e. 9% of project fund for livelihoods for asset less people and 10% for production system & micro-enterprises

x) Delegation of power of sanction of projects to States.

Source: Department of Land Resources, Government of India, ministry of Rural Development)

Providing Rural Amenities in Rural Areas (PURA)

PURA is a rural Development Programme announced by The President of India, Dr. A.P.J. Abdul Kalam, on the eve of 54th Republic Day of India i.e on 26th January 2004. The programme aims at providing amenities similar to urban areas to the rural people.

Mission: "Holistic and accelerated development of compact rural areas around a potential growth centre in a Panchayat (or group of Panchayats) through Public-Private Partnership (PPP) for provision of urban amenities in rural areas thereby improving the quality of life to bridge the rural-urban divide.

Primary Objective is to provide urban amenities in rural areas. Other objectives include : i) reduction of migration from rural to urban areas, and ii) ensuring in-situ livelihood opportunities.

Project area: A Gram Panchayat/ a cluster of geographically contiguous Gram Panchayats with population of about 25000-40000. It is a scheme to bridge rural-urban areas and achieve balanced socio-economic development by identifying the village clusters with growth potential and creating following types of connectivity within them:

- Road, transport and power connectivity
- Electronic connectivity (IT, Telecome)
- Knowledge connectivity (Educational training institute)
- Market connectivity

Amenities to be provide

i) Water supply
   - piped water supply through individual household connections
   - sustainability of water supply through water harvesting and water recharge activities.

ii) Sewerage
   - 100 % coverage of sewerage connections to individual households

iii) Solid waste management
   - 100 % coverage of SWM services to individual households
   - Scientific treatment of solid waste

iv) Village streets and drainage
   - 100% village streets paved along with storm water drains covering the entire rural population
   - 100% of village streets to have street lighting

v) Increase in employment
  - Increased economic activity for employment of the entire village population
  - Improving the standard of living to halt the migration of the population to the urban areas.

National Rural Health Mission

Recognising the importance of health in the process of economic and social development and improving the quality of life of our citizens, the Government of India launched National Rural Health Mission during 2005 to carry out necessary architectural correction in the basic health care delivery system. The mission adopts a synergistic approach by relating health to determinants of good health viz. Segments of nutrition , sanitation, hygiene and safe drinking water. It also aimed at mainstreaming the Indian systems of medicine to facilitate health care. The plan action includes increasing public expenditure on health, reducing regional imbalance in health infrastructure , pooling resources, integration of organisational structure optimisation of health manpower, decentralisation and district management of health programme, community participation and ownership of assets, induction of management and financial personnel into district health system, and operationalizing community health centres in to functional hospitals meeting Indian Public Health Standards in each Block of the Country.

Goals of the Mission

i) Improving the availability of and access to quality health care by people, especially for those residing in rural areas, the poor, women and children.
ii) Reduction in infant Mortality Rate (IMR) and Maternal Mortality Ratio (MMR)
iii) Universal access to public health services such as women's health, child health, water, sanitation and hygiene, immunisation, and nutrition.
iv) Prevention and control of communicable and non-communicable diseases including locally endemic diseases.
v) Enhancing access to integrated comprehensive primary health care.
vi) Population stabilisation, gender and demographic balance
vii) Revitalisation of local health traditions and mainstream AYUSH.
viii) Promotion of healthy life-style.

Strategy

i) Train and enhance capacity of Panchayat Raj Institutions (PRIs) to own , control and manage public health services.

ii) Promotion of female health activist (ASHA) to provide improved health care at household level

iii) Health plan for each village through Village Health Committee of the Panchayat.

iv) Strengthening sub-centre through a united fund to enable local planning and action

v) Strengthening existing PHCs and CHCs and provision of 30-50 beded CHC per lakh population for improved curative care to a normative standard (Indian Public Health Standard defining personnel, equipment and management standards),

vi) Preparpation and implementation of an inter- sectoral District Health Plan prepared by the District Health Mission, including drinking water, sanitation and hygiene, and nutrition.

vii) Integrating vertical Heath and Family Welfare Programmes at National, State, District and Block level.

viii) Techinical support to National ,State and District Health Missions for public health management.

ix) Strengthening capacities for data collection, assessment and review for evidence –based planning, monitoring and supervision.

x) Formulation of transparent policies for deployment and career development of human resources for health.

xi) Developing capacities for prepventive health care at all levels for promoting healthy life style , reduction in consumption of tobacco and alcohol, etc.

xii) Promoting non-profit sector particularly in undeserved areas.

National Food Security Mission (NFSM)

National Food Security Mission was launched in 2007-08 to increase the production of rice, wheat and pulses by 10, 8 and 2 million tonnes, respectively by the end of 11th Plan through area expansion and productivity enhancement; restoring soil fertility and productivity; creating employment opportunities; and enhancing farm level economy. The Mission is being continued during 12th Five Year Plan with new target of additional production of 25 million tonnes of food grains comprising of 10 million tonnes rice, 8 million tonnes of wheat, 4 million tonnes of pulses and 3 million tonnes of coarse cereals by the end of 12th Plan and promotion of commercial crops like cotton, jute & sugarcane.

The basic strategy of the Mission is to promote and extend improved techn-ologies, i.e., seed, micronutrients, soil amendments, integrated pest management, farm machinery and implements, irrigation devices resource conservation along with capacity building of farmers. The major interventions/activities covered under NFSM include cluster demonstrations of rice, wheat, pulses and coarse cereals, distribution of improved varieties/hybrid seeds, need based plant and soil management, resource conservation techniques /energy management, efficient water/application tools, cropping system based trainings and local initiatives; award for best performing districts etc. During 12th Plan, in 2014-15, NFSM is being implemented in 623 districts of 28 States.

Monitoring & Evaluation of NFSM

i) **National level:** A three-tier monitoring mechanism was inbuilt in NFSM at National, State and District levels. At National level General Council (GC) under the chairmanship of Union Agriculture Minister was constituted to oversee the implementation of NFSM and take policy decisions for mid-term corrections. National Food Security Mission Executive Committee (NFSMEC) under the chairmanship of Secretary (A&C) periodically reviewed the State Action Plan and the progress of the programme of each State. National Level Monitoring Teams (NLMTs) reconstituted for monitoring the National Food Security Mission (NFSM) activities in respect of NFSM States. Each team consists of experts in the field of rice, wheat, pulses and coarse cereals as per requirement, and the respective Directors of the Directorates of Crop Development of Ministry of Agriculture as Coordinator.

Altogether, there are eight (8) National Level Monitoring Teams (NLMTs).

ii) **State level:** The monitoring is undertaken by State Food Security Mission Executive Committee (SFSMEC) under the Chairmanship of Chief Secretary.

iii) **District level**: The monitoring is undertaken by District Food Security Mission Executive Committee (DFSMEC) under the chairmanship of District Collector.

The Mid-Term Evaluation of NFSM was conducted by an independent agency to assess the impact of the programme in increasing the productivity of rice, wheat, pulses and enhancement of farm income. The finding of the Mid-Term Evaluation revealed that NFSM has helped to widen the food basket of the country with significant contribution coming from the NFSM districts. Significant outputs were recorded under NFSM since inception of the programme in 2007-08. The Mission accomplished the target of additional production of 20 million tonnes within 4 years of its implementation.

The final evaluation of NFSM was assigned to independent agency to assess the impact of technological interventions of the programme in increasing the productivity of rice, wheat and pulses, etc.

Outcome of NFSM since inception

The focused and target oriented implementation of mission initiatives has resulted in bumper production of wheat, rice and pulses in the country. During 2012-13, the productions of rice, wheat and pulses have been achieved at the level of 105.24 million tonnes, 93.51 million tonnes and 18.34 million tonnes respectively. As per 4th Advance Estimates during 2013-14, the production of wheat increased from 75.81 million tonnes in 2006-07 (pre-NFSM year) to 95.91 million tonnes, i.e. an increase of 20.00 million tonnes. Similarly, the total production of rice increased from 93.36 million tonnes in 2006-07 to 106.54 million tonnes in 2013-14 i.e. an increase of nearly 13.00 million tonnes. The total production of Pulses also increased from 14.20 million tonnes during 2006-07 to 19.27 million tonnes during 2013-14 with an increase of 5 million tonnes.

Source: Annual Report,2014-15, Deptt. of Agriculture and Cooperation, Govt. of India

Mission for Integrated Development of Horticulture (MIDH)

During 12th Five Year Plan, with effect from 2014-15, Department of Agriculture & Cooperation launched Mission for Integrated Development of Horticulture (MIDH) by subsuming various Missions/Schemes on horticulture viz. (i) National Horticulture Mission (NHM), (ii) Horticulture Mission for North East and Himalayan States (HMNEH), (iii) National Bamboo Mission (NBM), (iv) National Horticulture Board (NHB), (v) Coconut Development Board (CDB), and (vi) Central Institute of Horticulture (CIH), Nagaland.

National Horticulture Mission (NHM)

This Centrally Sponsored Scheme launched in the year 2005-06, aims at the holistic development of horticulture sector by ensuring forward and backward linkage through a cluster approach with the active participation of all stake holders. All States and four Union Territories of Andaman & Nicobar Islands, Lakshadweep, Puducherry and Dadra & Nagar Haveli are covered under NHM whereas the states in the

North Eastern and Himalayan region are covered under the Horticulture Mission for North East and Himalayan States (HMNEH). 384 districts in 18 States and 4 Union Territories are covered under NHM. Sixteen National Level Agencies (NLAs) have also been included for providing support for developmental efforts which require inputs at the National level.

Supply of quality planting material through establishment of nurseries and tissue culture units production and productivity improvement programmes through area expansion and rejuvenation, technology promotion, technology dissemination, human resource development, creation of infrastructure for post harvest management and marketing in consonance with the comparative advantages of each State/region and their diverse agro-climatic conditions were major programmes implemented during 2013-14.

Horticulture Mission for North East and Himalayan States (HMNEH)

This Centrally Sponsored Scheme is being implemented since 2001-02 in all the eight North Eastern States and three Himalayan States namely Jammu and Kashmir, Himachal Pradesh and Uttarakhand with 100% central assistance.

Physical Progress: An area of 9539 ha. has been covered under various horticulture crops and 3114 ha. of old and senile plantation rejuvenated besides an area of 86.2 ha. has been brought under protected cultivation, 2804 ha. under IPM. Apart from this, 777 community water harvesting structures have been created and 3750 number of farmers have been trained under various horticulture activities.

National Bamboo Mission (NBM)

This scheme is being implemented in 27 States in the country since 2006-07. The Mission envisages promoting holistic growth of bamboo sector by adopting area- based, regionally differentiated strategy and to increase the area under bamboo cultivation and marketing. Under the Mission, steps have been taken to increase the availability of quality planting material by supporting the setting up of new nurseries/tissue culture units and strengthening of existing ones. To address forward integration, the Mission is taking steps to strengthen marketing of bamboo products, especially those of handicrafts items.

Coconut Development Board (CDB)

The Coconut Development Board was established by an Act of Parliament in 1979 and came into existence on 12.1.1981. The Board is implementing various programmes for the development of coconut sector which includes action plan like production and distribution of planting material, expansion of area under coconut and integrated farming in coconut holdings for productivity improvement and a technology mission on coconut.

National Horticulture Board (NHB)

The Board was established in 1984 as an autonomous registered society under the Department, with its headquarters in Gurgaon and 35 field offices located all over the country. Its main objectives are the creation of production hubs for commercial horticulture development, post-harvest infrastructure and cold chain facilities, promotion of new technologies, introduction and promotion of new crops, and promotion of growers' associations. The three major components of the National Horticulture Board are as follow :

i) Development of commercial horticulture through production and post-harvest management
ii) Investment subsidy for construction/ expansion/ modernization of cold storages and storages for horticulture produce
iii) Technology development and transfer for horticulture produce

Central Institute of Horticulture (CIH), Nagaland

Recognizing the importance for providing institutional support to the development of horticulture in the "North Eastern Region", the Government of India approved in January, 2006, a Central Sector Scheme for setting up of Central Institute of Horticulture in Nagaland with the following objectives:

- Capacity building by training of trainers, extension officers, farmers, entrepreneurs, processors and exporters;
- Demonstration of improved technologies such as use of improved varieties/ hybrids, adoption of INM/ IPM practices, Hi-tech farming, precision farming, protected cultivation, post harvest technologies, etc.;
- Follow on extension support in the field of horticulture;
- Promotion of organic cultivation of horticultural crops;
- Establishing convergence and synergy among programmes in the field of horticultural research and development; and
- Monitoring of Centrally Sponsored programmes in the area of horticulture.

Source: Annual Report,2014-15, Deptt. of Agriculture and Cooperation, Govt. of India.

National Mission on Oilseeds and Oil Palm (NMOOP)

The Centrally Sponsored Scheme of Integrated Scheme of Oilseeds, Oil Palm and Maize (ISOPOM), which was launched in 2004-05 and remained under implementation till March, 2014. Oil Palm Area Expansion (OPAE) programme, a sub-scheme of RKVY implemented during 2011-12 to 2013-14 have made significant contribution in increasing the oilseeds production and area expansion under oil palm. Implementations of these schemes have given fillip in augmenting the availability of vegetable oil in the country. The production of oilseeds has increased from 24.35 million tonnes in 2004-05 to 32.88 million tonnes in 2013-14. The highest production of oilseeds has been achieved during

2013-14. The oilseeds yield which was 885 kg. per hectare in 2004-05 increased to 1153 kg per hectare during 2013-14(as per 4th Advance Estimates. The schemes of ISOPOM, Tree Borne Oilseeds (TBOs) and Oil Palm Area Expansion (OPAE) programme have been restructured into National Mission on Oil Seeds and Oil Palm (NMOOP) during 12th Plan and launched during 2014-15.

Objectives of NMOOP

Mini Mission (MM): Target of 12th Plan

MM I on Oilseeds: Achieve production of 35.51 million tonnes and productivity of 1328 kg/ ha of oilseeds from the present average production & productivity of 28.93 million tonnes and 1081 kg/ha during the 11th Plan period respectively.

MM II on Oil Palm : Bring additional 1.25 lakh hectare area under oil palm cultivation through area expansion approach in the States including utilization of wastelands with increase in productivity of fresh fruit brunches (FFBs) from 4927 kg per ha to 15000 kg per ha.

MM III on TBOs: Enhance seed collection of TBOs from 9 lakh tonnes to 14 lakh tonnes and to augment elite planting materials for area expansion under waste land.

Strategy for NMOOP

The strategy to implement the proposed Mission will include increasing Seed Replacement Ratio (SRR) with focus on Varietal Replacement; increasing irrigation coverage under oilseeds from 26% to 36%; diversification of area from low yielding cereals crops to oilseeds crops; intercropping of oilseeds with cereals/pulses/ sugarcane; use of fallow land after paddy/ potato cultivation; expansion of cultivation of Oil Palm & TBOs in watersheds and wastelands; increasing availability of quality planting materials of Oil Palm & TBOs; enhancing procurement of oilseeds and collection & processing of TBOs. Intercropping during gestation period of oil palm and TBOs would provide economic return to the farmers when there is no production. The scheme would be implemented in a mission mode through active involvement of all the stakeholders. Fund flow would be monitored to ensure that benefit of the Mission reaches the targeted beneficiaries in time to achieve the targeted results.

Mini Mission-I (Oilseeds)

The scheme is being implemented through State Department of Agriculture. The expenditure on subsidies is mostly shared on 75:25 sharing basis between Central and State Government. Central Seed producing agencies and ICAR Institutions are provided 100% assistance for seed production and organization of Front Line Demonstrations (FLDs). Under this Mission, financial assistance is being provided for Seed Components (production & distribution of certified seeds & minikits, variety specific targeted seed production); Inputs (Plant Protection Equipments /eco-friendly light-trap, Bio-pesticides, Distribution of micronutrients, bio-fertilizers, improved farm implements, pipes, sprinklers, seed storage bins, seed treatment drums) and Transfer of Technology (Block demonstrations, Frontline demonstrations, farmers and extension workers training etc.).

Mini Mission-II (Oil Palm)

Interventions of MM-II are being shared in the ratio of 75:25 between the Central and the State Governments. In case of R&D 100% support is being provided to Directorate of Oil Palm Research (DOPR), Pedavegi, Andhra Pradesh. Under Mini Mission II (MM II) of NMOOP, financial support is being provided to the farmers @ 85% cost of the planting material and @ 50% cost of the other components like maintenance cost of new plantations for three years, installation of drip-irrigation system, diesel/electric pump-sets, bore-well/water harvesting structures/ponds, inputs for inter-cropping in oil palm, construction of vermi-compost units and purchase of machinery & tools etc.

Mini Mission-III (TREE BORNE OILSEEDS) (TBOs)

The strategy to implement Mini Mission-III will include expansion of cultivation of TBOs in watersheds and wastelands, increasing availability of quality planting materials of TBOs enhancing collection & processing of TBOs, and inter cropping during gestation period, etc. An action Plan has been approved for TRIFED for promotion of seed collection of TBOs and facilitating marketing of collected TBOs.

Source: Annual Report,2014-15, Deptt. of Agriculture and Cooperation, Govt. of India

National Mission for Sustainable Agriculture (NMSA)

National Mission for Sustainable Agriculture (NMSA) is one of the eight Missions outlined under National Action Plan on Climate Change (NAPCC). The Mission aims at promoting sustainable agriculture through seventeen deliverables focusing on ten key dimensions of Indian Agriculture. During 12th Five Year Plan, these measures have been embedded and mainstreamed into Missions/Progammes/ Schemes of Department of Agriculture & Cooperation (DAC) through a process of restructuring and convergence. NMSA as a programmatic intervention made operational from the year 2014-15 aims at making agriculture more productive, sustainable, and remunerative and climate resilient by promoting location specific integrated/composite farming systems; soil and moisture conservation measures; comprehensive soil health management; efficient water management practices and mainstreaming rainfed technologies.

Components of NMSA

i) Rainfed Area Development (RAD)

The major strategy in implementing RAD is promoting integrated farming system covering crops, livestock & fishery, plantation and pasture based composite farming for enhancing livelihood opportunities, ensuring food security and minimizing risks from crop failure through supplementary/ residual production systems.

ii) On Farm Water Management (OFWM)

It focuses primarily on enhancing water use efficiency by promoting efficient on-farm water management technologies and equipment. This will not only focus on application efficiency but, in conjunction with RAD component, for effective harvesting & management of rainwater. Assistance is being given for adopting water conservation technologies, efficient delivery and distribution systems etc.

iii) Soil Health Management (SHM)

SHM is aimed at promoting location as well as crop specific sustainable soil health management including residue management, organic farming practices by way of creating and linking soil fertility maps with macro-micro nutrient management, appropriate land use based on land type.

iv) Climate Change and Sustainable Agriculture Monitoring, Modelling & Networking (CCSAMMN)

CCSAMMN supports dissemination of climate change related information and knowledge by way of piloting climate change adaptation/ mitigation research/ model projects in the domain of climate smart sustainable management practices.

National Mission on Agricultural Extension & Technology (NMAET)

National Mission on Agricultural Extension & Technology consists of four submissions viz (i) Sub Mission on Agriculture Extension (SMAE); (ii) Sub Mission on Seed and Planting Material (SMSP); (iii) Sub Mission on Agricultural Mechanization (SMAM) and (iv) Sub Mission on Plant Protection and Plant Quarantine (SMPP). Various interventions/activities undertaken through these sub-missions are given below.

Sub Mission on Agricultural Extension

The 11th Plan Extension Schemes have been subsumed within the Sub Mission on Agricultural Extension (SAME) under the National Mission on Agricultural Extension and Technology (NMAET) being implemented during the 12th Plan with an objective to restructure and strengthen the agricultural extension machinery with a judicious mix of extensive physical outreach of personnel, enhancement in quality through domain experts & regular capacity building, interactive methods of information dissemination, Public Private Partnership, pervasive & innovative use of Information & Communication Technology (ICT)/ Mass Media, Federation of groups and convergence of extension related efforts under various schemes and programmes of Government of India and the State Governments. The SMAE aims to appropriately strengthen, expand and upscale existing Extension & Information Technology (IT) Schemes. The ongoing Extension Schemes include the Central Sector and Centrally Sponsored Schemes being implemented by the Extension Division/Directorate of Extension. Even in the case of Central Sector Schemes which have been subsumed within the Mission, a greater role has been envisaged for the States through their active involvement in planning, implementation and monitoring. The name of these schemes are given below:

i) Support to State Extension Programmes for Extension Reforms Scheme (ATMA Scheme)

The erstwhile Scheme 'Support to State Extension Programmes for Extension Reforms (ATMA)' implemented since 2005 has now been included as a component of the Sub-Mission on Agriculture Extension (SMAE) under NMAET with some cost revisions and additional components. It is now under implementation in 640 districts of 29 states & 3 UTs of the country.

ii) Mass Media Support to Agricultural Extension

This Scheme focuses on the use of Doordarshan and All India Radio (AIR) infrastructure for providing information and knowledge to the farming community in agriculture and allied sector. 180 Narrow casting Centres, 18 Regional Centres and 1 National Centre of Doordarshan telecast agricultural programmes in the name of Krishi Darshan for 30 minutes, five to six days a week. Programmes of Regional Kendras and some Narrowcasting Centres (NCs) are being repeated the next day on respective Regional Satellite Channel. Similarly, 96 Rural FM Radio Stations of All India Radio are being utilized to broadcast 30 minutes of programme for farmers 6 days a week under Kisanvani Programme.

iii) Establishment of the Agri-Clinics and Agri-Business Centres (ACABC)

The ACABC scheme is under implementation since 2002. The scheme aims at creating gainful self-employment opportunities to unemployed agricultural graduates, agricultural diploma holders, and intermediate in agriculture apart from science graduates with post-graduation in agriculture related courses for supporting agriculture development and supplementing the efforts of public extension. MANAGEis the implementing agency for training component under the scheme through a network of identified Nodal Training Institutes (NTIs) in various States. NABARD is implementing subsidy component under the scheme on the behalf of Government of India and is monitoring credit support to Agri-Clinics through Commercial Banks.

iv) Kisan Call Centers (KCC)

The KCC Scheme was launched on 21stJanuary 2004 to provide answer to farmers' queries on agriculture and allied sectors through toll free telephone lines. A country wide common eleven digit number '1800-800-1551'has been allocated for KCC. The replies to the queries of the farming community are being given in 22 local languages. KCCs operate from 14 locations in the country covering all the Sates and UTs. Calls are attended from 6.00 am to 10.00 pm on all 7 days of a week. Since inception of the scheme till 31st December, 2014 over 186.00 lakh calls have been registered in the KCCs. In order to make farmers aware of this facility, audio and video spots on Kisan Call Centres have been broadcasts/telecast through All India Radio, Doordarshan and private television channels. A Kisan Knowledge Management system (KKMS) has been created at the backend to capture details of the farmers calling KCCs provide correct, consistent and quick replies to the queries of farmers is being developed and by the putting therein validated information on agriculture and allied sectors. 8.21 The Kisan Call Centre scheme has been recently restructured and strengthened, with a good number of unique features viz. provision of IPPBX,100% call recording; call barging; voice mail service; customized IVRS; call conferencing through the experts; playing state specific advisories during call wait time and SMS to caller farmers giving a gist of answers given by the KCC Agent now known as Farm Tele Advisor. The farmer calling KCC can also register for receiving SMSs from experts on the subject area and their providing and also for receiving regular updates on mandi price of selected mandis and crops.

v) HRD Support

DAC has strengthened a network of training institutions in the country by supporting the National Institute of Agricultural Extension Management

(MANAGE) at Hyderabad; four Regional Extension Education Institutes (EEIs) at the regional level and the State Agricultural Management & Extension Training Institutes (SAMETIs) at the State level.

a) **MANAGE** : It is providing training support to senior and middle level functionaries of the State Governments. It is also providing necessary support to the states in implementation of Extension Reforms (ATMA) scheme.

b) **Extension Education Institutes (EEIs):** Four Extension Education Institutes namely, Nilokeri (Haryana), Rajendranagar, Hyderabad (Telangana), Anand (Gujarat), Jorhat (Assam) are functioning at the Regional Level. The objectives of EEIs are to improve the skills and professional competence of middle level Extension field functionaries of Agriculture and allied departments of the State Governments in the areas of (a) Extension Education; (b) Extension Methodology; (c) Information and Communication Technology; (d) Training Methodology; (e) Communication; (f) Extension Reforms Scheme; (g) Market led Extension; etc.

c) **Model Training Courses (MTCs):** Model Training Courses of eight days duration on thrust areas of Agriculture, Horticulture, Animal Husbandry, Fisheries Extension are supported by the Directorate of Extension (DOE) with the objective of improving the professional competence and upgrading the knowledge and developing technical skills of Subject Matter Specialists/ Extension workers of Agriculture and allied departments of the State Governments.

d) **National Gender Resource Centre in Agriculture (NGRCA)**: NGRCA has been set up as a unit of Directorate of Extension (DOE) of the DAC under the Scheme of Extension Support to Central Institutes/DOE. NGRCA reflects the national commitment of empowerment of women through 'strategy of mainstreaming and agenda setting'. The Centre acts as a focal point for the convergence of gender related activities and issues in agriculture and allied sectors within and outside DAC; addressing gender dimension to agriculture policies and programmes; rendering advocacy/ advisory services to the States /UTs to internalize gender specific interventions for bringing the farm women in the mainstream of agriculture development.

vi) National e-Governance Plan in Agriculture (NeGP-A)

The Government is implementing a Centrally Sponsored Scheme "National e-Governance Plan in Agriculture (NeGP-A)" in the entire country.The project envisages deployment of hardware and roll out of services down to the Block level. This centrally sponsored Mission Mode Project (MMP) scheme is being implemented in seven States, viz, Assam, Himachal Pradesh, Karnataka, Jharkhand, Kerala, Madhya Pradesh and Maharashtra from the last phase of the 11th plan (2010-11) it has now been approved for implementation in the remaining States and UTs during the current Plan period commencing from 2014-15 onward.

The Scheme aims to achieve rapid development of agriculture in India through the use of ICT for ensuring timely access to agriculture related information for the farmers of the country. The current IT initiatives/schemes under implementation by DAC which are aimed at providing information to the farmers on various activities in the agriculture value chain will be integrated so that farmers would be able to make proper and timely use of the available information. Such information is intended to be provided to farmers through multiple delivery channels such as Internet, Government Offices, Touch Screen Kiosks, Krishi Vigyan Kendras , Kisan Call Centres, Agri-Clinics, Common Service Centers, Mobile Phones (Broadcast, IVRS, interactive messaging using unstructured Supplementary Service Data and Voice Recognition).

Submission on Seed and Planting Material (SMSP)

Central Sector Scheme "Development and Strengthening of Infrastructure Facilities for the Production and Distribution of Quality Seeds" was under implementation on all India basis since 2005-06. The scheme is now subsumed into the new "Sub Mission on Seed and Planting Material (SMSP)" under the new centrally Sponsored Scheme "National Mission on Agricultural Extension and Technology (NMAET)". The Mission is intended to develop and strengthen the existing infrastructure for production and distribution of certified / quality seeds with a focused, time bound and integrated agenda to improve the availability of quality seeds for the farmers and to encourage the development of new varieties of plants.

Sub Mission on Agricultural Mechanization (SMAM)

Agriculture Mechanization is an essential input to modern agriculture to increase the productivity and for making judicious use of other inputs like seeds, fertilizers, chemicals & pesticides and natural resources like water, soil nutrients etc. besides reducing the human drudgery and cost of cultivation. Agriculture Mechanization also helps in improving safety and comfort of the agricultural worker, improvements in the quality and value addition of the farm produce and also enabling the farmers to take second and subsequent crops making Indian agriculture more attractive and profitable. It also helps the Indian farming to become commercial instead of subsistence. There is a linear relationship between availability of farm power and farm yield. Therefore, there is a need to increase the availability of farm power from 1.73 kW per ha to 2.0 kW per ha by the end of 12th FY Plan to cope up with increasing demand of food grains. Recognizing the need to mechanize the marginal and small farmers, and for inclusive growth of Farm mechanization Sector in the country, a Sub Mission on Agriculture Mechanization (SMAM) was launched in the year 2014-15 with the following objectives:

- Increasing the reach of farm mechanization to small and marginal farmers and to the regions where availability of farm power is low;
- Promoting 'Custom Hiring Centres' to offset the adverse economies of scale arising due to small landholding and high cost of individual ownership;
- Creating hubs for hi-tech & high value farm equipments;
- Creating awareness among stakeholders through demonstration and capacity building activities;
- Ensuring performance testing and certification at designated testing centers located all over the country.

Sub Mission on Plant Protection and Plant Quarantine (SMPP)

The objective of the Sub-Mission is to prevent crop loss through sustainable agriculture and protection of the India's bio-security. The Sub-Mission has 4 important components:

a) Strengthening and Modernization of Pest Management Approach (SMPMA),

b) Strengthening and Modernization of Plant Quarantine Facilities (SMPQF),

c) Monitoring of Pesticide Residues at National Level (MPRNL) and

d) National Institute of Plant Health Management (NIPHM).

National Crop Insurance Programme (NCIP)

Keeping in view the risks involved in Agriculture and to insure the farming community against various risks, Ministry of Agriculture introduced a crop insurance scheme in 1985 and thereafter brought improvements in the erstwhile scheme(s) from time to time based on the experience gained and views of the stakeholders, states, farming community etc. To enlarge the coverage in terms of farmers, crops and risks, National Agricultural Insurance Scheme (NAIS) was started w.e.f 1999. To make the crop insurance schemes more farmers friendly, a re-structured Central Sector Scheme namely "National Crop Insurance Programme (NCIP)" has been approved by merging the erstwhile

Pilot schemes of Modified National Agricultural Insurance Scheme (MNAIS), Weather Based Crop Insurance Scheme (WBCIS) and Coconut Palm Insurance Scheme (CPIS) with some improvements for full fledged implementation from Rabi 2013-14 season throughout the country. NAIS was to be discontinued after implementation of NICP from Rabi 2013-14 season. However, on the representations from States, it has been continued during 2013-14 and 2014-15.

The Scheme is optional for the State Governments and they can notify crops and areas according to provisions of the schemes. The Components under the Scheme are being implemented on "Area Approach Method" where yield of notified areas under MNAIS and Weather data of notified Reference Automatic Weather Stations (AWSs) under WBCIS are taken as one unit for assessment/ payment of claims for widespread calamities. However, claims are also being paid on the basis of losses at individual farms due to localized calamities like hailstorm and landslides under MNAIS and WBCIS (as add on/index-plus coverage). The penetration/coverage of these schemes in terms of number of farmers has reached about 30% of the total No. of land holdings in the country. The coverage of farmers under NCIP by terminal year of 12th Plan (i.e. 2016-17) has been projected to be at 50% with help of the improvements / changes made in NCIP component schemes of MNAIS, WBCIS &CPIS.

Salient features of NCIP

- Implementation is made compulsory for loanee farmers.
- Two indemnity levels of 80% & 90% would be available instead of three i.e. 70%, 80% & 90% under MNAIS.
- Under WBCIS, provision for add-on/index plus products for horticultural crops for compensating losses due to perils of hailstorm, cloudburst etc
- For successful implementation of WBCIS, 5000 AWS will be set-up in the country through the model of Private Public Participation(PPP).
- Pilots for use of modern technology like Remote Sensing Technology (RST)/ Satellite imageries to supplement the yield assessment through CCEs.
- Insurance eligibility condition of having at least 10 healthy palms by farmer has been reduced to 5 palms under CPIS. Increased Sum Insured under CPIS
- Loss intimation time has been increased from 7 days to 15 days under CPIS

National Agricultural Insurance Scheme (NAIS)

With a view to provide financial support to farmers in the event of loss / failure of any of the notified crop in the notified areas as a result of natural calamities (flood, drought etc.), pests and diseases, NAIS was introduced in the country from Rabi 1999-2000 season in place of erstwhile Comprehensive Crop Insurance Scheme (CCIS). NAIS was to be discontinued after implementation of NICP from Rabi 2013-14 season. However, on the representations from States, it has been continued during 2013-14 and 2014-15. The scheme is available to all the farmers (loanee and non-loanee) irrespective of their size of holding. Loanee farmers are covered on compulsory basis in a notified area for notified crops whereas for non-loanee farmers, scheme was voluntary. The Scheme covers all the food crops (cereals, millets and pulses), oilseeds and annual commercial/horticultural crops, in respect of which past yield data is available for adequate number of years. The administered premium rates are charged which range from 1.5% to 3.5% of sum insured for food and oilseed crops for normal sum insured and indemnity level. In the case of commercial/horticultural crops, higher sum insured & indemnity than the normal, actuarial rates are charged. Under the scheme, 10% subsidy in premium is available to small & marginal farmers.

Modified National Agricultural Insurance Scheme (MNAIS)

With a view to make the scheme simpler & farmer friendly, a Joint Group was constituted in 2004 under the Chairmanship of Additional Secretary in the Department of Agriculture & Cooperation to study the improvements required in the then existing crop insurance schemes. Based on the recommendations of the Joint Group and views/comments of various stakeholders, a pilot proposal on MNAIS was approved by Government of India for implementation on pilot basis in 50 districts from Rabi 2010-11 season. After evaluation of impact of Pilot, the scheme is being implemented as a full-fledged component of NCIP from Rabi 2013-14.

Weather based Crop Insurance Scheme (WBCIS)

With the objective to bring more farmers under crop insurance fold and to overcome the shortcoming regarding delay in settlement of claims etc. under NAIS, a pilot WBCIS was announced in the Union Budget for 2007-08 and was approved for implementation in 20 States on pilot basis. WBCIS is implemented as a full- fledged component scheme of NCIP from Rabi 2013-14 season. WBCIS intends to provide insurance protection to the farmers against adverse weather incidence, such as deficient and excess rainfall, high or low temperature, humidity etc. which are deemed to impact adversely the crop production. Under WBCIS, actuarial rates of premium are being charged. However, to make the scheme affordable to the farmers subsidy upto 50% of the premium is provided by the Government which is shared by Centre and State concerned on 50:50 basis. Actuarial rates of premium are capped at 10% during Kharif and 8% during Rabi for food crops & oilseeds. For annual commercial/ horticultural crops, cap of 12% on actuarial rates of premium is applicable. Both loanee & non-loanee farmers are covered under WBCIS irrespective of their size of holding. Like NAIS, the loanee farmers are covered on compulsory basis in a notified area for notified crops whereas for non-loanee farmers scheme is voluntary. Further, to provide competitive service to the farmers, private insurance companies have been involved for implementation besides the Agriculture Insurance Company of India (AIC) Ltd.

Coconut Palm Insurance Scheme (CPIS)

The Department of Agriculture and Cooperation has been implementing Coconut Palm Insurance Scheme (CPIS) on pilot basis from the year 2009-10 onwards in the selected areas of Andhra Pradesh, Goa, Karnataka, Kerala, Maharashtra, Odisha, Tamil Nadu and West Bengal. Now, the CPIS is being implemented as a full fledged component scheme of NCIP from Rabi 2013-14 season in all coconut growing States. The scheme is being administered by Coconut Development Board. Insurance coverage is being extended to the total loss of the individual palm in the age group of 4 to 60 years for dwarf & hybrid; and 7-60 years for tall variety, leading to either death of palm or the palm becoming useless due to various natural and other perils. The farmer should have at least 05 healthy nut bearing Palms in the age group of 4 to 60 years in contiguous area/plot and should have been enrolled by State Agriculture/Horticulture Department or Coconut Development Board (CDB) or any other such agency under rehabilitation/ development/expansion scheme. The Sum Insured is based on the average input cost of the plantation and the age of the specific plant. The Sum Insured varied from Rs. 900 per palm in the age group of 4-15 years to Rs. 1725 per palm in the age group of 16-60 years. The premium rate per palm ranged from Rs. 9.00 in the age group of 4 to 15 years to Rs. 14.00 in the age group of 16 to 60 years and it varied on sum insured per year, considering the age of specific palm. 50% of premium is contributed by Government of India; 25% by the concerned State Govt. and the remaining 25% by the farmer. The Insurance Company i.e. Agriculture Insurance Company of India (AIC) is implementing the scheme and responsible for making payment of all claims. The pilot CPIS is administered and implemented by the Coconut Development Board (CDB).

Source: Annual Report, 2014-15, Deptt. of Agriculture and Cooperation, Govt. of India.

Suggested Readings and References

1. Annual Reports, (2009-2017). Deptt. of Agriculture and Cooperation, Govt. of India.
2. Reddy, A.A. (1993). Extension Education, Sree lakshmi Press, Bapatla.
3. Dhama, O.P. and Bhatnagar, O.P. (2007). Education and Communication for Development. Oxford and IBH Pub. Co. Pvt. Ltd.
4. Mathialagan, P. (2007). Textbook of Animal Husbandry and Livestock Extension, International Book Distributing Co. 7, Meerabai Marg, Lucknow, India.
5. Singh, Katar (1999). Rural Development: Principles, Policies and Management, Second Edition, New Delhi, Sage Publications.
6. Verma, S.C. (1980). Direct Attack on Rural Poverty, Ministry of Rural Development, Delhi.
7. NIRD, Fifty Years of Rural Development in India (1998). NIRD, Hyderabad.
8. Desai, Vasant (2009). Rural Development in India, Himalaya Publishing House, Mumbai.
9. Ray, G.L. (2001). Extension, Communication and Management, 4th Edition, Naya Prokash, Calcutta.
10. Ministry of Agriculture, Government of India (2009). Report of the High Powered Committee on Cooperative.
11. Sharma, K.R.G. (2008). Veterinary Extension Education, BSPBS Publications, Hyderabad, Hyderabad.

22

ICAR Frontline Extension Programmes

1. All India Coordinated Project on National Demonstration Programme (NDP)
    a) Objectives of the National Demonstration:
    b) Operational Research Project
    c) The Specific Objective of the ORP:
2. Krishi Vigyan Kendra (KVK) (Farm Science Centre)
    a) The genesis of KVKs
    b) The Basic Concept of KVK
    c) Mandate of KVKs
    d) Objectives of KVKs
    e) Special Features of KVK
    f) Training Programmes of KVK
    g) Growth of KVKs
3. Lab-to-Land Programme (LLP)
    a) Objectives of LLP
4. National Agriculture Research Project (NARP)
5. National Agricultural Technology Project (NATP)
6. Technology Assessment and Refinement–Institute Village Linkage Programme (TAR- IVLP)
    a) Objectives of TAR - IVLP
7. Agricultural Technology Information Centres (ATICS)
    a) Objectives of ATIC
    b) Attributes of ATIC

8. National Agricultural Innovation Project
   a) The Basic Principles of NAIP
   b) Objectives of NAIP
   c) Components of NAIP
   d) Institutional Development Priorities of the NAIP
   e) Research & Development Priorities of the NAIP
   f) Agricultural Diversification
   g) Livestock and Fisheries Production
   h) Genetic Resources and Bio-prospecting
   i) Natural Resource Management
   j) Integrated Pest Management
   k) Value-addition and Post-harvest Processing
   l) Research on Policy Analysis and Market Intelligence
9. National Initiative on Climate Resilient Agriculture (NICRA)
   a) Background
   b) Objectives of the Project
   c) Project Components
   d) Strategic Research
   e) Technology Demonstration
   f) Early Outcome
   g) Sponsored and competitive grants
   h) Capacity building
   i) XII plan activities in NICRA
   j) Approach of the Scheme
10. Suggested Readings and References

ICAR Frontline Extension Programmes

It was recognized by Indian Council of Agricultural Research (ICAR) in the early sixties that agriculture development requires interdisciplinary and multi institutional approach. The integrated functioning of agricultural research, education and extension was for the first time recognized as the cardinal principle of agricultural development system, and accordingly agricultural research, education and extension function were integrated in the ICAR institutes and State Agricultural Universities (SAU). ICAR established a Section of Extension Education at its headquarter in 1971, which was later renamed as Division of Agricultural Extension to promote the transfer the agricultural technologies through the ICAR-SAU system. The present position, as on 31.03.2020, of ICAR institutes, Central Agriculture Universities and SAUs are as follows:

List of State Agriculture, Horticulture, Forestry and Fishery Universities

S.No.	Name of University
Andhra Pradesh	
1	Acharya NG Ranga Agricultural University, Guntur
2	**Dr. YSRHU (APHU), Venkataramannagudem**
Assam	
3	Assam Agricultural University, Jorhat
Bihar	
4	Bihar Agricultural University, Sabour, Bhagalpur
Chhattisgarh	
5	Indira Gandhi Krishi Viswa Vidhyalaya, Raipur
Gujarat	
6	Sardar Krushinagar Dantiwada Agricultural University, Dantiwada
7	Anand Agricultural University, Anand
8	Navsari Agricultural University, Navsari
9	Junagarh Agricultural University, Junagarh
Haryana	
10	Chaudhary Charan Singh Haryana Agricultural University, Hisar
11	**Haryana State University of Horticultural Sciences, Karnal**
Himachal Pradesh	
12	Ch. Sarwan Kumar Himachal Pradesh Krishi Viswavidyalaya, Palampur
13	**Dr. Yaswant Singh Parmar University of Horticulture & Forestry, Solan**
Jharkhand	
14	Birsa Agricultural University, Ranchi
Jammu & Kashmir	
15	Sher-e-Kashmir University of Agricultural Science & Technology, Srinagar
16	Sher-e-Kashmir University of Agricultural Science & Technology, Jammu
Karnataka	
17	University of Agricultural Sciences, Bangalore

18 University of Agricultural Sciences, Raichur
19 University of Agricultural Sciences, Dharwad
20 University of Horticulture Science, Bagalkot
21 University of Agriculture & Horticulture Sciences, Shimoga

Kerala

22 Kerala Agricultural University, Thrissur
23 Kerala University of Fisheries and Ocean Studies, Panangad, Kochi

Madhya Pradesh

24 Rajmata Vijayaraje Scindia Krishi VishwaVidyalaya, Gwalior
25 Jawaharlal Nehru Krishi Viswa Vidyalaya, Jabalpur

Maharashtra

26 Dr. Balaesahib Sawant Kokan KrishiVidyapeeth, Dapoli
27 Vasantrao Naik Marathwada Krishi Vidyapeeth, Parbhani
28 Matatam Phule Krishi Vidyapeeth, Rahuri
29 Dr. Punjabrao Deshmukh KrishiViswaVidyalaya, Akola

Orissa

30 Orissa University of Agricultural & Technology, Bhubaneswar

Punjab

31 Punjab Agricultural University, Ludhiana

Rajasthan

32 Maharana Pratap University of Agriculture & Technology, Udaipur
33 Swami Keshwanand Rajasthan Agricultural University, Bikaner
34 SKN Agriculture University, Jobner
35 Agriculture University, Kota
36 Agriculture University, Jodhpur

Tamil Nadu

37 Tamil Nadu Agricultural University, Coimbatore
38 Tamil Nadu Fisheries University, Nagapattinam

Telangana

39 Sri Konda Laxman Telangana State Horticultural University, Hyderabad
40 Professor Jayashankar Telangana State Agricultural University, Hyderabad

UttraKhand

41 G.B. Pant University of Agriculture & Technology, Pantnagar
42 VCSG Uttarakhand University of Horticulture & Forestry, Bharsar

Uttar Pradesh

43 Chandra Shekhar Azad University of Agricultural & Technology, Kanpur
44 Narendra Deva University of Agriculture & Technology, Faizabad
45 Sardar Vallabhbhai Patel University of Agriculture & Technology, Meerut
46 Banda University of Agricultural and Technology, Banda
47 Sam Higginbottom University of Agriculture, Technology & Sciences, Allahabad

West Bengal

48 Bidhan Chandra Krishi Viswa Vidhyalaya, Mohanpur
49 Uttar Banga Krishi Viswavidhyalaya, Cooch Behar

State Veterinary Universities

S.No.	Name of University
Andhra Pradesh	
1	Sri Venkateswara Veterinary University, Tirupati
Bihar	
2	Bihar Animal Sciences University, Patna
Chhattisgarh	
3	Chhattisgarh Kamdhenu Visvavidyalaya, Durg
Gujarat	
4	Kamdhenu University, Gandhinagar
Haryana	
5	Lala Lajpat Rai University of Veterinary & Animal Sciences, Hisar
Karnataka	
6	Karnataka Veterinary, Animal and Fisheries Sciences University, Bidar
Kerala	
7	Kerala Veterinary and Animal Sciences University, Pookode, Wayanand, Kerala
Madhya Pradesh	
8	Nanaji Deshmukh Pashu ChikitsaVisvaVidyalaya, Jabalpur
Maharashtra	
9	Maharastra Animal & Fisheries. Sciences University, Nagpur
Punjab	
10	Guru Angad Dev Veterinary and Animal Sciences University, Ludhiana
Rajasthan	
11	Rajasthan University of Veterinary & Animal Sciences, Bikaner
Tamil Nadu	
12	Tamil Nadu Veterinary & Animal Sciences University, Chennai
Telangana	
13	Sri PV Narsimha Rao Telangana Veterinary University, Hyderabad
Uttar Pradesh	
14	U.P. Pt. Deen Dayal Upadhyaya Pashu Chikitsa VigyanVishwaVidhyalaya Evem Go Anusandhan Sansthan, Mathura
West Bengal	
15	West Bengal University of Animal & Fishery Sciences, Kolkata

List of Deemed Universities

1. ICAR-Indian Agricultural Research Institute, New Delhi
2. ICAR-National Dairy Research Institute, Karnal
3. ICAR-Indian Veterinary Research Institute, Izatnagar
4. ICAR-Central Institute on Fisheries Education, Mumbai

List of Central Agricultural Universities

1. Central Agricultural University, P.O. Box 23, Imphal-795004, Manipur
2. Rani Laxmi Bai Central Agricultural University, Jhansi, Uttar Pradesh
3. Dr. Rajendra Prasad Central Agricultural University, Pusa (Samastipur)

List of ICAR Institutions

1. ICAR-Central Island Agricultural Research Institute , Port Blair
2. ICAR-Central Arid Zone Research Institute, Jodhpur
3. ICAR-Central Avian Research Institute, Izatnagar
4. ICAR-Central Inland Fisheries Research Institute, Barrackpore
5. ICAR-Central Institute Brackishwater Aquaculture, Chennai
6. ICAR-Central Institute for Research on Buffaloes, Hissar
7. ICAR-Central Institute for Research on Goats, Makhdoom
8. ICAR-Central Institute of Agricultural Engineering, Bhopal
9. ICAR-Central Institute for Arid Horticulture, Bikaner
10. ICAR-Central Institute of Cotton Research, Nagpur
11. ICAR-Central Institute of Fisheries Technology, Cochin
12. ICAR-Central Institute of Freshwater Aquaculture, Bhubneshwar
13. ICAR-Central Institute of Research on Cotton Technology, Mumbai
14. ICAR-Central Institute of Sub Tropical Horticulture, Lucknow
15. ICAR-Central Institute of Temperate Horticulture, Srinagar
16. ICAR-Central Institute on Post harvest Engineering and Technology, Ludhiana
17. ICAR-Central Marine Fisheries Research Institute, Kochi
18. ICAR-Central Plantation Crops Research Institute, Kasargod
19. ICAR-Central Potato Research Institute, Shimla
20. ICAR-Central Research Institute for Jute and Allied Fibres, Barrackpore
21. ICAR-Central Research Institute of Dryland Agriculture, Hyderabad
22. ICAR-National Rice Research Institute, Cuttack
23. ICAR-Central Sheep and Wool Research Institute, Avikanagar, Rajasthan
24. ICAR- Indian Institute of Soil and Water Conservation, Dehradun
25. ICAR-Central Soil Salinity Research Institute, Karnal
26. ICAR-Central Tobacco Research Institute, Rajahmundry
27. ICAR-Central Tuber Crops Research Institute, Trivandrum
28. ICAR-ICAR Research Complex for Eastern Region, Patna
29. ICAR-ICAR Research Complex for NEH Region, Barapani
30. ICAR-Central Coastal Agricultural Research Institute, Ela, Old Goa, Goa
31. ICAR-Indian Agricultural Statistics Research Institute, New Delhi
32. ICAR-Indian Grassland and Fodder Research Institute, Jhansi
33. ICAR-Indian Institute of Agricultural Biotechnology, Ranchi
34. ICAR-Indian Institute of Horticultural Research, Bengaluru
35. ICAR-Indian Institute of Natural Resins and Gums, Ranchi

36. ICAR-Indian Institute of Pulses Research, Kanpur
37. ICAR-Indian Institute of Soil Sciences, Bhopal
38. ICAR-Indian Institute of Spices Research, Calicut
39. ICAR-Indian Institute of Sugarcane Research, Lucknow
40. ICAR-Indian Institute of Vegetable Research, Varanasi
41. ICAR-National Academy of Agricultural Research & Management, Hyderabad
42. ICAR-National Institute of Biotic Stresses Management, Raipur
43. ICAR-National Institue of Abiotic Stress Management, Malegaon, Maharashtra
44. ICAR-National Institute of Animal Nutrition and Physiology, Bengaluru
45. ICAR-National Institute of Research on Jute & Allied Fibre Technology, Kolkata
46. ICAR-National Institute of Veterinary Epidemiology and Disease Informatics, Hebbal, Bengaluru
47. ICAR-Sugarcane Breeding Institute, Coimbatore
48. ICAR-Vivekananda Parvatiya Krishi Anusandhan Sansthan, Almora
49. ICAR-Central Institute for Research on Cattle, Meerut, Uttar Pradesh
50. ICAR-National Institute of High Security Animal Diseases, Bhopal
51. ICAR-Indian Institute of Maize Research,New Delhi
52. ICAR- Central Agroforestry Research Institute , Jhansi
53. ICAR-National Institute of Agricultural Economics and Policy Research, New Delhi
54. ICAR- Indian Institute of Wheat and Barley Research, Karnal
55. ICAR- Indian Institute of Farming Systems Research, Modipuram
56. ICAR- Indian Institute of Millets Research, Hyderabad
57. ICAR- Indian Institute of Oilseeds Research, Hyderabad
58. ICAR- Indian Institute of Oil Palm Research, Pedavegi, West Godawari
59. ICAR- Indian Institute of Water Management, Bhubaneshwar
60. ICAR-Indian Institute of Rice Research, Hyderabad
61. ICAR- Central Institute for Women in Agriculture, Bhubaneshwar
62. ICAR-Central Citrus Research Institute, Nagpur
63. ICAR-Indian Institute of Seed Research, Mau

List of ICAR Directorates/Project Directorates

1. ICAR-Directorate of Groundnut Research, Junagarh
2. ICAR-Directorate of Soybean Research, Indore
3. ICAR-Directorate of Rapeseed & Mustard Research, Bharatpur
4. ICAR-Directorate of Mushroom Research, Solan
5. ICAR-Directorate on Onion and Garlic Research, Pune
6. ICAR-Directorate of Cashew Research, Puttur
7. ICAR-Directorate of Medicinal and Aromatic Plants Research, Anand
8. ICAR-Directorate of Floricultural Research, Pune, Maharashtra
9. ICAR-Directorate of Weed Research, Jabalpur
10. ICAR-Project Directorate on Foot & Mouth Disease, Mukteshwar
11. ICAR-Directorate of Poultry Research, Hyderabad
12. ICAR-Directorate of Knowledge Management in Agriculture (DKMA), New Delhi
13. ICAR-Directorate of Cold Water Fisheries Research, Bhimtal, Nainital

List of National Bureaux of ICAR

1. ICAR-National Bureau of Plant Genetics Resources, New Delhi
2. ICAR-National Bureau of Agriculturally Important Micro-organisms, Mau, Uttar Pradesh
3. ICAR-National Bureau of Agricultural Insect Resources, Bengaluru
4. ICAR-National Bureau of Soil Survey and Land Use Planning, Nagpur
5. ICAR-National Bureau of Animal Genetic Resources, Karnal
6. ICAR-National Bureau of Fish Genetic Resources, Lucknow

List of National Research Centres of ICAR

1. ICAR-National Research Centre for Banana, Trichi
2. ICAR-National Research Centre for Grapes, Pune
3. ICAR-National Research Centre for Litchi, Muzaffarpur
4. ICAR-National Research Centre for Pomegranate, Solapur
5. ICAR-National Research Centre on Camel, Bikaner
6. ICAR-National Research Centre on Equines, Hisar
7. ICAR-National Research Centre on Meat, Hyderabad
8. ICAR-National Research Centre on Mithun, Medziphema, Nagaland
9. ICAR-National Research Centre on Orchids, Pakyong, Sikkim
10. ICAR-National Research Centre on Pig, Guwahati
11. ICAR-National Research Centre on Plant Biotechnology, New Delhi
12. ICAR-National Research Centre on Seed Spices, Ajmer
13. ICAR-National Research Centre on Yak, West Kemang
14. ICAR-National Centre for Integrated Pest Management, New Delhi
15. National Research Centre on Integrated Farming (ICAR-NRCIF), Motihari

Source: ICAR, Government of India

The unit of extension education at the ICAR headquarters therefore was intended to enforce this functional relationship down the line in the ICAR institutes, SAUs, and other institutions of the country. In order to sanitize the process of integration, few frontline extension education projects were launched by the ICAR in different years. For better understanding, brief details of these projects are given below.

All India Coordinated Project on National Demonstration Programme (NDP)

On the recommendation of a panel of scientists constituted by the minister of food and agriculture, a nationwide programme of demonstrations, known as National Demonstration (ND) on major food crops was launched in the 1964.The rationale behind the scheme was that unless the scientists could demonstrate what they advocated, their advice might not be heeded by the farmers. The conceptual frame work of national demonstration was that it was a nationwide project with a uniform design and pattern. It differed from other demonstrations in the following four major respects.

i) There was a specific yield-target and there was no separate control plot near the demonstration. The idea behind this principle was that the entire living memory of the farmers about the yield potential of the crop as well as the entire block in which the demonstration had been laid out would serve as the control.

ii) The area of the demonstration plot was about one hectare(it could be one acre if bigger plots were not available), so that the feasibility of raising a good crop could be strikingly and unquestionable demonstrated.

iii) The farmers in whose plots the demonstrations were laid out were the actual cultivators with small holdings, so that the high yields obtained were not attributed to the effects of affluence.

iv) The agricultural scientists conducted these demonstrations in association with local extension agencies and workers.

Initially, the national demonstration's project was implemented in 100 selected districts of 23 states in the country. During 1966, 1000 national demonstrations in rice alone were conducted as part of the celebration of 'International Rice Year'. The demonstrated conducted during 1965-67 were single crop demonstrations. From 1967 onwards, the ICAR reoriented the programme by introducing multiple cropping which aimed at maximizing production per unit area per unit time. In 1968, the demonstrations were also introduced in the non-irrigated areas. In 1970, it was further emphasized that these demonstrations would be used as training grounds. The concepts of entire farming demonstrations, introduced in 1980-81, was conducted with a few selected farmers only.

Objectives of the National Demonstration

The national demonstrations were intended to show the genetic production potentiality of new technologies and to influence both farmers and the extension agencies. The specific objectives of the project were as follows:

1. To demonstrate convincingly to farmers extension personnel the genetic production potentialities of major crops per unit area of land per unit time and encourage them to adopt and popularize these technologies for accelerating production.
2. To fully exploit these demonstrations for the purpose of training farmers and extension workers in improved cultivation practices

3. To provide research workers an opportunity to get firsthand knowledge of the problems being faced by farmers in adopting high yielding varieties and practising recommended package of practices.
4. To determine the income and employment generation potentialities of the crops/subjects under demonstration, and educate the farmers and extension agents about them.
5. To influence the extension systems (the State Department of Agriculture, voluntary organizations, etc.) in the country by demonstrating the yield-gaps and pointing out operational constraints.

An analysis of the results of national demonstrations conducted during 1977-80 revealed that the production of wheat could be raised 4 times, rice by 3 times, maize by 3 ½ times, sorghum by 5 times, and pearl millet by 5 times.

Operational Research Project

The experience with the national demonstration project highlighted the issue that the demonstration of a particular technology or a combinations of technologies in an area on watershed basis would prove more effective in convincing farmers and providing them greater scope for identifying constraints ,many of which are community based. The ICAR lunched a project during fifth five year plan (1975) known as Operational Research Project (ORP) which aimed at disseminating the proven technology in a discipline/ area among farmers on a watershed basis covering the whole village or cluster of villages and concurrently studying constraints (technological, extension or administrative) as barriers to the rapid spread of improved technical know-how. The ORP considered two kinds of problems. Firstly, the common agricultural problems affecting the farming community requiring group or community action like vaccination, plant protection. Secondly, problems related to the total resource development of the watershed area. Resource development like raising production of agriculture as well as livestock production.

The Specific Objective of the ORP

i) To test , adopt and demonstrate the new agricultural technology on farmers field in a whole village or in a cluster of few contiguous villages/ watershed area.
ii) To determine the profitability of the new technologies and there pace of spread among the farmers.
iii) To identify the constraints both technological as well as socio-economic which are barriers to rapid change.

iv) To demonstrate group action as a method of popularizing the modern technologies at a faster rate.

Krishi Vigyan Kendra (KVK) (Farm Science Centre)

The genesis of KVKs

The genesis of KVKs can be traced to the Second Education Commission (1964-66), under the Chairmanship of Dr. D.S. Kothari, which inter alia recommended the establishment of 'agricultural polytechnics' to provide vocational education in agriculture to school drop-outs and other rural youths. After careful deliberation by the Union Ministry of Education, Ministry of Agriculture and the Planning Commission and as a follow-up of the Kothari Commission recommendations, the Indian Council of Agricultural Research (ICAR) appointed a committee under the Chairmanship of Dr. Mohan Singh Mehta of Seva Mandir, Udaipur in 1973 for formulating an institutional design for Krishi Vigyan Kendra (KVK) to provide vocational training in agriculture. The committee submitted its report in 1974.

The Basic Concept of KVK

- The centre will impart learning through work-experience and hence will be concerned with technical literacy, the acquisition of which does not necessarily require the ability to read and write.
- The centre will impart training only to those extension workers who are employed and to the practicing farmers and fishermen. In other words, the centre will cater to the needs of those who are already employed or those who wish to be self-employed
- There will be no uniform syllabus for the KVKs. The syllabus and programme of each KVK will be flexible in nature and tailored according to the felt needs, natural resources and thepotential for agricultural growth in that particular area.

The three fundamental principles which form the backbone of the KVK programme are : i) agricultural production as the prime goal, ii) work-experience as the main method of imparting training, and iii) priority to the weaker section of the society.

As per the Dr. Meheta committee recommendation, the bulk of trainees may be either drop out from schools or the illiterate rural people. To them, some general education may be imparted to make them not only good rural people but also alert citizen as well. Need based training courses are designed for different types of clientele especially for the deserving weaker section of the society like the tribal farmers, small and marginal farmers, agricultural labourers, drought and flood affected farmers, etc. Training programmes are developed on the basis of information received through family and village survey.

Mandate of KVKs

In the beginning, the mandate of KVK was confined only to provide skill based training to the farmers, farm women and rural youth in crop production, horticulture, livestock production, fisheries, home science, farm machinery and implements and other allied vocations such as apiculture, mushroom cultivation etc. Besides, various extension activities such as field demonstration, field days, farmers' fairs, exhibitions, radio/TV talks, film show, publication of farm leaflets, etc. were also carried out for creating awareness and to disseminate the agricultural technology. With the consolidation of other front-line extension projects of the ICAR during the Eighth Five Year Plan, such as National Demonstration Project (NDP), Operational Research Project (ORP) and Lab to Land Programme (LLP), the mandate was enlarged and revised (i) to take up on-farm testing for identification of technologies in terms of location specific sustainable land use, (ii) to organize frontline demonstrations on various crops to generate production data and to organize training to update the extension personnel with emerging advances in agricultural research on regular basis, and (iii) to organize short and long term vocational training courses in agriculture and allied vocations for the farmers and rural youth with emphasis on "learning by doing" for higher production on farms and generating self-employment.

Objectives of KVKs

The main objective of the KVK is to provide a strong training support for bringing about production breakthrough in agriculture. The specific objectives are as follows:

i) To plan and conduct survey of the operational area through Participatory Rural Appraisal(PRA) methods and characterize physical and human resources with special reference to identifying the technological and training needs of the farming community.

ii) To compile all relevant recommendations/package of practices for the district to be meaningfully utilized in the training programmes and the follow-up extension activities.

iii) To plan and conduct production-oriented and need-based short and long duration training courses both on the campus as well as in the villages for various target groups with priority on the weaker and resource poorer sections.

iv) To organize Farm Science Clubs in order to inculcate in the younger generations a scientific temper and an interest on agriculture and allied sciences and for scientific farming through supervised individual and group projects.

v) To develop and maintain the campus farms and demonstration units on scientific lines as the facilities for providing work experience to the trainees, dissemination of the latest technical know-how and also as a means to achieve financial sustainability in due course of time.

vi) To provide practical training facilities of the Kendra to the teachers and the students of vocational agriculture of the higher secondary schools.

vii) To provide added training facilities in the area for home making and nutrition education for rural communities and gradually enlarging the training facilities to encompass other important areas such as home/rural crafts and cottage industries with the requirements of the integrated rural development in collaboration with the concerned organizations.

viii) To implement all such schemes of the ICAR and other related organizations which intend to strengthen the training and technology dissemination programmes as well as follow-up extension activities of the centre.

ix) To undertake on-farm testing of the technologies developed by the National Agricultural Research System (NARS) in agriculture and allied fields for their suitability and identifying the constraints.

x) To demonstrate the potentialities of various technologies and recommend for their adoption in maximizing yield/income per unit of time and area under different resource conditions.

Special Features of KVK

i) Technically competent and experienced trainers

ii) Need based courses

iii) Practical facilities for training

iv) Work experience as training device

v) Un-uniform syllabus

vi) Training without certificate and diplomas

vii) Limited areas of jurisdiction

viii) Flexibility in approach

ix) Strong forward and backward institutional linkage

x) Training of trainers

xi) Continued monitoring and evaluation of the activities

Training Programmes of KVK

The KVKs organize two types of training programmes i.e. On-campus and Off-campus training. No certificate or diploma is awarded irrespective of the duration of the courses. On-campus training programmes are organized on the campus of the KVK whereas off-campus training are conducted out of campus of KVK, either at villages, block, district training centre. Depending on the need, interest and categories of trainees, both short duration and long duration trainings are conducted by KVK. Short duration training programme may be of one day to ten days where as long duration training may of two weeks to twelve weeks or in some special cases it may be up to six months.

Growth of KVKs

The KVK project is sponsored by the ICAR and is implemented by the ICAR institutes, agricultural universities, selected voluntary organizations and some State Department of Agriculture. The first KVK was established by the Indian Council of Agriculture Research in 1974 at Puducherry (Pondicherry) under the administrative and supervisory control of Tamilnadu Agriculture University. By the end of Fifth Five Year Plan, 19 KVKs were established. In view of its growing utility and the demand, 89 KVKs were established by the end of the Sixth Five Year Plan (1980-85). During Seventh Five Year Plan, 20 more KVKs were established. The number of KVKs went up to 183 when 74 new KVKs were established during 1990-91 and 1991-92 by the Council. By the end of Eighth Five Year Plan, there were 261 KVKs in the country. The number of KVKs increased to 290 at the end of IX Five Year Plan (2001-02) by establishment of 29 KVKs. It was decided to establish the remaining 51 KVKs (sanctioned during IX Five Year Plan) during the X Five Year Plan, out of which 15 KVKs were sanctioned during 2002-03. Later, a major decision to establish 201 new KVKs (on 100% funding basis) was taken to have at least one KVK in each district of the country. On the occasion of Independence Day Speech on 15th August 2005, the Hon'ble Prime Minister of India announced that by the end of 2007 there should be one KVK in each of the rural districts of the country. This has taken the total number of KVKs to 551 at the end of Tenth Plan.

During IX Five Year Plan, 53 Zonal Agricultural Research Stations (ZARS) were strengthened to function as KVKs for which funds were provided under National Agricultural Technology Project (NATP). It was decided to continue their functioning as full-fledged KVKs during X Five Year Plana so, to be financed out of Plan Budget of KVKs after the termination of NATP. All these KVKs have also started functioning as full-fledged KVKs from 1stApril, 2004. By 2013, there were 630 KVKs in the country, of which 428 were under State

Agricultural Universities (SAUs) and Central Agricultural University (CAU), 51 were under ICAR institutes, 99 were under NGOs, 35 were under State Governments, and remaining 17 were under other educational institutions (2013).

The head of the KVK is the Programme Coordinator. Subject Matter Specialists form the core technical staffs of KVK and they are drawn from the discipline like agronomy, horticulture, animal husbandry, home science, fisheries and extension education. A Local Management Committee (LMC) with representatives from the agriculture university, ICAR, relevant Government Departments, PRI, progressive farmers, etc, is formed for each KVK for providing guidance on its working. The success of the KVK is judged by the extent to which it has been able to fulfill its obligations specified in the mandate. The achievement of the KVK is measured in terms of : i) training courses organized ii) number of beneficiaries covered under different activities, , iii) follow-up field extension activities organized, and iv) the impact of these activities on the farming community in general and agricultural production in particular.

Over the years, the KVKs have emerged as a national network of training organizations at the base level for imparting training to farmers, farm women, rural youth and extension functionaries on the improved knowledge and skills generated through research at the State Agricultural Universities, ICAR and State Governement institutions, among others.

Trainers' Training Centre (TTCs) : TTCs have been established in specialized subjects mainly in the ICAR institutes for in-service training of the teachers/ trainers of KVKs and such other non-degree level institutions. The centers offer in-service training courses for the trainers/instructors of the extension training centres, farmers' training centres, agricultural schools and teachers dealing with work-experience and vocational course.

State and Union-Territory wise distribution of KVKs in India (as on 31.03.2020)

S.No.	State	No. of KVKs
1	Himachal Pradesh	13
2	Jammu and Kashmir	21
3	Punjab	22
4	Uttarakhand	13
5	Delhi	1
6	Haryana	18
7	Rajasthan	44
8	Uttar Pradesh	83
9	Bihar	44
10	Jharkhand	24

11	A & N Islands	3
12	Odisha	33
13	West Bengal	23
14	Assam	26
15	Arunachal Pradesh	16
16	Sikkim	4
17	Manipur	10
18	Meghalaya	7
19	Mizoram	8
20	Nagaland	11
21	Tripura	7
22	Maharashtra	49
23	Gujarat	30
24	Goa	2
25	Chattisgarh	28
26	Madhya Pradesh	53
27	Tamil Nadu	32
28	Puducherry	3
29	Andhra Pradesh	24
30	Telangana	16
31	Karnataka	33
32	Kerala	14
33	Lakshadweep	1
Total		**716**

(Source: ICAR, Government of India)

Lab-to-Land Programme (LLP)

The Lab-to-Land Programme(LLP) was launched in 1979 by the ICAR as a part of its Golden Jubilee celebration. The overall objective of the progrmme was to improve the economic condition of the small and marginal farmers and the landless labourers, particularly scheduled castes and scheduled tribes by transfer of improved technology developed by the agricultural universities, research institutes, etc.

Objectives of LLP

The specific objectives of the lab-to-land programme were as follows:

i) To study and understand the background and resources of the selected farmers and land less agricultural laborers . to introduce low cost relevant agricultural and allied technologies on the farmers houses for increasing their employment , production and income.

ii) To assist the farmers to develop feasible farm plan keeping in view the availability of technologies, need and resources of the farmers and the resources which could be made available in the future from external agencies.

iii) To guide and help the farmers in adopting improved technologies as per there farm plans and demonstrate to them the economic viability of those technologies as well s methods of cultivation and farm management.

iv) To organize training programmes and other extension activities in relation to their adopted practices and prepare them for active participation in agricultural development programmes of the state department of agriculture.

v) To make the farmers aware of the various opportunities and agencies which they could utilize to their economic advantage.

vi) To develop functional relations and linkages with the scientists and the institutions for future guidance, advisory services and help.

vii) To utilize this project as a feedback mechanism for the agricultural scientists and extension functionaries.

The programme was initiated with 75,000 farm families over the whole country, and it was implemented by agricultural universities, ICAR institutions, State departments of agriculture and some selected voluntary organizations.The programme operated in anumber of phases and a phase ran for a period of two years with a particular set of farmers.

With effect from 1st April, 1992 all the first-line transfer of technology projects of the ICAR, viz,ND, ORP and LLP have been integrated into KVKs.

National Agriculture Research Project (NARP)

NARP was launched in 1978 by ICAR with the assistance of world bank with the main objective to provide solutions to the location specific problems faced by the State by reorganizing the research in agriculture. Through this project, the regional research capacity of the State Agriculture Universities was improved and strengthened. ICAR provided financial support to SAUs to develop suitable infrastructure to carry out area specific research in agriculture under different agro-climatic zone.

National Agricultural Technology Project (NATP)

National Agriculture Technology Project was launched by ICAR in 1998 with the assistance of world bank. The main objective was to enhance the performance and effectiveness of research system in responding to the location specific needs of the farmers. The basic premise of the NATP is that research and extension programmes should be farmer-centered and demand driven. The NATP had three major components i.e. Agriculture Research Management, Research and Innovation in Technology Dissemination. The innovation in technology dissemination component of NATP was with Division of Agriculture Extension. This component has four sub-components:

i) Institute Village Linkage Programme (IVLP)
ii) Remandating of Selected Zonal Agricultural Research Srtation (ZARS)
iii) Agricultural Technology Innovation Centre (ATIC)
iv) Strengthening of Directorate of Extension and Zonal Co-ordination Units.

Technology Assessment and Refinement-Institute Village Linkage Programme (TAR-IVLP)

In the earlier programmes, the strategy followed in designing and implementing transfer technology projects has been based more on the supply of technological information than on the consideration of limitations of the small farmers at the farm level. The usual approach has been that any technology, which produces the best results at the experimental level, is superior, and that is what should be offered to the farmers. Failure to consider the actual circumstances under which small farms operate has seriously affected the appropriateness of these technologies. What was felt a technology generation and transfer mechanism and a methodology that would make it possible to recognize and classify the different types of small farmers. Then, and only then, the organizational design can generate and make available to farmers an appropriate technology, which they could adopt. A more holistic approach in terms of diagnosis of problems, identification of technological interventions based on farmers knowledge and technology identification for various production systems was needed to address the special production issues of small farmers. It was in this concept, a programme captioned TAR-IVLP was evolved to address the above elements to arrive at appropriate technologies. The programme got its fillip and momentum since 1999 when it was brought under the fold as part of NATP.

Objectives of TAR - IVLP

i) To introduce technological interventions with emphasis on stability and sustainability along with productivity and profitability taking into account environmental issues in well-endowed and small production systems.
ii) To introduce and integrate appropriate technologies to increase the productivity with marketed surplus in commercial and off farm production systems.
iii) To monitor socio-economic impact of technological interventions for different production systems.
iv) To identify extrapolation domain for new technology/technology modules based on environmental characterization as at meso and mega levels.

The project was implemented by Central Agricultural Research Institutes/State Agricultural Universities through a multidisciplinary core team of scientists numbering 4-5 from the implementing institution led by a Team Leader (Principal Investigator). The TAR-IVLP also envisages an optional team of scientists drawn from other institutes to look into specific issues.

Agricultural Technology Information Centres (ATICS)

Agricultural Technology Information Centre (ATIC) was conceived and put into practice since 1998-99 under National Agricultural Technology Project (NATP) sponsored by World Bank and implemented through 40 ICAR Institutes and State Agricultural Universities (SAUs) located in various parts of the country.

Objectives of ATIC

ATIC is established with the objectives to provide all basic needs of the farmers through a single window service. This unique system not only serves the farmers but also other stakeholders of the farming practices to provide solution to their location specific problems and make available all the required technological information together with technology inputs and products for testing and use by them. The important objectives are:

1. To provide a single window delivery system for the products and species available from an institution to the farmers and other interested groups as a process of innovativeness in technology dissemination at the institute level;
2. To facilitate direct access to the farmers to the institutional resources available in terms of technology, advice, products, etc., for reducing dissemination losses; and
3. To provide mechanism for feedback from the users to the institute.
4. To sale and distribute improve products
5. To provide published literature
6. To overcome technology dissemination loss
7. Research generation to the institute/ SUs

Attributes of ATIC

1. Availability and accessibility of new technologies
2. Relevance of new technologies
3. Responsiveness of new technologies to the needs of different categories of farmers
4. Varied requirements for different categories of farmers and
5. Sustainability of such unit within overall institutional framework.

National Agricultural Innovation Project (2006)

Agriculture growth was on the ascendancy till the mid-nineties but after that the growth slowed down. Since 1996-97, the growth rate of agricultural GDP was on an average, 1.75 % per year in contrast with the rate of 4% that was required. On the other hand, the farmer has been facing rising input costs, declining returns from the inputs, uncertain market, increasing role of market in agriculture and blurring of distinction between the domestic market and the international market. To assist the farmer in these changing contexts, new strategies and innovative solutions are urgently required which in turn will require technological support. Hence, the agricultural research system which generates technologies has to conduct the business of agricultural research in an innovative way. The World Bank aided National Agricultural Innovation Project (NAIP) has been conceived by ICAR in 2006 to pilot this innovation in conducting agricultural research.

The Basic Principles of NAIP

1. To give the agricultural research and technology development system an explicit development and business perspective through innovative models. In other words, the agricultural research system should be able to support agriculture as a business venture and also as a means of security of livelihood of the rural Indian while maintaining excellence in science.
2. To make the National Agricultural Research System a 'pluralistic' system where every Organisation having stake in agricultural research: public, private or civil society, has to play a role.
3. Working in well defined partnership groups with clear common goals and understanding on sharing responsibilities and benefits.
4. Funding through competition so that a wide choice of excellent innovative ideas come in from the stakeholders themselves.
5. Work with focus, plan and time frames.
6. Develop well-tested models for application of agricultural research and technology for profitability of farming, income generation and poverty alleviation.

The overall objective of the NAIP is to facilitate an accelerated and sustainable transformation of the Indian agriculture so that it can support poverty alleviation and income generation through collaborative development and application of agricultural innovations by the public organizations in partnership with farmers' groups, the private sector and other stakeholders.

Objectives of NAIP

a) To build the critical capacity of the ICAR as a catalyzing agent for management of change in the Indian NARS

b) To promote 'production to consumption systems research' in priority areas / themes to enhance productivity, nutrition, profitability, income and employment.

c) To improve livelihood security of rural people living in the selected disadvantaged regions through technology-led innovation systems encompassing the wider process of social and economic change covering all stakeholders.

d) To build capacity to undertake basic and strategic research in frontier areas of agricultural sciences to meet challenges in technology development in the immediate and predictable future.

The NAIP is planned for six years (2006-12) to allow time for piloting, learning and scaling up, wherever possible.

Components of NAIP

The NAIP will function through four components:

1. The ICAR as the Catalyzing Agent for the Management of Change in the Indian NARS
2. Research on Production to Consumption Systems (PCS)
3. Research on Sustainable Rural Livelihood Security (SRLS) and
4. Basic and Strategic Research in the Frontier Areas of Agricultural Sciences (BSR).

Institutional Development Priorities of the NAIP

Competitiveness and access to information are of greater relevance to poor-population groups to prevent them from further marginalization. The quantum of new information and the rapid rate at which the existing knowledge is becoming obsolete may pose a threat to the traditional and indigenous knowledge of our country.

Thus, the NAIP shall strive for striking a balance between utilization of the existing/ indigenous knowledge, creation of new knowledge and protection of useful traditional knowledge through documentation, validation, dissemination and utilization.

India's agricultural sector is composed of a large number of small individual entrepreneurs. Farmers are becoming increasingly dependent on other entrepreneurs for services, inputs, implements, marketing and processing. The capacity of these large numbers of entities to adjust to the rapid changes in the institutional, economic and political environments, and inter-collaborations is highly crucial for the success of agricultural development.

Capacity building and strengthening of partnerships will be major elements in all the Components of the NAIP. Capacity building applies to individual farmers, farmers' groups/ organizations, and agrarian institutions and businesses, which support them. Partnerships refer to collaborations among public sector institutions, farmers' organizations, self-help groups, NGOs and the private sector. The NAIP has a built-in awareness that women farmers, whose number and contributions are significant in the Indian agriculture, have to be increasingly involved in the development process. Participatory mode of technology development, learning and action taking shall be the essential ingredients for capacity building and project management in the NAIP.

With the increasing importance of marketing in the Indian agriculture, enhancing the business skills of agricultural research institutions assumes high significance. There is a need to develop business development units/ groups as models in potential institutions for business planning, and market development for commercialization of agro-technologies.

Research & Development Priorities of the NAIP

The broad thrust areas mentioned below are the national and sectoral-level thrusts, as reflected in the National Agricultural Policy and the Tenth Five-Year Plan of India (2002-07), including its Mid-Term Appraisal Report, recommendations of the National Commission of Farmers and several consultations held with a wide array of stakeholders.

1. Agricultural Diversification

For making the Indian agriculture profitable, sustainable and competitive, we target a multi-faceted approach with greater appreciation for various site-specific needs and compulsions of the farming systems, agro-climatic conditions, endowments of land and water resources, rural infrastructure, and the market demand both within and outside the country. Facilitating services and support systems, covering, credit, extension, marketing, prices, etc. are critical for successful diversification. This would require efficient field operations/ hatchery management, facilitating and improving processing, post-harvesting management, marketing, quality assurance and strengthening of infrastructure for rapid multiplication of disease-free planting material. On-farm experimentation would be accorded high priority for testing and disseminating technologies suitable for increasing food, feed, fodder and fuel (rural energy) security, and improving the livelihoods of resource-poor farmers.

2. Livestock and Fisheries Production

Emerging as "sunrise sectors". Livestock in India is largely owned by small and marginal farmers and landless people in rural areas, especially in the dry land areas. So this sector's rapid growth provides direct benefits to the poorer households. Further, the contribution of women in these sectors is substantial. Focused attention on genetic up gradation, nutrition, management, disease surveillance and control, production of feeds, diagnostic kits and vaccines, post-harvest handling and processing and marketing of livestock and aquaculture produce, by-produce and wastes will certainly bring prosperity to poor and gains to the country.

Studies on monitoring and control of trans-boundary livestock diseases have important implications for human health, international trade and compliance with hygiene and sanitary requirements of the importing country.

3. Genetic Resources and Bio-prospecting

Regular improvements in germplasm (plants and animals, including fish and microbes) and nutritional value of staple foods, besides management of diseases and pests of crops and livestock need to continually attempted.

i) **Genetic resources** (plant, animal and microbial) constitute one of the most important and invaluable natural resources and their proper documentation and effective utilization is an important endeavour. The importance of undertaking such an activity with the help of local communities, NGOs, etc. cannot be overemphasized.

ii) **Bio-prospecting** will have to lay the foundation for effective mining and targeting the transfer of genes for specific traits. The vast microbial gene pool has to be explored and utilized for crop and animal improvement.

This is capital- and knowledge-intensive sector, but at the same time warrants strong public-public and public-private partnerships. Interactions between research institutions and the industry need to be strengthened for realizing the full potential of frontier sciences.

4. Natural Resource Management

In view of the increasing water scarcity and the growing competition for water-use in agriculture, household and industry, efficient and sustainable management of water resources, with focus on watersheds and local-level community management is needed. Through its Consortia approach, the NAIP will aim to combine short- and possibly long-term economic benefits (farmers' interests) with long-term environmental concerns (public interest) and favorable institutional development.

i) **Soil health** has been affected adversely owing to depletion of organic carbon, imbalanced use of nutrients, micronutrient deficiency, etc. IPNM approach with appropriate policies, precision agriculture, etc. may be explored to tackle the inadequate replenishment of nutrients to the soil.

ii) **Global warming** is becoming an important issue for sustainable agriculture. Understanding its effects and developing adaptation and mitigation strategies should receive attention.

Selected areas having competitive advantage and technologies that support modern organic farming may be generated/ strengthened. This research will not only contribute to enhanced nutritional and environmental security but also improve export prospects of agri-products.

5. Integrated Pest Management

Pesticides are often not accessible to small-scale farmers and skill and knowledge in the sound use of pesticides is lacking. Pesticide-misuse is therefore a significant health and economic hazard to producers, consumers and the environment. The evolution of new races, pathotypes, strains and biotypes of the pathogens and insect-pests worsens the scenario further. In this context, to manage such biotic stresses, efficient and effective integrated approaches are required. Consortia within the NAIP may take up elaboration and validation of **IPM policies and practices** for the ecologically-tolerable and economically-sustainable use of pesticides.

6. Value-addition and Post-harvest Processing

Value-addition to and post-harvest processing of agri-produce is an area of immense significance to meet the global competition. At present, only 7% of the output of the agricultural sector is provided value-addition and 2% of the volume of perishables is processed. In view of the small and scattered farm holdings and a majority of farmers being resource-poor, strengthening of co-operatives, self-help groups, and contract farming assumes significance. **Processing technologies** need to follow the changing consumption patterns. Establishing **local storage** and **small-scale processing capacity** to minimize post-harvest losses is important.

7. Research on Policy Analysis and Market Intelligence

In the scenario of globalization and emergence of **increasingly competitive, fast-changing and quality-conscious markets** the importance of market intelligence to predict the trends and develop models for forecasts cannot be overemphasized. Integration of markets within the country and with world markets, supported by appropriate policies, needs to be seriously considered.

National Initiative on Climate Resilient Agriculture (NICRA)

Background

Climate change has become an important area of concern for India to ensure food and nutritional security for growing population. The impacts of climate change are global, but countries like India are more vulnerable in view of the high population depending on agriculture. In India, significant negative impacts have been implied with medium-term (2010-2039) climate change, predicted to reduce yields by 4.5 to 9 percent, depending on the magnitude and distribution of warming. Since agriculture makes up roughly 16 percent of India's GDP, a 4.5 to 9% negative impact on production implies a cost of climate change to be roughly up to 1.5 percent of GDP per year. The Government of India has accorded high priority on research and development to cope with climate change in agriculture sector. The Prime Minister's National Action Plan on climate change has identified Agriculture as one of the eight national missions. With this background, the ICAR has launched a major Project entitled, **National Initiative on Climate Resilient Agriculture (NICRA)** during 2010-11 with an outlay of Rs.350 crores for the XI Plan.

Objectives of the Project

- To enhance the resilience of Indian agriculture covering crops, livestock and fisheries to climatic variability and climate change through development and application of improved production and risk management technologies
- To demonstrate site specific technology packages on farmers' fields for adapting to current climate risks
- To enhance the capacity building of scientists and other stakeholders in climate resilient agricultural research and its application.

Project Components

Both short term and long terms outputs are expected from the project in terms of new and improved varieties of crops, livestock breeds, management practices that help in adaptation and mitigation and inputs for policy making to mainstream climate resilient agriculture in the developmental planning. The overall expected outcome is enhanced resilience of agricultural production to climate variability in vulnerable regions. The project is comprised of four components.

1. Strategic research on adaptation and mitigation
2. Technology demonstration on farmers' fields to cope with current climate variability
3. Sponsored and competitive research grants to fill critical research gaps
4. Capacity building of different stake holders

Strategic Research

The strategic research has been planned at leading research institutes of ICAR in a network mode covering crops, horticulture, livestock, natural resource management and fisheries sectors. To begin with, the project is focusing on crops like wheat, rice, maize, pigeonpea, groundnut, tomato, mango and banana; cattle, buffalo and small ruminants among livestock and both marine and freshwater fish species of economic importance. The major research themes are:

- Vulnerability assessment of major production zones
- Linking weather based agro-advisories to contingency planning
- Assessing the impacts and evolving varieties tolerant to key climatic stresses (drought, heat, frost, flooding, etc.) in major food and horticulture crops
- Continuous monitoring of greenhouse gases in open field conditions in major production systems
- Evolving adaptation and mitigation strategies through enhancing water and nutrient use efficiency and conservation agriculture
- Studying changes in pest dynamics, pest/pathogen-crop relationships and emergence of new pests and pathogens under changing climate
- Adaptation strategies in livestock through nutritional and environmental manipulations
- Harnessing the beneficial effects of temperature in inland and marine fisheries through better understanding of the spawning behaviour.

The research was initiated during 2011-12 in all the above themes. The major emphasis during the year was on building state of art research infrastructure like high throughput phenotyping platforms, free air temperature elevation systems in open fields, environmental growth chambers with CO2and temperature controls and special caloric metric system to study livestock response to heat stress. These are some of the unique facilities being set up for the first time in Asia. In all the target crops like rice, wheat, maize, pigeonpea, tomato and mango, core sets of genetic resources were assembled and field phenotyped at different institutions with a view to identify sources of tolerance to climatic stresses and related genes and traits. For the first time, all the germplasm of wheat with NBPGR has been multiplied for field phenotyping and currently under evaluation. Country wide studies have been initiated to understand the impact of temperature on flowering behaviour in mango. A nationwide pest surveillance and monitoring system has been put in place for all the target crops for major pests and diseases wherein real time incidence is being monitored along with weather parameters to build pest warning models. Methods for measurement of green house gas emissions in the marine ecosystem have been standardized. Carbon sequestration potential through agro forestry systems across the country is being quantified. Monitoring of experiments on conservation agriculture in different production systems is initiated to assess the adaptation and mitigation potential of CA practices. The vulnerability of all the rural districts in the country (about 540) is being quantified in terms of exposure, sensitivity and adaptive capacity in order to prepare a vulnerability atlas.

Technology Demonstration

The technology demonstration component deals with demonstrating proven technologies for adaptation of crop and livestock production systems to climate variability.

This component is implemented in selected vulnerable districts of the country through location specific interventions by Krishi Vigyan Kendras in a participatory mode. The project is implemented in 100 districts (see map) involving over one lakh farm families across the country. These districts are selected based on the following criteria besides the strength of the KVKs:

- Drought proneness based on 30 years rainfall data (Source : IMD)
- Cyclone proneness based on frequency as recorded by IMD/State Disaster Management agencies.
- Flood proneness based on IMD data and NDMA maps.
- Vulnerability to heat wave and cold wave based on IMD grid data on temperatures.
- Actual incidence of floods and droughts as recorded by AICRPAM centers

The interventions in the village panchayats are finalized following a participatory approach through the Village Climate Risk Management Committee (VCRMC), after the PRA to assess the climate related problems in the village and baseline survey. The program was launched formally in all the villages by involving the state line department functionaries and leaders of the panchayats to ensure local ownership of the project from the beginning and convergence of related schemes currently in operation in the panchayat. In each village, the interventions are made in the following four modules:

Module I: Natural resources: This module consists of interventions related to in-situ moisture conservation, water harvesting, supplemental irrigation, improved drainage in flood prone areas, conservation tillage where appropriate, artificial ground water recharge and water saving irrigation methods.

Module II: Crop Production: This module consists of introducing drought/temperature/flood tolerant varieties, advancement of planting dates of rabi crops in areas with terminal heat stress, water saving paddy cultivation methods (SRI, aerobic, direct seeding), frost management in horticulture through trash burning, community nurseries for delayed monsoon, custom hiring centres for timely planting, location specific intercropping systems with high sustainable yield index.

Module III: Livestock and Fisheries: Use of community lands for fodder production during droughts/floods, improved fodder/feed storage methods, preventive vaccination, improved shelters for reducing heat stress in livestock, management of fish ponds/tanks during water scarcity and excess water, etc.

Module IV: Institutional Interventions: This module consist of institutional interventions either by strengthening the existing ones or initiating new ones relating to seed bank, fodder bank, commodity groups, custom hiring centre, collective marketing, introduction of weather index based insurance and climate literacy through a village level weather station.

The unique features of this project are setting up of custom hiring centers in all the 100 villages and formation of Village Climate Risk Management Committees. For each intervention, it is planned to work out the carbon, water and energy foot prints.

Early Outcome

The project has made significant initial impact and was well received in most of the districts. Technologies such as on-farm water harvesting in ponds, supplemental irrigation, introduction of early maturing drought tolerant varieties, paddy varieties tolerant to sub-mergence in flood prone districts, improved drainage in water logged areas, recharging techniques for tube wells, site specific nutrient management and management of sodic soils, mulching, use of zero till drills were enthusiastically implemented by the farmers in NICRA villages across the country. In Belgaum district village level agro-advisory system was piloted successfully. The intervention which found tremendous support across the country was the custom hiring centres. One hundred such centres are opened across the country and this intervention posed several research problems which were not anticipated like lack of tractors in some tribal villages and the difficulty in using tractor drawn implements. In the first year itself, between Rs. 5000 to

50,000 revenue has been generated in many villages and the VCRMCs as an Institutional mechanism is able to manage these centres.

Overall, the project has generated high enthusiasm among farmers and raised hopes that by combining technology solutions with community mobilization, we can help small and marginal farmers to cope with current climate variability, to some extent.

Sponsored and competitive grants

Under this component, critical researchable issues like impact on plant pollinators, fisheries in esturian habitats, hail storm management, hill and mountain eco-system, small ruminants and socio economic aspects of climate change etc. are provided research grants.

Capacity building

Since climate change is an emerging area of science, capacity building of young scientists on simulation modeling, high through put phenotyping, greenhouse gasses measurement, etc. is being taken up through training programs organized in India and sponsoring scientists abroad. Simultaneously, more than 100 training programs have been organized across the country covering 50000 farmers to create awareness on climate change and variability.

XII plan activities in NICRA

State of the art infrastructure is being built at the major research institutes of the ICAR to take up long term basic and strategic research on the impact of climate change on crops and livestock, modeling future climate impacts on agriculture, water resources and development of location specific adaptation and mitigation options. To address critical gaps in the initiative, specific additional projects have been sanctioned within the scheme under sponsored/competitive mode from institutions within and outside NARS. These projects are addressing critical areas like arid zone, hill and mountain eco system, climate impact on pollinators, hail-storm management and socio-economic impacts of climate change including adaptation financing.

In the limited time of one year, efforts are being made to build state of the art of infrastructure, set up the best equipments for basic research, initiate large scale screening of crop/horticulture germplasm for heat, drought and flooding stresses, characterize livestock breeds in relation to climatic stresses and study the impact of climate variability on spawing in marine and freshwater fisheries.

Considering that the climate variability impact the food production in future it is important that we continue to address this critical area in XII Five Year Plan with significant emphasis. Hence, the scheme is being formulated to build up on the initiative taken during XI Five Year Plan, by strengthening the theme areas, viz., phenotyping/breeding programs in crops, horticulture and livestock, simulation modeling to understand the impacts at regional level and national level, address crops and regions which could not be covered in the XI Plan and expand the technology demonstration to more vulnerable districts.

Approach of the Scheme

The unique features of the Scheme to be implemented in XII Five Year Plan are:

- Strengthening the existing net-work research on adaptation and mitigation (food crops, horticulture, livestock and fishery) with more infrastructure and capacity building
- Setting up of high through put phenotyping platforms and temperature, CO2, ozone gradient facilities at identified locations/ institutions including North East region.
- Strengthening research on climate sensitive crops like cotton, maize, sugarcane, onion, etc. which are critical for India's farm GDP/exports but not covered in the XI Plan
- Projected impacts on water availability at the river basin level and participatory action research at large number of sites on evolving coping strategies through water saving technologies
- Evolving a national level pest and disease monitoring system to assess the changing pest/disease dynamics under changed climate (both in crops and livestock)
- Strengthening crop simulation and climate scenario down-scaling modeling capabilities at major Institutes and a dedicated unit at IARI, New Delhi
- Piloting the operationalization of the district/block level agromet advisory services through KVKs/district line departments and contingency plans during droughts and floods
- Expanding the technology demonstration and dissemination to 130 vulnerable districts of the country. (Source: http://www.nicra-icar.in)

Suggested Readings and References

1. Annual Reports (2009-2017). Department of Agriculture and Cooperation, Govt. of India
2. Annual Reports (2008-2016). Indian Council of Agriculture, Government of India

3. Reddy, A.A. (1993). Extension Education, Sree lakshmi Press, Bapatla.
4. Dhama, O.P. and Bhatnagar, O.P. (2007). Education and Communication for Development. Oxford and IBH Pub. Co. Pvt. Ltd.
5. Mathialagan, P. (2007). Textbook of Animal Husbandry and Livestock Extension, International Book Distributing Co. 7, Meerabai Marg, Lucknow, India.
6. Ray, G.L. (2001). Extension, Communication and Management, 4th Edition, Naya Prokash, Calcutta.
7. Sharma, K.R.G. (2008). Veterinary Extension Education, BSPBS Publications, Hyderabad, Hyderabad.
8. Supe S.V. (1987). An Introduction to Extension Education, Oxford and IBH Publishing Co. Pvt. Ltd. New Delhi.
9. Choudhary, B.N. (1999). Krishi Vigyan Kendra – A Guide for the KVK Managers, ICAR, New Delhi.

23

Livestock Development Programmes/Schemes

1. Gausalas
2. Gosadans
3. Key Village Scheme (KVS)
4. Intensive Cattle Development Project (ICDP)

   a) Difference between KVS and ICDP
5. Operation Flood
   a) Phase I (1970 to 1981):
   b) Phase II (1981 to 1985):
   c) Phase III (1985 to 1996):
6. Special Livestock Breeding Programme (SLBP)
7. Technology Mission on Dairy Development
8. National Programme for Bovine Breeding and Dairy Development (NPBB&DD)
9. Rashtriya Gokul Mission
   a) Objectives:
   b) Components Rashtriya Gokul Mission
10. National Mission on Bovine Productivity
    a) Objectives:
    b) Components of the Scheme
11. National Programme for Dairy Development (NPDD)
12. Assistance to Cooperatives
13. Strengthening Infrastructure for Quality & Clean Milk Production
14. Dairy Entrepreneurship Development Scheme

   a) Objective of the scheme
   b) Pattern of Assistance
   c) Activities covered
   d) Eligible Beneficiaries

15. National Livestock Mission (NLM)
   a) Sub-Mission on Livestock Development:
      i) Risk Management and Insurance
      ii) Entrepreneurship Development and Employment Generation (EDEG)
      iii) Innovative project on Genetic Development of Sheep and Goat
      iv) Rural Backyard Development Programme for Sheep, Goat and Pigs
   b) Sub-Mission on Pig Development in North-Eastern Region
   c) Sub-Mission on Fodder and Feed Development,
   d) Sub-Mission on Skill Development, Technology Transfer and Extension

16. Livestock Health & Disease Control
   a) Assistance to States for Control of Animal Diseases (ASCAD)
   b) Professional Efficiency Development (PED)
   c) National Project on Rinderpest Surveillance and Monitoring (NPRSM)
   d) Foot & Mouth Disease Control Programme (FMD-CP)
   e) National Animal Disease Reporting System (NADRS)
   f) Peste des Petits Ruminants Control Programme (PPR-CP)
   g) Brucellosis Control Programme (Brucellosis - CP)
   h) Classical Swine Fever Control Programme (CSF-CP)
   i) Establishment and Strengthening of Existing Veterinary Hospitals and Dispensaries (ESVHD)

17. National Dairy Plan
   a) Objectives
   b) Major components funded under the scheme

18. Supporting Dairy Cooperatives and Farmer Producer Organizations Engaged in Dairy Activities

19. Suggested Readings and References

Livestock Development Programmes/Schemes

Gausalas

Recognizing the potential of Gaushalas (about 10000) in the country which were engaged in rehabilitation of disowned cattle, the government of India in 1952 set up the Central Council of Govsamvardana (CCG). Some of these gaushalas were providing quality indigenous / crossbreds / heifers / bulls at many places like Nasik, UrliKanchan, Amirtsar, Indore and Ahmednagar. One gaushala at Bombay had completed a century of devoted work in 1986 and had established two institutes, one for research and another for fodder research and grassland development. The Sabarmathi Ashram gaushala founded in 1915 by Mahatma Gandhi near Ahmedabad is now being managed by NDDB and has a training center for AI service including embryo transfer.

Objectives

- To preserve the Indian cows and progeny and to breed and upgrade them for supplying plenty of unadulterated milk and milk products to the people and distribute the best female calves to the villagers.
- Prepare best pedigree Indian Bulls and supply to villagers for breeding and upgrading village cows.
- Production of best healthy bullocks for draught work and preserve male calves for distribution to agriculturists.

Gosadans

The Government of India appointed a 'Cattle Preservation and Development Committee' on 19th November, 1947 under the chairmanship of Sardar Datar Singh, Vice President of the Indian Council of Agricultural Research. The Committee recommended establishment of 'Gosadans' where 'uneconomic' cattle could be housed cheaply and allowed to die naturally. In pursuance of this recommendation a scheme for establishment of 160 Gosadans in the country was included in the first Five Year Plan with an outlay of Rs. 97.15 lakhs with the idea to segregate the old, unproductive and useless cattle from the good ones so as to control promiscuous breeding and also to relieve pressure on the limited resources of feeds and fodder available for the productive stock. One Gosadan was designed to house 2000 cattle in a land of about 4000 acres. The scheme could not achieve the projected targets. Only 17 Gosadans could be started during the plan period. Gosadans established in the States of Bihar, UP, Pepsu, Coorg, Bhopal, Kutch, Vindhya Pradesh, Tripura and Saurashtra, these Gosadans could have only 5293 cattle against the capacity of 34,000. Lack of funds with the State Governments for meeting their share of expenditure, non-availability of suitable land, absence of legislative measures for the compulsory removal of unproductive cattle from owner's premises, transport difficulties etc. are the reasons generally advanced as to why the 'Gosadan' scheme could not succeed then.

Key Village Scheme (KVS)

The Key Village Scheme was launched in August 1952. This was the first step initiated by Independent India for systematic cattle improvement with the comprehensive programme of :

- Introduction of superior bulls
- Castration of undesirable inferior bulls
- Use of artificial insemination
- Milk recording
- Improved fodder production
- Prevention and treatment of diseases
- Distribution of mineral feed supplements

Artificial Insemination (AI) was included as an integral part of the technical programme. It envisaged establishment of Key Village Blocks in breeding tracts of bovines and each block consisted of one AI center and four key village units to cover about 10,000 breedable cows and buffaloes. The scheme was evaluated at different phases and by 1962 it was very well realized that it failed to evince the desired impact and that too a large number of dairy plants were unable to collect sufficient quantities of milk.

The reasons for failure include establishment of centers in the states where there were no recognized breeds, creating confusion in the personnel of Animal Husbandry Departments (AHDs) by introducing lot of modifications in the scheme, inadequate attention paid to the fodder development and in establishment of marketing cells.

Intensive Cattle Development Project (ICDP)

The implementation of Key Village Scheme(KVS) in 1952 in the First Five Year Plan as a component of livestock development was considered as the first systematic attempts to improve the productivity of cattle and buffalo in the country. The objective of the scheme was rapid multiplication of crossbred cattle for meeting the acute shortage of bull for the grading up of the indigenous cattle population. The KVS was initially concentrated on establishing the bull breeding farms in the major cattle tracts of the country. The initial phase of the programme was very general in nature and no serious attempts were made to improve the productivity of the animals. The other aspects of the cattle development such as nutrition, fodder development, disease control and health aspects were not given adequate attention and as a result the KVS could achieve any breakthrough in the first three plan periods. On realizing the above lacunae, the Intensive Cattle Development Project (ICDP) almost on the similar lines of Intensive Agriculture District Programme was initiated in 1963-64 with much wider objectives of having a package of improved practices for the cattle owner to achieve breakthrough in dairy development. The ICDP was started as a Special Development Programme during Third Five Year Plan. It was envisaged to locate the projects in the breeding tracts of indigenous breeds of cattle and buffaloes. The package of improved practices included under this project were:

1. Cattle breeding
2. Castration of scrub bulls
3. Veterinary aids and disease control
4. Registration and milk recording
5. Introduction of high yielding milch cattle
6. Subsidies and incentives for milk production
7. Feed and fodder development including demonstration, distribution of fodder seeds, silage making and popularization of chaff cutters
8. Dairy extension

Difference between KVS and ICDP

Aspect	KVS	ICDP
Year of Implementation	1952 (First Five Year Plan)	1963-1964 (Third Five year plan)
Aim	Improvements in production potentiality of milch animals	To increase production of milk and productivity of cows and buffaloes
Area of operation	Key Village blocks- Breeding tracts of bovines; each block had one AI centre and four Key village Units to cover 10,000 breedable female cattle and buffalo	ICDP covers one district with a semen bank, four Regional AI centres and about 100stockmen centre to cover 1,00,000 breedable female and cattle and buffaloes.
Activities	Improved breeding through AI, improved feeding, effective disease control and organized marketing etc.	Bench mark survey and diary extension were added to the activities of KVS.

No of centres	Started in many parts of India where recognized breeds were available. Later it was extended to areas where recognized breeds were not there.	Started as a central scheme with four Central ICDPs-Gurgaon and Karnal in Haryana. Bikaner in Rajasthan and Meerut in Uttar Pradesh. Later it was extended to many districts as state government project
Year of closure	1962	Closed in phases and now ICDPs were merged with existing schemes of the A H Departments.
Reason for failure	Centre were opened where there were no recognized breeds of cattle and buffaloes.	Considerable time lag in providing organizational structure and various inputs; shortage of funds, wastage of semen.

The programme was launched in the milk shed areas which had good potential and conditions to respond to cattle development programmes. Each ICDP was expected to cover one lakh breedable female bovine population and to provide necessary inputs and technical services. The ICDP was considered as the most determined effort to increase milk production and productivity of cows and buffaloes. However, the Programme Evaluation Organization (1970-71) in its evaluation report indicated that the ICDPs also did not succeed in accomplishing their objectives.

Operation Flood

The National Dairy Development Board started biggest dairy development programme in the country in 1970 named as 'Operation Flood'. This programme with its whopping success was called as 'White Revolution' The main architect of the white revolution in the country was Dr.Verghese Kurien, also known as father of White Revolution. In 1949 Mr. Kurien joined Kaira District Co-operative Milk Producers' Union (KDCMPUL), now famous as Amul voluntarily leaving a government job of dairy engineer. Kurien has since then built this organization into one of the largest and most successful institutions in India. The Amul pattern of cooperatives had been so successful, in 1965, then Prime Minister of India, Shri Lal Bahadur Shastri, created the National Dairy Development Board (NDDB) to replicate the program on a nationwide basis citing Kurien's "extraordinary and dynamic leadership" upon naming him chairman.

Phase I (1970 to 1981)

The basic objectives under this phase were to increase the capacity of dairy processing facilities, resettlement of city cattle in rural areas, development of basic transportation and storage network to facilitate regional and seasonal balancing of milk supply and demand, development of milk procurement systems in rural areas, to improve the productivity of animals, to assure the rural milk producers of a year round stable milk market and to establish 14 milch animal centres. This phase was financed by the sale of skimmed milk powder of 1,26,000 MT and butter oil 42,000 MT donated by the European Economic Community through the World Food Programme. Through sale of these commodities, funds to the tune of Rs.1164 millions were generated and were utilized for creating infrastructure facilities necessary for dairy development. The major achievements in the first phase were increase in milk production from 21 million tons in 1970 to 30 million tons in 1979-80, reaching the target of 29 lakh litres per day in processing of milk for supply to the four metropolitan cities: Delhi, Mumbai, Kolkatta and Chennai, establishment of dairy cooperatives in 18 major milk shed areas and establishment of 14 milch animal centres and the Institute of Rural Management at Anand (IRMA). Operation Flood , phase- 1, was originally meant to be completed in 1975, actually spanned the period of about nine years from 1970–79, at a total cost of Rs.116 crores.

Phase II (1981 to 1985)

Operation Flood's Phase II (1981-85) increased the milksheds from 18 to 136; 290 urban markets expanded the outlets for milk. By the end of 1985, a self-sustaining system of 43,000 village cooperatives covering 4.25 million milk producers had become a reality. Domestic milk powder production increased from 22,000 tons in the pre-project year to 140,000 tons by 1989, all of the increase coming from dairies set up under Operation Flood. In this way EEC gifts and World Bank loan helped to promote self-reliance. Direct marketing of milk by producers' cooperatives increased by several million litres a day.

Phase III (1985 to 1996)

Phase III (1985-1996) enabled dairy cooperatives to expand and strengthen the infrastructure required to procure and market increasing volumes of milk. Veterinary first-aid health care services, feed and artificial insemination services for cooperative members were extended, along with intensified member education. The gains obtained in the earlier phases were further consolidated in Phase III. Some of the significant achievements were;

- Increase in the production of milk leading to an increase in the per capita availability of milk to 193 grams per day in 1994 from 107 grams in 1975.
- Supply of milk to about 300 million consumers spread in 550 cities and towns at a reasonable price.

- Procuring milk daily from 10 million producers spread in 74,000 villages and earning an incremental income of about Rs.2500 crore from sale of milk.
- Establishment of a nationwide network of multi - tier milk producers' co-operative societies.
- Modernization and expansion of dairy industry.
- Indigenous production of dairy equipments.

Operation Flood's Phase III consolidated India's dairy cooperative movement, adding 30,000 new dairy cooperatives to the 42,000 existing societies organised during Phase II. Milksheds peaked to 173 in 1988-89 with the numbers of women members and Women's Dairy Cooperative Societies increasing significantly. Phase III gave increased emphasis to research and development in animal health and animal nutrition. Innovations like vaccine for Theileriosis, bypass protein feed and urea-molasses mineral blocks, all contributed to the enhanced productivity of milch animals.

From the outset, Operation Flood was conceived and implemented as much more than a dairy programme. Rather, dairying was seen as an instrument of development, generating employment and regular incomes for millions of rural people. "Operation Flood can be viewed as a twenty year experiment confirming the Rural Development Vision" (World Bank Report 1997.)

Special Livestock Breeding Programme (SLBP)

The Special Livestock Breeding Programme was launched in 1975-76.by Government of India basing on the recommendations of National Commission on Agriculture (NCA). The main objectives of the programme are - to provide employment opportunities to the weaker sections of the rural poor and to supplement their income. - to increase the production of livestock products like milk, eggs, wool etc. The programme includes crossbred heifer rearing scheme and setting up of sheep, poultry and piggery production units. The expenditure on SLBP is to be shared on 50:50 basis between Central and State Governments and cent per cent by Central Government to union territories. Thirty per cent of the beneficiaries selected under the programme are to come from SC/ST communities. For setting up of sheep, poultry and piggery units, subsidy is provided at the rate of 25% to small farmers and 33.33% to marginal farmers and agricultural labourers and 50% in case of tribal beneficiaries. The scheme also aims at assisting the landless agricultural labourers, marginal and small farmers in improving the quality of crossbred heifer calves. The female calves in the age group of 4 to 10 months are included in the scheme. Balanced calf feed is supplied on subsidy to the owners of these selected calves up to 32 months or till the age at first calving whichever is earlier. The calves included in the scheme are also insured by the Department of Animal Husbandry. The purpose of supplying calf feed to reduce the age at first calving is defeated in many cases because the calf feed is offered by the beneficiaries to their cows for milk production rather than to their calves. In some cases the calf feed is being sold by the beneficiaries to the other cattle owners.

Technology Mission on Dairy Development

To accelerate the phase of Dairy Development in the country, the Government of India launched Technology Mission on Dairy Development in August 1988. The Mission has assigned 29 need based research programme to research institute of ICAR, State Agricultural Universities and NDDB. It also emphasized the optimization of resource use for cattle improvement in terms of breeding farms, bull mother farms, semen freezing and artificial insemination facilities, veterinary health care facilities etc. available with the State animal husbandry departments and under Operation Flood. In addition, the research establishments under the Indian Council of Agricultural Research (ICAR) and State Agricultural Universities (SAUs) have also been linked up in the process to provide the research/ technological support.

National Programme for Bovine Breeding and Dairy Development (NPBB & DD)

A restructured scheme titles "National Programme for Bovine Breeding and Dairy Development' (NPBB&DD) was launched in February 2014 with a budgetary allocation of Rs.1800 crore for implementation during 12th Plan, by merging of four ongoing schemes namely: (i) Intensive Dairy Development Programme (IDDP), (ii) Strengthening infrastructure for Quality and Clean Milk Production (SIQ-CMP), (iii) Assistance to Cooperative (A to C) and (iv) National Project for Cattle and Buffalo Breeding (NPCBB).

This has been done with a view to integrate milk production and dairying activities in a scientific and holistic manner, so as to attain higher levels of milk production and productivity, to meet the increasing demand for milk in the country. The Scheme has two components (a) National Programme for Bovine Breeding (NPBB) and (b) National Programme for Dairy Development (NPDD).

The component National Programme for Bovine Breeding has focus on extension of field AI Net work through "MAITRI-Multi-purpose AI Technician in Rural India", monitoring of AI programme, development and conservation of indigenous breeds, streamlining storage and supply of Liquid Nitrogen, procurement of disease free high genetic merit bulls for AI, supply of breeding bulls of high genetic merit for natural service, strengthening bull mother farms, and establishment of Breeders' Associations and Societies to encourage conservation and development of recognized indigenous breeds of the country.

Objectives

The objectives of National Programme for Bovine Breeding and Dairy Development are as under:

1. to ensure quality Artificial Insemination services at farmers' doorstep;
2. to bring all breedable females under organised breeding through Artificial Insemination or natural service using germplasm of high genetic merits;
3. to conserve, develop and proliferate selected indigenous bovine breeds of high socio-economic importance;
4. to provide quality breeding inputs in breeding tracts of important indigenous breeds so as to prevent the breeds from deterioration and extinction;

Rashtriya Gokul Mission

Indigenous bovine breeds of India are robust and possess the genetic potential to play a crucial role in the national economy. In the absence of a specific programme on development and conservation of indigenous breeds, their population has been declining and their performance is below the potential at present. For development and conservation of indigenous cattle and buffalo breeds, the Government of India launched Rashtriya Gokul Mission, implemented under Department of Animal Husbandry, Dairying & Fisheries as a part of National Programme for Bovine Breeding (NPBB) in December 2014 with the aim to conserve and develop indigenous breeds in a scientific and holistic manner by setting aside Rs.500 crores.

Objectives

The Rashtriya Gokul Mission is being implemented with the objectives of:

1. To undertake breed improvement programme for indigenous cattle breeds so as to improve their genetic makeup and increase the stock.
2. To enhance milk production and productivity of indigenous bovine breeds.
3. To upgrade nondescript cattle using elite indigenous breeds like Gir, Sahiwal, Rathi, Red Sindhi, Tharparkar, Kankrej and Hariana.
4. Arrange quality Artificial Insemination (A.I) services at farmers' doorstep
5. Bring all breedable females under organised breeding through Artificial Insemination using germplasm of high genetic merit disease-free bulls.
6. Increasing population of high genetic merit female population

Components Rashtriya Gokul Mission

Major components under the scheme are as under:

i) Conservation of Indigenous Breeds

a) Establishment of "Gokul Gram" or integrated cattle development centre

b) Establishment of National Kamdhenu Breeding Centre

c) Pashu Sanjivni - Identification and issue of Health Cards to in-Milk bovines

ii) Breed Improvement by Modern Reproductive Techniques

a) Establishment of sexed semen production

b) Establishment of Embryo Transfer Technology (ETT) & In-Vitro Fertilization (IVF) laboratories

c) E-Pashuhaat Portal

d) Establishment of National Bovine Genomic Centre for Indigenous Breeds.

iii) Awareness Program

a) Award to Farmers ("Gopal Ratna") and Breeders' Societies/Organisation ("Kamdhenu")

b) Organisation of Fertility Camps.

iv) Enhancement of Production and Productivity by Traditional methods

a) Field performance Recording

b) Progeny Testing

c) Pedigree Selection.

v) Extension of AI Coverage

a) Artificial insemination (AI) coverage

b) Establishment of MAITRI centres

c) Strengthening of field AI network

d) Strengthening of Liquid Nitrogen(LN) storage, transport and distribution system

e) Strengthening of AI training infra structure

f) Manpower development

g) Evaluation of Semen stations

National Mission on Bovine Productivity

The Livestock sector, besides contributing to the national economy, plays a key role in providing livelihoods to seventy million rural households. India is a global leader amongst dairying nations. The dairy cooperatives of the country have the singular distinction of providing seventy five percent of their sales on the average to the farmers. In order to improve productivity and enhance milk production, thereby making dairying more remunerative to the farmers a New Scheme namely "National Mission on Bovine Productivity" has been initiated in November 2016 with an allocation of Rs. 825 crore (₹ 575.80 crore as Central Share and ₹ 249.20 crore as State Share) over a period of three years and imple-mentation of spill over activities of the project beyond the project period. The National Mission on Bovine Productivity (NMBP) is implemented as a part of Rashtriya Gokul Mission under Umbrella Scheme White Revolution-Rashtriya Pashudhan Vikas Yojna.

Objectives

The scheme NMBP is implemented with the following major objectives with special reference to farmers from socio-economically weaker sections and doubling their income:

i) To enhance milk production and productivity of bovine population by increasing population of disease free high genetic merit female population and check on spread of diseases.

ii) To improve quality of dairy animals, milk and milk products.

iii) To increase trade of livestock and livestock products by meeting out sanitary and phytosanitory (SPS) issues.

iv) To create e-market portal for bovine germplasm for connecting breeders and farmers, specially from socioeconomically weaker sections.

v) To increase farmers' income as a part of goal set by Hon'ble Prime Minister for doubling farmers' income by 2022.

Components of the Scheme

The NMBP will be implemented with following four components:

i) Pashu Sanjivni: An Animal Wellness Programme encompassing provision of Animal Health cards (Nakul Swasthya Patra) along with UID identification and uploading data on National Data Base;

ii) Advanced breeding Technology: Including Assisted Reproductive Techniques- IVF/MOET and sex sorted semen technique to improve availability of disease free high genetic merit female bovines;

iii) Creation of "E-Pashu Haat": An e-market portal for bovine germplasm for connecting breeders and farmers and

iv) National Bovine Genomic Centre for Indigenous Breeds (NBGC-IB).

National Programme for Dairy Development (NPDD)

A restructured scheme titled "National Programme for Bovine Breeding and Dairy Development" (NPBB&DD) was launched in Feb-2014 with budgetary provision of Rs. 1800 Crore for implementation during 12th Plan, by merging of four ongoing schemes namely Integrated Dairy Development Programme (IDDP), Strengthening Infrastructure for Quality & Clean Milk Production (SIQ-CMP), Assistance to Cooperatives (A to C) and National Project for Cattle & Buffalo Breeding (NPCBB). NPBB&DD have two components (a) National Programme for Bovine Breeding (NPBB) and (b) National Programme for Dairy Development (NPDD). The IDDP, CMP and A to C has been discontinued from April, 2017.

Objectives of NPDD

The NPDD focuses on creating/ strengthening of infrastructure for Production of quality milk, Procurement, Processing and Marketing of Milk & Milk Products by the State Implementing Agency (SIA) i.e. State Cooperative Dairy Federations/ District Cooperative Milk Producers' Union.

Assistance to Cooperatives

The Central Sector Scheme 'Assistance to Cooperatives' was launched in January 2000 with the objective to revitalize the sick dairy cooperatives having accumulated cash losses. It provides grant in aid to such cooperative Milk Unions on 50:50 sharing basis between Central and the State Government. The rehabilitation plans were prepared with the objective to make net worth of the cooperative become positive within a period of seven years. The scheme has now been subsumed under the scheme "National Programme for Bovine Breeding and Dairy Development" launched in February 2014.

Strengthening Infrastructure for Quality & Clean Milk Production

In order to improve the quality of milk & milk products in Domestic market and to increase the export of milk products in the International market, the Department had started a Centrally Sponsored scheme namely Strengthening Infrastructure for Quality & Clean Milk Production in October, 2003. The scheme has been subsumed under the new scheme titled "National Programme for Bovine Breeding and Dairy Development" launched in Feb., 2014.

Dairy Entrepreneurship Development Scheme (DEDS)

Dairy Entrepreneurship Development Scheme (DEDS) was started in September, 2010 with the objective to generate self-employment opportunities in dairy sector in the country. This scheme is being implemented through NABARD which provides financial assistance to commercially bankable projects with loans from Commercial, Cooperative, Urban and Rural banks with a back ended capital subsidy of 25% of the project cost to the beneficiaries of general category and 33.33% of the project cost to SC & ST beneficiaries.

Objective of the scheme

To generate self-employment and provide infrastructure for dairy sector, to set up modern dairy farms and infrastructure for production of clean milk, to encourage heifer calf rearing for conservation and development of good breeding stock, to bring structural changes in the unorganized sector, so that initial processing of milk can be taken up at the village level, to upgrade traditional technology to handle milk on a commercial scale, to provide value addition to milk through processing and production of milk products.

Pattern of Assistance

A back ended capital subsidy of 25% of the project cost to the beneficiaries of general category and 33.33% of the project cost to SC & ST beneficiaries. Entrepreneur contribution (Margin) for loans beyond Rs.1 lakh (Subject to any revision in RBI guidelines) -10% of project cost (Minimum). Bank Loan - Balance portion.

Activities covered

Establishment of small dairy unit from 2 to 10 milch animals, Rearing of heifers (upto 20 calves), Vermi-Compost, Purchase of Milking Machines, Milko testers & BMCs (upto 5000 litres capacity), Purchase of Milk Processing equipments for manufacture of indigenous milk products, Transportation & Cold Storage facilities, Establishment of private veterinary clinics, Setting up of Milk Parlour for enhancement of milk production, Procurement, Cold chain and Transportation facilities, Processing and Marketing of milk & milk products.

Eligible Beneficiaries

An individual entrepreneur, farmer, Group of farmers, Self Help Groups, Dairy Cooperative Societies, District Milk Unions and Panchayati Raj Institutions are eligible under the scheme. An applicant may avail assistance for all components under the scheme but only once for each component. More than one member of a family can be assisted under the scheme provided they set up separate units with The distance between the boundaries of two such farms should be at least 500 m.

National Livestock Mission (NLM)

For sustainable and continuous growth of livestock sector by emulating the success achieved in Dairy and Poultry sectors, across species and regions, the National Livestock Mission has been launched in 2014-15 with an approved outlay of R2,800 crore during XII Plan. This Mission is formulated with the objectives of sustainable development of livestock sector, focusing on improving availability of quality feed and fodder, risk coverage, effective extension, improved flow of credit and organisation of livestock farmers / rearers, etc. with the following four Sub-Missions:

i) Sub-Mission on Livestock Development,

ii) Sub-Mission on Pig Development in North Eastern Region,

iii) Sub-Mission on Fodder and Feed Development,

iv) Sub-Mission on Skill Development, Technology Transfer and Extension.

NLM broadly covers all the activities required to ensure quantitative and qualitative improvement in livestock production systems and capacity building of all stakeholders. The major outcomes of the Mission envisaged are mainstreaming of livestock rearing as business models and linkages for successful business ventures to achieve 5-6% annual growth rate, optimal utilization of scarce nutritional resources – reducing the gap in demand and availability of fodder, conservation and improvement of indigenous breeds, higher productivity and production in a sustainable and environment friendly manner, enhanced livelihood opportunities, especially in rainfed areas and for landless, small and marginal farmers, increased awareness, improved risk coverage and better availability of quality animal products to consumers overall socio-economic upliftment of livestock rearers.

Following are the main activities under the above four sub Mission of NLM.

Sub-Mission on Livestock Development

Risk Management and Insurance

The objective of the Risk Management & Insurance as component of sub-mission on livestock development of NLM is to management of risk and uncertainties by providing protection mechanism to the farmers against any eventual loss of their animals due to death and to demonstrate the benefit of the insurance of livestock to the people. The 'Risk Management & Insurance' as component of sub-mission on livestock development of NLM is being implemented in all the Districts of the Country from 1.05.2014 and in case if new Districts are carved out of the existing Districts, than the new districts will also be covered. The indigenous / crossbred milch animals, pack animals (Horses, Donkey, Mules, Camels, Ponies and Cattle/Buffalo. Male) and other livestock (Goat, Sheep, Pigs, Rabbit, Yak and Mithun) will be under the purview of the 'Risk Management & Insurance'. Benefit of subsidy is to be restricted to 5 animals per beneficiary per household for all animals except sheep, goat, pig and rabbit. In case of sheep, goat, pig and rabbit the benefit of subsidy is to be restricted based on 'Cattle Unit' and one cattle unit is equal to 10 animals i. e. for sheep, goat, pig and rabbit. Therefore, the benefit of subsidy to sheep, goat, pig and rabbit is to be restricted to 5 'Cattle Unit' per beneficiary per house hold. If a beneficiary has less than 5 animals / 1 Cattle Unit can also avail the benefit of subsidy. The funds under the scheme are being utilized for payment of premium subsidy, honorarium to the Veterinary practitioners and publicity.

Entrepreneurship Development and Employment Generation (EDEG)

Under the Sub-mission of Livestock Development of NLM, the Component-Entrepreneurship Development and Employment Generation (EDEG), efforts have been initiated through NABARD for establishment of poultry, pig and sheep/ goat rearing & breeding units in various States to encourage entrepreneurship development. Till March, 2019, a total number of 12054 beneficiaries have been assisted for establishment of poultry (1412), sheep/ goat (9919), piggery (683) and salvaging of male buffalo calves (40) units for Entrepreneurship Development and Employment Generation among women, poor and marginal farmers. A portal named "ENSURE" was launched by Hon'ble Minister of Agriculture and Farmers Welfare, on 11th December, 2018. With the launch of the ENSURE, a subsidy-based Scheme EDEG of NLM the existing process of subsidy delivery.

Innovative project on Genetic Development of Sheep and Goat

In 2017-18, the Department of Animal Husbandry, Dairying and Fisheries introduced an "**Innovative project on Genetic Improvement of Sheep and Goat** (GISG)" on pilot basis for up-gradation of indigenous sheep and goat. It is envisaged that with the implementation of the ***Innovative project of Goat and Sheep*** there will be the triple advantages of higher population of high genetic merit coupled with increased farmers income per animal and at the same time addressing the meat, milk and wool demand of the country. In 2017-18, Gujarat, Rajasthan and Uttar Pradesh were assisted for Genetic Improvement in Goats and funds to the tune of Rs. 1800.27 lakh, Rs. 1217.4 lakh and Rs.

564.294 lakh were released to the States respectively. Similarly in 2017-18, Tamil Nadu, Telangana, Rajasthan, Karnataka and Himachal Pradesh were assisted for genetic improvement of Sheep and funds to the tune of Rs. 315.246 lakh, Rs. 586.18 lakh, Rs. 87.5 lakh, Rs. 75.12 lakh and Rs. 161.524 lakh for sheep were released to the States respectively. In 2018-19 the State of Punjab has been assisted for Genetic Improvement of Beetal Goat and fund to the tune of Rs. 19.83 lakh has been released to the State.

Rural Backyard Development Programme for Sheep, Goat and Pigs

In 2018-19 the Department of Animal Husbandry, Dairying & Fisheries has introduced a scheme named Rural Backyard Development Programme for Sheep, Goat and Pigs to assist and encourage poor/marginal farmers for doing animal husbandry with improve breeds of animals, to enhance productivity of Sheep, Goat and Pigs, to increase farmer's income, to ensure better nutrition and also to utilize agriculture food waste. This project involves distribution of Sheep/ Goat Unit involving 10 (ten) nos. of high yielding young female of age group 4-5 months and 1 (one) no. of high yielding young male of age group 5-6 months to farmers. In 2018-19, so far 2760 farmers have been benefitted in Rural Backyard Goat Development Schemes in the State of Himachal Pradesh, Odisha, Kerala, Mizoram, Manipur and Meghalaya and funds to the tune of Rs. 1256.04 lakh has been released to these States. In addition to this 150 farmers have been assisted in Rural Backyard Sheep Development Scheme and for this purpose Rs. 59.40 lakh has been released to the State of Odisha. Furthermore 2774 farmers have been supported in Rural Backyard Pig Development Scheme in the State of Kerala, Odisha, Manipur, Meghalaya, Mizoram, and Nagaland and funds to the tune of Rs. 487.242 lakh has been released to these States for this purpose.

Sub-Mission on Pig Development in North-Eastern Region

There has been persistent demand from the North Eastern States including Sikkim seeking support for the all- round development of pigs. Therefore, in the North Eastern Region, pig development is being implemented as a Sub-mission of the NLM. This is envisaged to be done by incorporation of superior germplasm of high genetic merit through import and then crossing them with the low productive indigenous breeds to eventually result in cross breds which would perform and yield better harvest to the pig rearers. During the year 2018-19 till December, 2018, an amount of Rs. 247.186 lakh has been released to the State of Meghalaya, Mizoram, Nagaland, Sikkim for import of Pig germplasm under the "Innovative Pig Development Project for North East (IPDPNE)". During the year 2018-19 till December, 2018, an amount of Rs. 278.40 lakh has been released to the States of Mizoram, Nagaland and Sikkim for Strengthening of six Pig breeding farms, 3,45,000 Health cover for Pigs and import of 24 Pig germplasm under the Sub Mission on Pig Development in NER.

Sub-Mission on Fodder and Feed Development

To overcome the shortage of feed and fodder and to improve the nutritive value, this department is implementing the sub-mission on Feed and Fodder Development. It is to mention that India with only 2.29% of the land area of the world, is maintaining about 10.71% of the livestock population of the world. The major reasons for shortage of feed and fodder are increasing pressure on land for growing food grains, oil seeds and pulses. Further, on account of diversified use of agricultural residues, the grazing lands are gradually diminishing. The area under fodder cultivation is also limited. Majority of the grazing lands have either been degraded or encroached upon restricting their availability for livestock grazing. The area under fodder cultivation is only about 4% of the cropping area, and it has remained static for long period of time. Owing to the importance of food crops and other cash crops it is very unlikely that the area under fodder cultivation would increase substantially. Though the availability of feed and fodder has improved in the last decade, still a lot is required to be done to bridge the gap between the demand and availability of fodder in the country, particularly during the lean periods and crisis situations. To overcome the shortage of feed and fodder and to improve the nutritive value of feed fodder, a sub-mission on Feed and Fodder Development in the National Livestock Mission from 2014-15 onwards. Under the National Livestock Mission there are Eight Regional Fodder Stations which are located in different agroclimatic zones of the country with the following objectives.

a. Introduction of fodder crops in existing crops rotation.

b. Demonstration of superior package of practices for use of fertilizers, water and soil management in production of cultivated fodder crops, studies of these practices with regards to new and promising species of fodder crops and grasses.

c. Evolution of fodder calendars suitable to the region.

d. Demonstration for improvement and management of village grazing land and natural grass land and study their proper utilization in combination with forage crops.

e. Demonstration of different methods of fodder conservation and utilization.

f. Production of high quality foundation seeds of forage crops for further multiplication and distribution.

g. Conducting training programmes to educate State Government officials and dairy farmers.

h. Organizing farmers' fair/field days.

The Eight Regional Fodder Stations are at Hessarghatta, Bengaluru (Karnataka), Mamidipally, yderabad (Andhra Pradesh), Dhamrod, Surat (Gujarat), Hisar (Haryana), Suratgarh (Rajasthan), Suhama (Jammu &Kashmir), Alamadhi, Chennai (Tamil Nadu) and Kalyani (West Bengal). These stations have produced 304 tonnes of fodder seeds, conducted 9516 demonstrations, and organized 200 training programmes and 200 farmers' fairs/field days, during this financial year till March, 2019.

Sub-Mission on Skill Development, Technology Transfer and Extension

Under National Livestock Mission (NLM), a Sub Mission on Skill Development, Technology Transfer & Extension has been launch with the objective to adoption of new technologies and practices require linkages between stakeholders. The sub-mission will provide a platform to develop, adopt or adapt the technologies including frontline field demonstrations in collaboration with farmers, The Components of the Sub Mission are:

1. IEC Support for Livestock Extension,
2. Training and capacity Building,
3. Livestock Farmers Groups/Breeder's Association,
4. Organization of Livestock Mela / Show,
5. Regional Livestock fair,
6. Operationalisation of Farmers Field Schools,
7. Exposure Visit for livestock Extension facilitators,
8. Exposure Visit of farmer and Staff

Livestock Health & Disease Control

In order to effectively tackle the issue of livestock health, the Government of India is supplementing the activities of the State Governments / Union Territories by way of providing assistance through 'Livestock Health & Disease Control Scheme (LH&DC). During 2015-16, the scheme has been categorized under State plan with change funding pattern. Now, the scheme has been clubbed under umbrella scheme " White Revolution – Rastriya Pashudhan Vikas Yojana" as "Veterinary Services" and funding pattern has been changed to 60:40 between Centre and State (90:10 for the 8 North Eastern and 3 Himalayan States and UT's 100%. The scheme is having following components:

1. Assistance to States for Control of Animal Diseases (ASCAD)
2. Professional Efficiency Development (PED)
3. National Project on Rinderpest Surveillance & Monitoring (NPRSM)
4. Foot and Mouth Disease Control Programme (FMD-CP)
5. National Animal Disease Reporting System (NADRS)
6. Peste des Petits Ruminants Control Programme (PPR-CP)
7. Brucellosis Control Programme (Brucellosis - CP)
8. Establishment and Strengthening of existing Veterinary Hospitals and Dispensaries (ESVHD).
9. Classical Swine Fever Control Programme (CSF-CP).

The details of the components are as under:

Assistance to States for Control of Animal Diseases (ASCAD)

Under this component, assistance is provided to State/Union Territory Governments for control of economically important diseases of livestock and poultry by way of immunization, strengthening of existing State Veterinary Biological Production Units, strengthening of existing Disease Diagnostic Laboratories and in-service training to Veterinarians and Paraveterinarians. Under this programme funds are also provided for immunization against canine rabies and control of endo-parasites in cattle & buffaloes. The state biological production units are also being strengthened to make then GMP compliant under this scheme.

Professional Efficiency Development (PED)

Professional Efficiency Development envisages establishment of Veterinary Council of India at Centre and State Veterinary Council at State level in those States/Union Territories,which have adopted the Indian Veterinary Council Act, 1984. The objective of the Scheme is to regulate veterinary practice, the maintenance of Register of veterinary practitioners. Towards this purpose, there is a provision of setting up of Veterinary Council of India in centre and State Veterinary Councils in all States/UTs where Indian Veterinary Council Act, 1984 have been extended. Presently, all States except Jammu & Kashmir and all UTs have adopted the Indian Veterinary Council Act, 1984.

National Project on Rinderpest Surveillance and Monitoring (NPRSM)

The main objective of the scheme is to strengthen the veterinary services to maintain required vigil to sustain the country's freedom from Rinderpest & Contagious Bovine Pleuro-pneumonia (CBPP) infection. Under the programme, surveillance of various animal disease including Syndromic diseases with more focus on Contagious Bovine Pleuropneumonia (CBPP) and Bovine Spongiform Encephalopathy (BSE) are being undertaken throughout the country to maintain India's freedom status from these diseases. This physical surveillance is done with the help of the staff of Animal Husbandry Department of the States & Union Territories to maintain the freedom status.

Foot & Mouth Disease Control Programme (FMD-CP)

Foot and Mouth Disease is a highly contagious viral disease primarily of cattle, buffaloes and pigs. However other animals namely sheep, goats and several other species of wild and captive animals are also susceptible to the disease. Therefore, to prevent economic losses due to Foot and Mouth Disease and to develop herd immunity in cloven-footed animals, a location specific programme called 'Foot and Mouth Disease Control Programme (FMD-CP)' is being implemented in the country. The intensive Foot & Mouth Control Programme was under implementation since 10th Five Year Plan (2003-04) initially in selected 54 districts covering 8 States and 6 UTs. The programme was further extended to cover more States in phases gradually during 11th and 12th Five Year Plans. As of now the programme is being implemented covering all the States and Union Territories of the country. The major activities of the intensive programme component is for vaccination of all the eligible cattle and buffaloes at six monthly interval, Publicity and Mass Awareness Campaign, including orientation of the State functionaries for implementation of schemes, Sero-surveillance/monitoring of animal population on random basis, procurement of cold cabinets, assessment of the randomly collected samples of vaccines for their quality, virus typing in case of outbreaks and recording/regulation of animal movement from unvaccinated areas through temporary quarantine/ check-posts. To assess the effectiveness of the vaccination programme, serum samples of 10 cattle and 10 buffalo (at random) before vaccination and 21 - 30 days post vaccination from 10 villages at random from each district for each round of vaccination is collected and screened for level of serotype specific neutralizing antibodies. A total of 400 serum samples per district per round of vaccination are collected at random and tested.

National Animal Disease Reporting System (NADRS)

In order to streamline the system of animal disease reporting from States/UTs, a web based Information Technology system for reporting the diseases from the field level has been implemented known as National Animal Disease Reporting System (NADRS). It is a part of the Centrally Sponsored Scheme, "Livestock Health and Disease Control" and has been executed through National

Informatics Centre (NIC). The main objective of NADRS is to record and monitor livestock disease situation in the country with a view to initiate preventive and curative action in a timely and speedy manner. The NADRS involves a computerized network, linking each Block, District and the State/ UT Headquarters in the country to the Central Project Monitoring Unit in the Department of Animal Husbandry, Dairying and Fisheries at New Delhi. NADRS is a web based System which will report the occurrence of animal diseases data from the Block & District level Veterinary Units.

Peste des Petits Ruminants Control Programme (PPR-CP)

The Peste des Petits Ruminants (PPR) is a viral disease characterized by high fever, inflammation of the gastro-intestinal tract leading to necrosis and ulceration of the mucous membrane and diarrhea. The PPR infection causes huge losses in the rural economy, both in terms of morbidity and mortality in sheep and goats. The PPR Control Programme involving intensive vaccination of susceptible animals has been started in 2010 on 100% central assistance basis. The programme involves vaccinating all susceptible goats & sheep and three subsequent generations. Under first phase, States of Kerala, Tamil Nadu, Karnataka, Andhra Pradesh, Maharashtra, Goa and UTs of Lakshadweep, Daman & Diu, Dadra & Nagar Haveli, Andaman & Nicobar Islands and Pondicherry were covered. In the second phase, the programme has been implemented in all States during 2014- 15. It is expected that by the end of 12th Plan, the disease is expected to be brought under control.

Brucellosis Control Programme (Brucellosis - CP)

Brucellosis, an economically important zoonotic disease has become endemic in most parts of the country. It causes abortions and infertility in animals. Prevention of abortions will add new calves to the animal population leading to enhanced milk production. This new component has started in 2010 and central assistance is provided to States/UTs for mass vaccination of all female calves of age between 6-8 months in the areas, where incidence of the disease is high.

Classical Swine Fever Control Programme (CSF-CP)

In order to control the Classical Swine Fever disease in pigs, a new component namely, 'Classical Swine Fever Control Programme (CSF-CP)' has been added in the existing scheme of Livestock Health and Disease Control during 2014-15. Funds on 90% central share basis are provided to the States for carrying out the vaccination of entire eligible pig population in a phased manner starting in NE states.

Establishment and Strengthening of Existing Veterinary Hospitals and Dispensaries (ESVHD)

In order to assist the States to set up infrastructure for new veterinary hospitals and dispensaries and to strengthen/equip the existing ones, the Government of India is providing funds on 60:40 (Centre: State) sharing basis except NE and Himalayan States, where the grants are provided on 90:10 basis.

National Dairy Plan (NDP)

National Dairy Plan Phase-I (NDP-I) is a scientifically planned multi-state initiative to increase productivity of milch animals and thereby increase milk production to meet the rapidly growing demand for milk through scientific breeding and feeding and to provide rural milk producers with greater access to the organised milk processing sector. It is a Central Sector Scheme for a period of 2011-12 to 2018-19. NDP I is implemented with a total investment of about ₹ 2242 crore comprising ₹ 1584 crore as International Development Association (IDA) credit, ₹ 176 crore as Government of India share, ₹ 282 crore as share of End Implementing Agencies (EIAs) that will carry out the projects in participating states and ₹ 200 crore by National Dairy Development Board and its subsidiaries for providing technical and implementation support to the project. Board of Executive Directors of the International Development Association has approved a US$ 352 million credit on 15 March 2012 and Department of Animal Husbandry, Dairying and Fisheries, Government of India issued administrative approval of central sector scheme NDP I vide office memorandum F.No. 22-23/2011-DP dated 16 March 2012.

Objectives

NDPI is a scientifically planned multi-state initiative with the following Project Development

Objectives

1. To help increase productivity of milch animals and thereby increase milk production to meet the rapidly growing demand for milk
2. To help provide rural milk producers with greater access to the organised milk-processing sector

These objectives would be pursued through adoption of focused scientific and systematic processes in provision of technical inputs supported by appropriate policy and regulatory measures.

Project Area

NDP I is being implemented in 18 major milk producing states namely Andhra Pradesh, Bihar, Gujarat, Haryana, Karnataka, Kerala, Madhya Pradesh, Maharashtra, Odisha, Punjab, Rajasthan, Tamil Nadu, Uttar Pradesh, West Bengal, Telangana, Uttarakhand, Jharkhand and Chhattisgarh which together account for over 90% of the country's milk production. Coverage of NDP I will however be across the country in terms of benefits accruing from the scheme.

Major components funded under the scheme

Breed Improvement

Production of High Genetic Merit (HGM) cattle and buffalo bulls, Strengthening of "A" and "B" graded Semen Stations, Pilot Model for Viable Doorstep AI delivery Services.

Animal Nutrition

Ration Balancing Programme, Ration Balancing Programme, Fodder Development Programme.

Village Based Milk Procurement System

Strengthening and Expanding Milk Procurement System at Village level.

Supporting Dairy Cooperatives and Farmer Producer Organizations Engaged in Dairy Activities

Department of Animal Husbandry, Dairying & Fisheries Ministry of Agriculture & Farmers Welfare Government of India has approved a new Central Sector Scheme "Supporting Dairy Cooperatives and Farmer Producer Organizations engaged in dairy activities" from 2016-17 with a corpus of Rs. 300 crore to be kept in perpetuity with National Dairy Development Board to be used for providing soft loans for working capital to enable State Dairy Cooperative Federations to provide a stable market access to farmers. The scheme is being implemented by National Dairy Development Board.

Objectives of the Scheme

1. To assist the State Dairy Cooperative Federations by providing soft working capital loan to tide over the crisis on account severely adverse market conditions or natural calamities.
2. To provide stable market access to the dairy farmers.
3. To enable State Cooperative Dairy Federations to continue to make timely payments of dues to the farmers.

4. To enable the cooperatives to procure milk at a remunerative price from the farmers, even during the flush season.

Suggested Readings and References

1. Annual Reports, (2010-2019). Department of Animal Husbandry, Dairying and Fisheries Ministry of Agriculture & Farmers Welfare.
2. Government of India Annual Reports (2008-2016). Indian Council of Agriculture, Government of India.
3. Sharma, K.R.G. (2008). Veterinary Extension Education, BSPBS Publications, Hyderabad, Hyderabad.
4. Mathialagan, P. (2007). Textbook of Animal Husbandry and Livestock Extension, International Book Distributing Co. 7, Meerabai Marg, Lucknow, India.
5. Dhama, O.P. and Bhatnagar, O.P. (2007). Education and Communication for Development. Oxford and IBH Pub. Co. Pvt. Ltd.
6. Choudhary, B.N. (1999). Krishi Vigyan Kendra – A Guide for the KVK Managers, ICAR, New Delhi.

Index

A

B

C

D

E

F

J

K

L

M

N

O

P

Q

R

S

T

U

V

W

Z